SPINE IN SPORTS

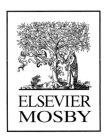

Edited by

Ted A Lennard MD, FAAPMR
Department of Physical Medicine and Rehabilitation
Springfield Neurological and Spine Institute
Springfield, Missouri
and Clinical Assistant Professor
Department of Physical Medicine and Rehabilitation
University of Arkansas for Medical Sciences, Little Rock, Arkansas

H Mark Crabtree MD, FACS
Neurosurgical Physician
Springfield Neurological and Spine Institute
Missouri

ELSEVIER
MOSBY

ELSEVIER
MOSBY

Mosby is an affiliate of Elsevier, Inc

First published 2005

ISBN 0 323 03574 4

British Library Cataloguing in Publication Data
A catalogue record for this book is available from the British Library

Library of Congress Cataloging in Publication Data
A catalog record for this book is available from the Library of Congress

Notice
Medical knowledge is constantly changing. Standard safety precautions must be followed, but as new research and clinical experience broaden our knowledge, changes in treatment and drug therapy may become necessary or appropriate. Readers are advised to check the most current product information provided by the manufacturer of each drug to be administered to verify the recommended dose, the method and duration of administration, and contraindications. It is the responsibility of the practitioner, relying on experience and knowledge of the patient, to determine dosages and the best treatment for each individual patient. Neither the Publisher nor the editor assume any liability for any injury and/or damage to persons or property arising from this publication.
The Publisher

Printed in China
Last digit is the print number : 9 8 7 6 5 4 3 2 1

Working together to grow
libraries in developing countries

www.elsevier.com | www.bookaid.org | www.sabre.org

ELSEVIER   BOOK AID International   Sabre Foundation

The Publisher's policy is to use **paper manufactured from sustainable forests**

SPINE IN SPORTS

We were saddened to hear of the death of Dr. Scott Nadler on December 26, 2004. Our heartfelt sympathy is extended to his family and friends. Scott was a prolific writer, astute clinician, excellent teacher, and most of all a family man who was admired by all.

We will miss you Scott.

TAL
HMC

Commissioning Editor: Dolores Meloni
Project Development Managers: Andrea Alphonse and Henrietta Preston
Project Manager: Anne Dickie
Senior Designer: Stewart Larking
Illustration Manager: Mick Ruddy
Design Manager: Andy Chapman
Illustrator: Mandy Miller
Marketing Managers (UK/USA): Verity Kerkhoff and Laura Meiskey

Contents

Contents

List of contributors

Frederick Boop, MD
Associate Professor of Neurosurgery
and Pediatric Neurosurgeon
Semmes Murphey Clinic
Memphis, Tennessee

Matthew Chalfin, MD
University of Medicine and Dentistry of
New Jersey –
New Jersey Medical School
Newark, New Jersey

Robert Clendenin, MD
Director of Physical Medicine
TN Ortho Alliance
Nashville, Tennessee

Frank JE Falco, MD
Mid Atlantic Spine
Newark, Delaware

Thomas D Fulbright, MD
Clinical Assistant Professor of Surgery
University of Tennessee School of Medicine
Chattanooga Unit
Chattanooga, Tennessee

Michael Furman, MD
Clinical Assistant Professor
Department of Physical Medicine and
Rehabilitation
Temple University School of Medicine
Philadelphia, Pennsylvania

Laurie L Glasser, MD
Associate Professor
Orthopaedic Institute of Central New Jersey
Sea Girt, New Jersey

David C Karli, MD
Spinal Physical Medicine and Rehabilitation
Specialist
Steadman-Hawkins Clinic
Vail, Colorado

Frank King, MD
Huntington Beach
California

James J Laskin, PT, PhD
Director, New Directions Wellness Center
and Professor of Physical Therapy
Department of Physical Therapy
The University of Montana
Missoula, Montana

Julian Lin, MD
Assistant Professor of Neurosurgery and
Pediatrics
Department of Neurosurgery
University of Illinois College of Medicine at
Peoria
Peoria, Illinois

John Metzler, MD
Instructor, Physical Medicine and
Rehabilitation
Department of Orthopaedic Surgery
Washington University School of Medicine
St. Louis, Missouri

Scott F Nadler, DO
Formerly Assistant Professor
Department of Physical Medicine and
Rehabilitation
University of Medicine and Dentistry of
New Jersey –
New Jersey Medical School
Newark, New Jersey

J Keith Nichols, MD
Associate Director of Physical Medicine
TN Ortho Alliance
Nashville, Tennessee

Ricardo Nieves, MD
Medical Director of the Rehabilitation Medicine
Unit
Spine Pain Sports Med PC
Carlsbad, New Mexico

Heidi Prather, DO
Assistant Professor and Chief of Section
Physical Medicine and Rehabilitation
Department of Orthopaedic Surgery
Washington University School of Medicine
St Louis, Missouri

Luke Rigolosi, MD
Department of Physical Medicine and
Rehabilitation
University of Medicine and Dentistry of
New Jersey –
New Jersey Medical School
Newark, New Jersey

Stephen Roman, MD
Trenton Orthopedic Group
Mercerville, New Jersey

Ross Sugar, MD
Assistant Clinical Professor
Emory Department of Rehabilitation
and Associate
Georgia Pain Physicians PC
Marietta, Georgia

Samuel Thampi, MD
Attending Pain Management, Anesthesiology
North Shore Pain Service
Valley Stream, New York

Robert Tillman, PT, MOMT
Professor of Orthopedic Manual Therapy
Senior Instructor for the Ola Grimsby Institute
and President of Orthopedic Rehabilitation and
Specialty Centers
Little Rock, Arkansas

Bryan Williamson, MS, PT, ATC
Outpatient Physical Therapy Department
Skaggs Community Hospital
Branson, Missouri

Robert E Windsor, MD
Program Director, Emory/Georgia Pain
Physicians Pain Management Training
Program
Georgia Pain Physicians PC
Marietta, Georgia

Lee R Wolfer, MD, MS
Chief, Division of Physical Medicine and
Rehabilitation
St. Luke's Hospital
San Francisco, California

Jeffrey L Woodward, MD, MS
Private Physician
Springfield Neurological and Spine Institute
LLC
Springfield, Missouri

Peter Yonclas, MD
Department of Physical Medicine and
Rehabilitation
University of Medicine and Dentistry of
New Jersey –
New Jersey Medical School
Newark, New Jersey

Preface

The diagnosis and treatment of sports injuries has changed over the last decade. These changes have included surgical advances in minimally invasive techniques, multidisciplinary approaches to complex problems, improved imaging studies, and preventive strategies that encompass strength training, agility, and nutritional concepts. The sports medicine literature is abundant with the fundamentals of individual sports and their impact on peripheral joints and soft tissues. By comparison, this same information appears insufficient when relating individual sports to the spine. This text was developed, in part, to address this difference and to specifically evaluate individual sports and their effect on the spine.

Our goal for this book, in part, was to evaluate spine biomechanics that are commonly seen by the physician, therapist, or trainer during individual sports. In most chapters, general spine movements unique to a particular sport are analyzed and the subtle and obvious impacts observed during these movements discussed. It is our belief that a solid understanding of these biomechanics helps the practitioner to make informed decisions when evaluating the spine disorder in the athlete.

This text, *Spine in Sports,* is divided into three sections. The first section features a discussion about general spine health and biomechanics. The second section divides major categories of spinal injuries based on age group: mainly pediatric and senior adults. Spinal disorders unique to these populations and how they affect sports are discussed. The final section features individual sports – biking, running, tennis, volleyball, weightlifting, wheelchair activities, martial arts, basketball, football, and gymnastics. The predominant stresses placed on the spine were carefully evaluated for each of these sports. Common injury patterns, treatment options, and prevention techniques are discussed. We specifically sought out experts in their specialties, who have both personal experience and treatment expertise with each sport discussed, to author these chapters. In addition, various specialties and viewpoints are represented, including surgical and nonsurgical, academic and clinical, physician and therapist.

We would like to thank each author for contributing their expertise to this text. Countless hours of research and writing are required by each of these contributors to produce such a volume. In addition, our thanks go out to the publisher, numerous transcriptionists, medical artists, mainly Suzanne Lennard, and our families who tolerated us during this project. We hope this text deepens your understanding of the spine in sports.

Ted A Lennard, MD
H Mark Crabtree, MD

Dedications

Ted Lennard – to my wife, Suzanne, and daughters, Selby, Claire, Julia and Maura

Mark Crabtree – to my wife, Tammy, and sons, Nathan, Brandon and Ryan

Section One

General spine fitness and preparation for sports

CHAPTER

1

Principles of Spine Fitness in the Athlete

David C Karli
Lee R Wolfer

INTRODUCTION

The spine is the core from which our movements originate. Athletic performance is dependent upon a stable spine with well-coordinated neuromuscular patterns of movement. A stable spine is maintained by three subsystems with passive, active, and neural components, as described by Panjabi[1] (Fig. 1.1). The

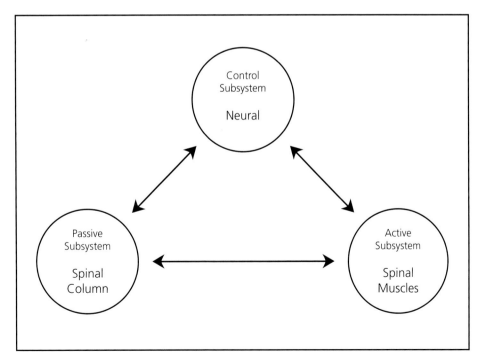

Figure 1.1
The spinal stability system as outlined by Panjabi. (Adapted from Panjabi.[1])

passive subsystem includes intrinsic spinal anatomy comprising vertebrae, intervertebral discs, facet articulations, joints capsules, and extensive ligamentous attachments. The active subsystem includes the muscles and tendons acting on the intrinsic elements. The neural subsystem comprises afferent sensory receptors distributed throughout all tissues, an efferent arm, which executes motor actions, and a control center, which integrates sensorimotor function. Coordination of these subsystems is critical to the generation of movement.

The lumbopelvic region acts as a focal point through which our center of gravity travels. Specifically, the center of mass during standing and with movement has been determined to lie approximately 5 cm anterior to the second sacral vertebra. This concept is important because movement of the body as a whole requires transfer of force from the center of mass through the extremities. Athletic performance requires efficient and coordinated transfer of these forces. The reason a 170 lb pitcher can generate a 90 mph fastball is due to an ability to generate power by efficient transfer of forces from ground to leg, to lumbopelvis, to trunk, to upper extremity, and, finally, to the ball. This concept has been described as the functional kinetic chain.

This chapter outlines a physiatric approach to the spine in sports, wherein is contained the core principles for achieving athletic and fitness goals. This functional model is well outlined in the 1997 World Health Organization definitions of impairment, activity, and participation (Box 1.1). These core principles include understanding spine biomechanics, flexibility, strength, conditioning, core strengthening, stabilization, and cross training. We also describe the concept of functional movement and the importance of developing more efficient movement patterns before focusing on strength training and sports-specific skills. These core principles provide the building blocks for enhancing athletic performance. This applies to all levels of sports participation, from the weekend gladiator to the elite athlete.

Yet another important concept is prehabilitation. Training to prevent injury and enhance performance defines prehabilitation. Most times, spine fitness is not addressed until after the onset of back pain. Many athletes develop inefficient movement patterns due to asymmetries of flexibility and strength. By identifying and correcting these inefficiencies, the practitioner may help the athlete prevent injury, disability and improve performance (Box 1.2). This chapter outlines an approach towards assessment of the musculoskeletal system in the athlete, through baseline health-related fitness testing, functional movement screening, and developing an exercise prescription to correct the deficits.

> **Box 1.1** World Health Organization definitions
>
> *Impairment*: any loss or abnormality of body structure or of a physiological or psychological function.
> *Activity*: the nature and extent of functioning at the level of the person.
> *Participation*: the nature and extent of a person's involvement in life situations in relationship to impairments, activities, health conditions, and contextual factors.
>
> *Source*: from WHO International Classification of Impairments, Activities, and Participation, 1997. Geneva: World Health Organization.

> **Box 1.2** Factors influencing injury, rehabilitation, and return to sport
>
> Prior injury
> Age
> Type of injury
> Level of competition
> Overall fitness (e.g., flexibility deficit)
> Time of sporting season
> Equipment

EPIDEMIOLOGY OF SPINAL-RELATED PAIN IN ATHLETES

Injury is a realistic complication of intense exertional activity. High-velocity bodily movements, collision and repetitive forceful muscle contractions push the limits of tissue integrity. Athletic performance continues to improve with advances in training and nutrition. Enhanced performance places muscles, tendons, soft tissues and bony articulations at high risk for failure.

The spine links the torso to the extremities. This link ensures a coordinated transfer of power from the ground through the body, producing movement and performance. Due to anatomical relationships, spinal elements are subject to tremendous stresses during athletic activity. This includes normal physiologic curvatures, which preferentially load posterior spinal structures and intervertebral discs. Zygoapophyseal joints, the pars interarticularis, and disc structures are tissues that most commonly demonstrate pathology in the athlete. In particular, the lumbar segments accept the greatest stresses in the form of ground reaction forces, which are high due to gravitational effects and body weight. Episodes of pain are typically related to one of two mechanisms: acute trauma or, more commonly, repetitive stress fatigue injury. Sports involving potentially high-impact axial loading of the cervical spine have resulted in rare episodes of high-profile injuries to the spinal canal and cord.

In the general population, back pain is one of the most common complaints prompting physician visits. The lifetime prevalence of spinal-related pain in population studies ranges from 60% to 80%.[2] Recovery from episodic acute back pain occurs in 70% of cases within 3 weeks, 90% within 3 months, and 95% within 6 months. In 4% of the general population back pain becomes chronic. Up to 70% of patients have recurrent episodic back pain. Treatment costs and secondary disability-related costs create an enormous societal financial burden.

During athletic activities, the spine is subject to rapid, repetitive, sometimes high-impact loading. As the beneficial effects of exercise continue to be recognized and marketed, an increase in the number of people participating in higher-impact exercise and athletics has followed. This trend has included older populations and seniors. In addition, quality and quantity of training and prepartication preparation varies greatly. These factors have resulted in subsequent increases in the total number of injuries, including injuries to the spinal column.

Attempts at quantifying the incidence of spinal-related pain have been difficult. As is seen in the general population, most episodes of back pain in athletes resolve spontaneously, without specific treatment. This leads to underreporting of the condition, and difficulty documenting the condition among trainers and health care practitioners. Numerous authors have estimated that approximately 10–15% of sports injuries are related to the spine.[3] Authors Dreisinger and Nelson reported an incidence between 1.1 and 30% of back pain in athletes, depending specifically on the sport involved. A study by Tall and Devault recorded spinal injury with associated neurologic deficit in 0.6–1% of all athletic injuries.[3] Most studies comparing contact and noncontact at various levels of competition reveal a soft tissue source that is self-limited. Those injuries with significant neurologic sequellae are usually associated with direct axial forces, and are closely related to the mechanism of injury as opposed to a specific sport.

The lumbar spine is the most frequent site of injury in gymnastics, football, weightlifting, wrestling, dance, rowing, swimming, amateur golf, and ballet.[4] In professional golf and aerobic dance, the lumbar spine is the second most common site of injury.[4] Lumbar spine pain is also a significant source of disability in general dance, skating, tennis, baseball, jogging, cycling, and basketball. Sport-specific epidemiologic studies have shown that 30% of football players and 15% of basketball players have lost time from play due to low back pain.[4] Among professional men's tennis players, 38% have missed at least one tournament because of low back pain.[4] In a 10-year review of traumatic cervical spine injuries in children, 10% were attributed to athletics.[4]

Similar to recovery data from the general population, a significant majority of acute-onset back and neck pain in the athletic population are self-limited injuries that respond well to conservative management. These recovery patterns are influenced by factors unique to the athletic population. Discrepancies exist when comparing athletes and nonathletes as well as adolescent versus adult athletes. Epidemiologic studies suggest that a majority of back injuries in both athletes and nonathletes are soft tissue related. In these instances, a specific pain generator is often unidentifiable. A significant majority of cases have an unestablished diagnosis at the time of initial presentation. With this in mind, numerous studies have identified high-risk sports and athletic activities that predispose athletes to these types of injuries. Recall that back injuries in upper level or professional athletes are likely to be underreported due to fear in the athletes that they will miss competition time or financial incentives. The general population, however, may be more likely to report even minor spinal-related pain to gain access to workers' compensation or disability benefits. Motivation to recover may also be different in these two populations for similar reasons.

Adolescent athletes also face different challenges from the mature athlete. Skeletal immaturity, growth, decreased body mass, training and nutritional deficiencies all set up a unique potential for spinal pathology. Discrepancies between bony and soft tissue growth set up excessive tightness in the lumbosacral fascia and hamstrings, leading to hyperlordosis and increased stress through the posterior elements. Immature skeletal endplates can lead to tissue failure and herniation of nucleus pulposis into the vertebral body. Pars defects are more commonly encountered in the skeletally immature athlete, especially in those subject to repeated lumbar hyperextension.[5]

FOUNDATIONS OF SPINE FITNESS

Functional spinal biomechanics

As the axis from which the extremities originate, the spine has several critical functions: (1) support, (2) mobility, (3) housing and protection, and (4) control. As a supporting structure, the spine creates a framework from which gross bodily movements can occur, acting as a dynamic but stable conduit to conduct forces throughout the body. Spinal segments act as the origin for the protective bony rib cage, and numerous attachment points for soft tissue structures within the axial body habitus. The spine houses and protects the spinal cord and associated neural structures, and has a critical role in maintaining postural alignment against the effects of gravity.

Spinal anatomy has often been categorized as a series of "motion segments," or a tandem series of functional units, working as a whole to create a physiologic range of motion.[6] Each motion segment is composed of two adjacent vertebral bodies, and the intervertebral tissues including disc, ligament, joint, and muscle. This unit is the smallest segment of the spine, exhibiting all of the biomechanical properties of the entire spinal column.

Actions producing movement within this functional segment relate to multiple degrees of freedom (three translations and three rotations). Translation occurs when applied shear forces induce parallel movement of one vertebra on its adjacent counterpart. Rotation occurs in response to torque and involves a spinning motion of a vertebra about a stationary axis. Loads and torque applied to motion segments along multiple axes produce primary and coupled translations and rotations, which generate complex spinal flexibility characteristics. Bony anatomical discrepancies and primary physiologic curvatures among different segments of the spine create unique motion limitations specific for that functional segment. Cervical motion segments are anatomically structured to accommodate a wide range of flexion, extension, side bending, and rotation. Thoracic segments and the bony elements of the rib cage create significant motion limitations in multiple planes, to fulfill a role as a more static framework and protector for the chest cavity. Lumbar segments are tailored towards weight-bearing and stabilization of forces created by the lower extremities, allowing for flexion and extension but limiting other planes of motion.

Soft tissues associated with the spine play critical roles in support and mobility. Ligaments act as passive restraints to spinal motion, whereas muscles are both passive and active restraints. A vertebral column stripped of all tissues except bone, intervertebral disc and ligaments is only capable of supporting around 40 lbs of axial load before collapse. Addition of the rib cage and pelvis increases weight-bearing capacity to around 70 lbs. Active extrinsic support from the supporting muscle tissue is required to accommodate demands of life and exercise.

Two key muscle groups – flexors and extensors – act as spinal stabilizers and functional mobilizers of the spine. These muscle groups are most critical in the load-bearing lumbosacral vertebral segments. In this region, spinal flexors are differentiated into two layers. The deep, short lever arm layer includes a thick psoas group. A second, longer lever arm group includes anterior and oblique abdominals muscles. The longer moment arm gives these muscles a distinct mechanical advantage. In part, these outer layer muscles provide stabilization indirectly by allowing internal visceral structures to act as a hydraulic strut when they are contracted and intra-abdominal pressures increase. A complex of paraspinal muscles make up the spinal extensors. Due to an extremely small lever arm, these muscles have limited actions as spinal stabilizers. They are essential in controlling spinal flexion via eccentric activation. This allows for controlled collapse of the spine until the ligamentous system is under full stretch, where they can take over stabilization. In the frontal plane, movements and stabilization are controlled primarily by the quadratus lumborum muscle.

Flexibility

Introduction

Among athletes, coaches, and health professionals, average to above-average flexibility is universally considered a critical component for achieving and maintaining optimal sports performance as well as for injury prevention. Although basic science studies have supported this assertion, clinically there is conflicting evidence on the role of flexibility in injury prevention, rehabilitation and sports performance.[7] There is a lack of critically reviewed scientific evidence to suggest that enhanced flexibility improves performance or reduces injury risk. Despite this, flexibility remains an accepted and relatively standard element within fitness and athletic training, as well as most rehabilitation protocols. In addition, within exercise-oriented cultures, flexibility-based fitness programs such as yoga and Pilates continue to gain popularity. According to the American College of Sports Medicine, numerous benefits are ascribed to improved flexibility (Box 1.3).

Definition

Flexibility can be quantified as either static or dynamic.[9] Static flexibility is the range of motion (ROM) of a joint or series of joints. The individual is in a relaxed state for these measurements. An individual's flexibility is primarily affected by connective tissue. Quantification of resistance to movement shows tendons contribute 10%, ligaments 47%, and fascia 41%.[10] Range of motion reflects a chain of elements from the joint (which may be arthritic or have a bony deformity), to the ligamentous joint capsule, to the tendon, to extra- and intramuscular fascial layers, and then finally to the muscle itself.

Dynamic flexibility is defined as the ease of movement within the joint ROM.[7] Dynamic flexibility is affected both by the static flexibility of a given muscle and by the strength of the corresponding antagonist muscle. For example, a football place kicker must have the hip extensor flexibility to achieve the necessary range for adequate force generation and then have adequate hip flexor and knee extensor strength to follow through with the kick.

Clinically speaking, there are generally accepted static ranges of motion for given joints.[9] However, there is a spectrum of norms if one considers the difference between adequate flexibility for activities of daily living in a sedentary individual versus the ideal range needed for a professional ballet dancer to achieve optimal flexibility for mastery of technique and injury prevention.[11] Optimal flexibility depends on multiple factors, including the specific joint and individual factors, sports-specific demands, and so forth.[11]

Each sport has a specific pattern of muscle use that must be taken into account for prehabilitation, sports performance, risk of injury, and rehabilitation for return to sport. Demands for flexibility also vary considerably across sports. Certain obvious comparisons contrast the optimal range of flexibility needed in ballet, gymnastics, or figure skating versus running, skiing, or football. Injuries can occur from either too much (hyper) or too little (hypo) flexibility, depending on the stress placed on the muscles and joints. Muscles strains, as opposed to joint sprains, are associated with a relative lack of flexibility. A lack of hamstring flexibility is associated with low back pain. Joint sprains are more common with excessive flexibility: e.g., pitchers may gain flexibility but lose stability and thereby develop anterior glenohumeral joint laxity and chronic subluxation. In gymnasts there is a well-described increased risk of spondylolisthesis due to repetitive hyperextension movements.

Factors affecting flexibility

Many factors have been explored in the literature as having effects on flexibility. Extensive literature exists on factors affecting flexibility; however, only selected factors will be addressed in this chapter. Flexibility is influenced by both intrinsic and extrinsic factors: age, gender, genetic predisposition, temperature, neurophysiologic and biomechanical properties of a given muscle, antagonist muscle strength, and so forth.[12] Factors such as neurophysiologic and biomechanical properties may be modifiable with training and activity.

Age. Generally, it is believed that age is inversely correlated with flexibility. The young are thought to be the most flexible, whereas the elderly are thought to be the least flexible. With careful review of the literature, however, it is evident that there is not a simple linear decline of flexibility with aging. One of the largest studies performed evaluated ability to touch toes in over 4500 youth, from kindergarten to 12th grade.[13] The patterns of flexibility found by these authors have been borne out over time. Overall, studies reveal that young children (ages 5–8) are the most flexible; subsequently, however, flexibility then decreases until puberty. Micheli[14] documented decreased flexibility during growth spurts when bone growth outpaces muscle elongation. Clinically, this relationship is associated with overuse injuries among active youth and Osgood–Schlatter's disease. During adolescence, flexibility increases. After adolescence, flexibility remains level for a short time and then begins to decrease. Barnekow-Bergkvist[15] followed males and females from age 16 to 34 and showed decreased absolute flexibility in both genders. It is important to note that many of these studies may be confounded by not adjusting age for maturation stage. In a study of high school boys, Pratt[16] demonstrated that the maturational age by Tanner staging is correlated with flexibility as opposed to chronological age.

In older individuals, flexibility decreases are affected by intrinsic changes to the collagen, which include increased collagen fiber diameter, crystalline content, and intra- and intermolecular cross-links. These changes make the tissues less compliant and mobile.[10,17] Older individuals also have significantly less water content in their tissues. In older individuals, extrinsic factors such as sedentary lifestyle, effects of disease, and deconditioning also contribute to decreased flexibility. Fortunately, numerous studies have shown that older individuals can maintain or improve their flexibility through a regular stretching program.[18,19]

Gender. Factors contributing to differences in flexibility by gender have been better substantiated by the research literature and specific anatomic and physiologic differences. For example, the pelvic bones of women are broad and shallow, allowing greater hip and pelvic ROM, as opposed to men whose bones are narrow and heavy.[10] Secondly, the hormonal changes associated with pregnancy are thought to increase joint laxity and general flexibility. A female's lower center of gravity may also allow greater trunk flexion.[20]

Extrinsic gender-biased and sex-role dominant psychosocial factors encourage females to pursue traditionally "feminine" activities such as dance and gymnastics and discourage them in pursuing more "masculine" activities such as weightlifting, football, baseball, and so forth. The opposite social pressures are exerted on males. Such social forces shape a person's vocational and avocational decisions and therefore influence body type and exercise habits. These psychosocially instigated influences are potential confounding factors in any gender-based flexibility research study.

Genetic predisposition. There are a number of hereditary disorders, such as Marfan's syndrome and Ehlers–Danlos syndrome, with defective collagen biosynthesis. Affected individuals with these syndromes are pathologically flexible. Homocystinuria can cause joint hypermobility. In the less-severe category, there are also individuals who exhibit genetic hyperlaxity which may or may not predispose them to injury.

Temperature. Muscle and connective tissues change their physical properties with elevated or reduced temperatures. Overall, elevated temperature facilitates greater range of motion. Many factors are involved, including reduced viscosity, increased collagen extensibility, and neural facilitation of stretching. Heat facilitates stretching by diminishing the muscle spindle reflex and increased firing of Golgi tendon organs.[21] Heat can be used therapeutically to decrease muscle spasm.

Clinically speaking, warm-up (by passive or active means), is recommended to enhance performance and prevent injury. Warm-up is universally recommended before beginning flexibility exercises. Box 1.4 lists the benefits ascribed to warming up.

Muscle physiology

Besides actin and myosin, myofibrils contain a third, recently rediscovered, filament called titin. Titin is thought to give myofibrils elasticity because of its intrinsic properties and position in the sarcomere. Titin has a high proline content and is organized into random coils instead of more rigid alpha-helices.[22] The elastic titin filaments connect the thick filaments to the Z-line of the sarcomere.[10] The titin filaments are positioned to maintain resting tension in the myofibrils. Various muscle types contain differing proportions of titin. For example, slow-twitch muscle fibers contain less titin than fast-twitch muscle fibers and are less flexible.[12] Titin is also found in different isoforms.[10] The elasticity of a muscle cell may be dependent on the type and amount of titin.

Box 1.4 Benefits associated with warming up

Increased body temperature

Increased blood flow through active muscles by reducing vascular bed resistance

Increased heart rate to prepare the cardiovascular system for work

Increased metabolic rate

Increases in the Bohr effect (facilitates exchange of oxygen from hemoglobin)

Increased speed at which nerve impulses travel, thereby facilitating body movement

Increased efficiency of reciprocal innervation (thus allowing opposing muscles to contract and relax more efficiently)

Increased physical working capacity

Decreased viscosity (or resistance) of connective tissue and muscle

Decreased muscular tension (improved muscle relaxation)

Enhanced connective tissue and muscular extensibility

Enhanced psychological performance

Source: adapted from Alter.[10]

Muscle biomechanics. When discussing joint flexibility we refer to the flexibility of the connective tissue that comprises tendons, ligaments, fascial layers, joint capsules, and muscle. Connective tissue is made of collagenous fibers in a protein–polysaccharide ground substance with both elastic and plastic properties.[11] With stretching there is lengthening due to both properties; however, when the stretching force is removed, the elastic elements return to their resting length and the plastic elements stay elongated. Plastic deformation causes lasting changes in the length of connective tissues, which is enhanced by elevated temperature and the application of low force loads for long periods of time. These physiologic properties of connective tissue form the basis for the recommendation to warm-up the body before stretching and to use static stretching techniques. However, static stretching may not actually significantly increase the length of the muscle; instead, it may be that regular stretching decreases the excitability of the stretch reflex and increases stretch tolerance.[10]

Neurologic factors. Muscle flexibility is a dynamic process mediated by input from three major sensory receptors: the muscle spindles, Golgi tendon organs, and articular (joint) mechanoreceptors. Muscle spindles are composed of small muscle fibers encased within a fusiform (spindle-shaped) capsule or sheath of connective tissue. The ends of the muscle spindles are attached to the extrafusal fibers such that when the muscle is stretched so is the spindle. There are two types of muscle spindles, primary and secondary, which react to change in rate of elongation and to change in absolute length, respectively. The spindle reflex is activated during muscle elongation and prevents over-stretching by causing the extrafusal fibers to contract and shorten the muscle. Conversely, the spinal reflex, mediated by the Golgi tendon organ, promotes muscle elongation.[12]

The Golgi tendon organ (GTO) is located at the aponeuroses or muscle–tendon junctions. As opposed to muscle spindles, which are found parallel to the myofibrils, the GTO is in line with the force vectors from muscle to bone and therefore in series with the muscle. The GTO is a mechanoreceptor innervated by a single fast-conducting Group Ib afferent nerve fiber.[23] The function of GTOs, on a simplistic level, is autogenic inhibition. GTOs are thought to serve a protective function against muscle contraction forces that would cause damage at the musculotendinous junction. Past a certain threshold stimulus, the GTOs shut down the agonist and synergistic muscles and facilitate the antagonist muscles. Of course, this mechanism is often overridden in athletes because of higher center influence to optimize performance.

The third major sensory receptor subtype is the joint receptor, located in all the synovial joints of the body. The receptors are classified as types I–IV, based on various morphologic and behavioral attributes of the nerve endings. Mechanoreceptors sense stretch pressure and distension on joints.

Ergonomic factors. Researchers found that prolonged sitting in school leads to decreased hamstring flexibility.[24] Such ergonomic factors may confound age-related changes in flexibility, in that it is actually the sedentary lifestyle that results in decreased flexibility rather than actual age-related changes in the muscle. Pheasant[25,26] evaluated the ergonomics of sitting and describes a hypothesis for the loss of hamstring flexibility. In the classic, slouched sitting position, the hamstring muscles are relatively slack because the pelvic is rotated backwards behind the pubic symphysis. With upright posture, balancing on the ischial tuberosities, the hamstrings are taut. Pheasant hypothesizes that with prolonged poor seated posture, the hamstrings adapt and shorten.

Flexibility and strength training

The standard conception is that increased strength training leads to decreased flexibility. There is often an anecdotal bias in this observation: persons engaged in resistance training may not perform regular flexibility exercises and may focus only on "mirror muscles," which can create muscular asymmetries in strength and flexibility. In fact, with proper weightlifting, flexibility can be improved with resistance training.

To enhance flexibility using resistance training, the muscle is trained utilizing its full ROM and accentuating the negative work or eccentric phase of the lifting technique.[10] In an eccentric contraction, the muscle elongates as it contracts; in concentric contraction, the muscle shortens as it contracts. During an eccentric contraction, there are fewer muscle fibers contracting, thus placing a greater stress and therefore greater stretch per fiber.[10] This is why focusing on eccentric contractions during weight lifting causes such sore muscles.

Flexibility and breathing

Only a rare few publications in the literature on flexibility address breathing and flexibility and try to answer the question of whether or not proper breathing can facilitate stretching. Proper breathing is the core part of hatha yoga. Many different breathing techniques are used in the mainstream to elicit the relaxation response and as a part of meditation. Breathing exercises are also a core part of the armamentarium for managing chronic pain. Lewitt[27] describes the term synkinesis in sports medicine, which refers to a movement being linked with expiration or inspiration. Few studies have looked at the effects of breathing on flexibility. According to Alter,[10] a correct breathing pattern can be coupled with movements that facilitate flexibility. For example, with forward trunk flexion, expiration decreases the size of the thoracic cavity, moves the diaphragm upwards, reduces tension on the erecter spinae, intercostals, and abdominal muscles, and ultimately increases flexion. Controlled breathing also can elicit a relaxation response which can decrease the excitability of the myotactic stretch reflex. Overall, there appears to be no negative consequence of coordinating breathing with stretching. Athletes can be instructed to inhale in extension poses and exhale for forward flexion and lateral bending postures.

Flexibility and injury

The prevailing beliefs among healthcare professionals and athletes is that better flexibility means lower risk of musculoskeletal injury. In particular, being flexible is thought to protect against muscle strains and overuse injuries. The biomechanical explanation is that the more compliant (less stiff) a muscle is, the more it can be stretched (greater strain) and thereby less chance of strain injury.[7] According to Gleim and McHugh,[7] who extensively reviewed the epidemiology of sports injury, there is "no strong evidence proving that flexibility stretching is associated with rates of strains, sprains or overuse injuries that can be applied across all sports or levels of competition." Gleim and McHugh[7] state that sports injury is a "multifactorial problem" difficult to study without very large studies. This is not to say that a flexibility benefit does not exist: studies to date have not been able to definitively bear this out. Basic science research in the animal model has shown that active warm-up with isometric contractions increases elasticity and raises the force and length at which the muscle will fail.[28] A fatigued muscle was found to be more susceptible to strain injury.[29] Smith et al[30] studied adolescent figure skaters and revealed an association between anterior knee pain and tight hamstrings and rectus femoris muscles. Interestingly, in the case of elite runners, the less flexible runners were more economical and thus more efficient than their more flexible counterparts ($r = 0.53$–0.65). The authors speculated that increased stiffness perhaps meant less need for postural muscles or more stored energy from the elastic recoil of the stiff muscles.[31] As can be seen from the preceding paragraph, much research needs to be done to elucidate the links between flexibility and injury.

Stretching techniques

Various stretching techniques are recommended (Box 1.5). Usually, simple static stretching is recommended for most patients. The more complicated techniques require greater patient education and often are more effective when performed with a partner. Blanke[11] describes the common techniques. Static stretching involves moving slowly to the point of moderate discomfort (not pain) of a joint ROM and

Focus: major muscle groups

Warm-up first: slow 5–10 light exercise (jog or walk)

Frequency: 3–7 days per week

Repetitions: 3–5 times

Type: slow, sustained static stretches (PNF, AIS recommended when educated by trained professionals)

Duration: hold between 10 and 30 seconds

Don't strain: the goal is to feel a slight pull, not pain. Muscles will adapt to progressive slight overload over time.

Cool-down after exercise bout: recent studies advocate light preparatory stretching and a more intense post-workout stretch afterwards. One theory is that stretching after working out allows quicker removal of energetic wastes and decreases delayed-onset muscle soreness.

then holding the position for 10 seconds to 1 minute. The goal with moving slowly is to avoid eliciting the stretch reflex which would inhibit elongation. Next, an athlete can use static stretching with contraction of the antagonist (reciprocal inhibition). This technique adds isometric contraction of the antagonist muscle, which further reduces the stretch reflex (i.e., when stretching the hamstrings, one would isometrically contract the quadriceps for 5–30 seconds). Static stretching can also be performed with contraction of the agonist (proprioceptive neuromuscular facilitation, PNF). In PNF, the joint is moved to the end of its ROM and then the agonist muscle is contracted (varying strength contraction force) for 5–30 seconds. The goal is to contract the muscle being stretched. These stretching maneuvers can then be combined for even greater effect. In this method, the athlete performs static stretching with contraction of the agonist followed by contraction of the antagonist (PNF). First, the muscle being stretched is contracted; then the agonist is relaxed and the antagonist muscle is contracted for 5–30 seconds. Purportedly, this method has an additive effect on stretching the muscle.

Ballistic stretching is not generally recommended because of the increased risk of injury when a joint is moved to the end of its ROM by jerking or bouncing movements. Ballistic stretching is effective but there is an increased likelihood of muscle strain, connective tissue sprain or bone avulsion when a joint is moved beyond its comfortable ROM. On a neurophysiologic level, slow, steady stretching is recommended over ballistic stretching because it is less likely to elicit the stretch reflex. Muscles contain spindles that are sensitive to the amount and rate of elongation of the muscle. When a muscle is stretched quickly and intensely, especially near the end of a joint's ROM, the muscle spindle sends a stimulus to the spinal cord that causes the muscle being stretched to contract. This is a protective reflex against stressing a muscle and joint beyond its comfortable ROM.

Flexibility prescriptions

In summary, it is critical to include a warm-up and a cool-down period when designing a flexibility program. The cool-down period is thought to help with clearing the waste products from metabolism. Next, consider the appropriate stretching technique for the individual, e.g., static stretching versus PNF. As a rule, apply low loads over longer duration as opposed to high loads over short times to decrease the risk of injury. Trainers can identify the key stretches for particular sports: e.g., shoulder flexibility in swimmers. Finally, for dynamic flexibility, be sure to strengthen the antagonist muscles. The ACSM put forth guidelines for stretching in 1998.

Strength

Strength training remains a standard element of any core exercise program. As a working definition, strength represents the ability of skeletal muscle to develop force for the purpose of providing stability and mobility within the musculoskeletal system, so that functional movement can take place.[32]

Strength training principles have been developed and refined over many years. The rationale for these principles is based on an understanding of muscle cell physiology and cellular adaptations to training and progressive resistance loading. Force generation is dependent on the integrity of contractile and support tissue within the muscle cell. It also relies on central and peripheral neural interactions and metabolic support systems.

Skeletal muscle comprises two major fiber types, which differ in their histologic, biochemical, and metabolic makeup. Type I (slow oxidative) fibers are densely supported by a circulatory network that continually feeds the tissue with oxygen-rich blood. Energy production in these tissues is through aerobic oxidative pathways, which allow the fibers to work most efficiently in repetitive, low-impact, sustained contractions. Type II fibers are subdivided in types IIa and IIb. These fibers are best used for rapid, nonsustained, high-force contractions. Type IIa (fast oxidative glycolic) fibers use a combination of aerobic and anaerobic pathways, acting as an intermediary between type I and type IIb (fast gycolytic) fibers, which gain energy from anaerobic pathways – namely glycolysis. Type IIb fibers produce the highest force of contraction, but fatigue most easily. All muscles contain a variable ratio of types I and II fibers, making some muscles more resistant to fatigue, and others set up for power generation. A high distribution of type I fibers is found in postural muscles in which low-intensity, sustained muscle contractions hold the body stable and erect against gravity. Muscles with a high percentage of type II fibers produce rapid bursts of tension over short periods of time.

Neural control over muscle contraction is created by the motor unit. Neurons from the anterior horn of the spinal cord supply groupings of muscle fibers. Motor units are subdivided into smaller type I and larger type II groupings. These groupings are "recruited" into activation as a higher force of contraction is required. The normal sequence of motor unit activation recruits smaller units first, due to the lower threshold for firing of their associated alpha motor neurons, within the anterior horn. As the functional demand for higher force increases, larger, type II motor units are activated sequentially to fill the demand. This has important implications in training principles, as a submaximal effort will not induce a training effect of all type II motor units.

Muscle tissue can sustain different types of contractions, depending on the applied loads. Three distinct types of contractions can occur:

- concentric contraction is created when force generated within the muscle exceeds the magnitude of the applied external force, resulting in muscle shortening,
- isometric contraction occurs when the force generated within the muscle equals the force of the applied load and there is no resulting change in muscle length,
- an eccentric contraction is created when external force exceeds force developed by the muscle, and gross lengthening of the muscle results.

Muscle force potential is effected by a length–tension relationship, set up by specialized histology contained within the sarcomere unit. An optimal muscle length exists, at which the muscle can generate its greatest force. At this length, maximal cross-bridging occurs between actin and myosin proteins of the sarcomere. This position occurs at some midpoint of the contraction, with less force development at more lengthened and contracted positions.

A second performance relationship exists, defining an optimal velocity of muscle contraction. Actin and myosin cross-linking is affected by speed of contraction. The ratchet effect created by cross-bridging, and recycling of ATP, has an optimal frequency at which the greatest force and efficiency of the system occurs. During concentric contractions, greater force of contraction is created with decreasing speed, approaching maximal force at zero velocity, or a static isometric contraction. During eccentric contractions, exponential increases in force generation occur with increasing speed. This effect is felt to represent contributions by both the contractile mechanism and the elastic properties of muscle connective tissue.

A number of intrinsic and extrinsic factors affect muscle performance and strength. Intrinsic factors include general health parameters such as neurologic, metabolic, circulatory, and hormonal effects. The effects of aging on muscle tissue are also well established.[33] With age comes a progressive decline in muscle force potential. This results from a combination of factors, including progressive loss of muscle mass, mainly due to a decline in the number of motor neurons, leading to a decrease in motor unit recruitment and frequency of action potential generation. The efficiency of neuronal inputs also becomes less efficient. These factors all contribute to lessen the ability of aged muscle to rapidly develop maximal forces of contraction.[33]

Prolonged immobilization also has adverse effects on muscle performance. This applies to bedrest and habitual or seasonal inactivity as well as to cast immobilization with acute injury, a scenario often seen in the athlete. In the absence of muscular contraction, physiologic changes in muscle tissue result. Reduced neural input leads to decreased muscle size, fiber atrophy, alterations in metabolic pathways, reduction in capillary density, and connective tissue thinning. As a result, a smaller, weaker, less-efficient and less-elastic muscle is created. The rate of atrophy is rapid during the first few weeks of fixed immobilization, then plateaus and progresses more slowly.[34] Muscles immobilized in shortened positions will atrophy more than those in neutral or elongated positions. This is a result of a net loss of sarcomeres in a short immobilized muscle, and net gain of sarcomeres in an elongated, immobilized muscle, both adaptations to the respective positions. The end result is a change in normal length–tension relationships discussed earlier, and compromised performance. Both type I and type II fiber types are affected by these adaptations, with decreased type I fiber cross-sectional area occurring earlier than that seen in type II.

Muscle tissue adaptations to strength training

Muscle tissue responses to progressive loading have been investigated extensively. A series of neuro-muscular and histologic changes occur to increase force generation capacity. The initial trigger inducing these anabolic changes appears to be increased neural input from descending motor neurons. This induces the opposite effect of disuse or immobilization, a catabolic effect described previously.

In addition to hypertrophic changes in the contractile elements of muscle, animal studies show evidence of expansion of the synaptic area of the neuromuscular junction in response to heavy resistance training.[35] With augmented neural input, skeletal muscle hypertrophy ensues. This comes in the form of increased muscle fiber size and cross-sectional diameter, secondary to a remodeling of muscle histology. Sarcomeres and myofibrils are reproduced in both type I and type II fibers, depending on the stimulus intensity, with type I fibers being trained at lower intensity levels. In addition, metabolic changes lead to a conversion of type IIb fibers to type IIa fibers. A final effect occurs with proliferation and strengthening of connective tissue and supportive satellite cells.[36]

Systemic benefits of resistance training include increases in bone mass and bone mineral density (BMD). This effect is directly proportional to the magnitude of applied skeletal loading. This is apparent in studies comparing endurance athletes to athletes trained for power and explosion. Smith and Rutherford[37] compared male triathletes to rowers to nonathletes, with higher BMD seen in rowers over triathletes. Other positive effects of strength training include increases in lean body mass and a decreased percentage of body fat. Metabolic demands within skeletal muscle under exertion rely in part on oxidative phospho-rylation of free fatty acids, which are mobilized from adipose tissue.

Functional benefits of resistance training are evident in studies on elderly subjects, which demonstrate improvements in balance, coordination, gait, and higher level performance in athletic and occupational tasks. These changes are impacted by comorbidities, psychological status, and pretraining strength levels. Although no direct studies have been definitive, similar effects can be expected on a more subtle level in highly trained athletes, who have less general comorbidity, but may often be faced with more isolated dysfunction, as is seen with acute or chronic injury. These principles will apply on a more localized scale to the affected body part, which will be functioning suboptimally due to tissue damage, inflammation, and disuse.

Principles of strength training

Strength training can be tailored to selectively train and recruit different fiber types in muscles, by controlling and varying the load/intensity, speed, and duration of the exercise. Using basic principles of strength training, programs can be uniquely designed for a variety of athletic activities and athletes. These principles apply to all skeletal muscles in the body, including those structures intimately associated with the spinal column.

In its simplest applications, strength training involves inducing stress and microtrauma in muscle tissue by applying moderate to maximal contractions against a gradual increase over time in the applied load. This activity is interrupted by periods of rest with nutritional support of the muscle on an ongoing basis. Muscle undergoes reactive neurophysiologic and histologic changes, as described previously.

Resistance can be applied to contracting muscle tissue under static or dynamic conditions. Isotonic resistance exercise is a dynamic form of exercise with a change in muscle length through an achievable range of motion against a constant or variable load. Derivation of the term means "same or constant tension"; however, under real conditions, tension is variable during the movement. As the muscle shortens or lengthens against a fixed load, tension changes due to the effects of fixed gravity against a changing lever arm. Variable resistance exercise equipment has been developed to maintain a fixed load on contracting muscle through an entire physiologic range of motion, in order to load the muscle at all points during the contractions. Isotonic contractions can be performed concentrically, eccentrically, or both. A concentric contraction produces muscle shortening against a load. Eccentric contraction involves resisting muscle lengthening against an applied load. Most resistance programs involve a combination of both movements. The maximal possible muscle tension force is produced during an eccentric contraction.

Isokinetic resistance exercise is a second form of dynamic exercise, during which a rate-limiting device controls the velocity of muscle length change to a constant speed of movement. If maximal exertion is exhibited and maximal loading is applied, then near-maximal tension is created throughout the movement. Despite this increase in consistency of applied load, some variability of resistance still exists during the movement. This increase in consistency allows for improved safety with high-velocity power training.

Isometric resistance training is a static form of exercise, occurring when muscle tension is created without any gross change in muscle length or motion within the affected joint. Tension and force are created within the muscle tissue; however, no physical work is done in the absence of length change. Strength gains have been demonstrated with isometric training; however, this will only occur at the position at which the exercise is performed. Strength gains throughout a muscle range of motion requires dynamic progressive resistance loading through that range. Following injury, or in response to other situations requiring immobilization, isometric training can maintain or strengthen weakened tissues during the period of immobilization.

Identifying optimal target resistance and training intensity to ensure maximal strength gains has been a difficult task. Basic strength programs utilize a set of consecutive muscle contractions against an applied load, repeated over several sets of increasing intensity. DeLorme and Watkins devised a method for developing strength programs utilizing a repetition maximum (RM).[38] This is defined as the greatest load a muscle can move through a full range of motion a specific number of times. Investigators have recommended a baseline of 6 RM to 15 RM to improve strength.[39] Extensive research has demonstrated that muscle strength gains have been greatest when trained between 60 and 100% of a 1 RM.[38,39] Other methods of determination have utilized isokinetic dynamometers or myometers, which are somewhat more accurate in determining an optimal starting point to initiate a weight training program. A second variable in resistance training programs is the number of repetitions to promote strength gains. An optimal number of repetitions has yet to be definitively determined. Both load and repetitions can be progressively increased as part of training to improve strength and endurance. Many standard strength training programs involve training with 60–80% of a 1 RM through 8–12 repetitions over 3–4 sets. Great variability exists in defining optimal resistance and intensity with which to train.

Additional variables that can be manipulated within strength training are the duration of the program, the velocity with which movements are performed, and the ability to overload specific muscles to be trained by isolation. Physiologic and histologic changes of muscle in response to strength training occur over weeks to months. A balance exists between tissue breakdown (catabolism) and tissue buildup (anabolism). This is impacted by a number of factors, including nutritional support, rest, and stress. The velocity of concentric muscle contraction has an inverse relationship with the tension generated by the tissue. As velocity of contraction increases, potential force generation within the muscle decreases. The opposite is true for eccentric contractions, which have high potential force generation with higher velocity movements, often seen in multijoint, high-resistance power training. A variety of exercise movements exist for specific muscles. Often, different exercises selectively train a portion of a muscle, allowing greater specificity of training to tailor to an athlete's individual needs.

Strength training for the spine and supporting elements

Basic strength training principles apply to supporting muscles of the spine in the same way they do in muscles within the extremities. Several critical factors impact on these principles as they pertain to the spinal column. Earlier it was mentioned that the vertebra, intervertebral disc, zygapophyseal joints, and the ligamentous system of the spine create physiologic limitations in spinal range of motion, limiting potential resistance training movements. In addition, the deep muscles, which attach or originate from the spine, have very short lever arms, creating a disadvantage when attempting to apply loads across these muscles. Muscles controlling spinal movements tend to work as groups, making muscle isolation difficult to accomplish. Multiple degrees of freedom and planes of motion of spinal segments require complex training movements, which can be difficult to perform safely and correctly.

Typically, strength training programs targeting the spinal column focus on three core muscle groupings. All three groupings will be briefly described, with differentiation between cervicothoracic and thoracolumbar exercises which target the respective regions. Little scientific evidence exists to support selection of one form of spinal exercise over another. It must be recognized that spinal-related muscle groupings can be loaded and strengthened in more than one fashion. Popular programs utilize mat- or floor-based techniques, exercises using a physioball, machine-based movements, and free weight exercises. Examples of each type of approach will be discussed and presented.

The spinal extensor complex stems from a thick thoracolumbar fascia and extends cephalad along the entire dorsal spinal column, ending in the suboccipital region. This muscle grouping comprises several layers of long strap-like planes of muscle. The muscle planes act in combination to produce extension and/or rotation of spinal motion segments. These muscles also serve a postural role in maintaining upright position of the head and torso. In the upper back the more superficial rhomboid and trapezius muscles link the spinal column to the scapula. From there, the shoulder girdle musculature transmits functional movement to the upper extremity. Similarly, in the low back the gluteals, hip girdle, and hamstring muscles act in similar fashion, transmitting force through the lower extremities, and indirectly contributing to lumbar spinal extension. Standard strength training movements for the upper back and shoulder girdle are listed in Box 1.6. Lumbar extensor and associated hip girdle movements are listed in Box 1.7.

The spinal flexors oppose the extensor group, and work through more complex mechanisms. In the cervical spine the sternocleidomastoid muscles act obliquely to produce a combination of flexion and rotation of the head and neck. In the lower torso, multiple planes of muscles act as the key flexors of the torso. Superficially, the midline abdominals – namely the rectus abdominis – act as key stabilizers and flexors. Internally, the iliopsoas muscles act as flexors and rotators. Finally, the rectus femoris and superficial hip flexors also contribute in stabilizing and flexing the lower torso. Traditional lumbar flexor strength training movements are listed in Box 1.8.

A third group of accessory muscles serve key functions in lumbar spinal mechanics. The quadratus lumborum muscle arises off each side of the spinal column and inserts onto the posterior ilium. It acts as a weak extensor and major muscle to induce sidebending. In addition, it contributes to postural stabilization and control. A series of muscle sheets lateral to the rectus abdominus have gained recognition as important postural stabilizers in addition to their role as rotators and side-benders of the lumbar spine.[40] The large, posterior latissimus dorsi muscle also plays a role in controlling sidebending of the lower trunk (see Box 1.3).

Box 1.6 Upper spinal extensor and shoulder girdle strength training movements

Upright Row – Trapezius/Rotator Cuff
Barbell/Dumbbell Shoulder Shrug – Trapezius
T Bar/Bent Over Row – Rear Deltoid/Rhomboid
Seated Cable Row – Rear Deltoid/Rhomboid
Lateral Dumbbell Raises – Deltoids
Military Press – Deltoids/Trap
Cable Lat Pulldown – Latissimus/Rotator Cuff

Box 1.7 Lumbar spinal extensor and hip girdle strength training movements

Deadlift – Paraspinals/Gluteals
Roman Chair – Paraspinals/Gluteals
Squat/Leg Press – Gluteals/Quadriceps
Lumbar Extension Machine – Paraspinals
Multiaxis Hip Girdle Machine – Hip Flexion/Extension/Abduction/Adduction
Prone Leg Curl Machine – Hamstrings

Box 1.8 Lumbar spinal flexor and accessory muscle strength training movements

Prone Abdominal Crunch – Upper Abdominals
Hanging Bent Knee/Straight Knee Leg Raise – Middle/Lower Abdominals/Hip Flexors
Decline Bench Situp – Upper/Middle/Lower Abdominals
Sidelying Oblique Crunch – Abdominal Obliques
Rotary Torso Machine – Obliques/Latissimus/Paraspinals

Spinal stabilization

In addition to graded, progressive resistance strengthening techniques, recent trends in spinal rehabilitation have emphasized the functional importance of a spinal stabilization program to augment more traditional strengthening, flexibility training, and conditioning.[41] These principles can be applied to augment a general spine fitness program. They build upon the idea of a "neutral spine" position, whereby the spinal motion segments and shoulder/pelvic positioning are restored to their natural balance and alignment. Using the lumbar spine as an example, this ensures better distribution of force through the spinal elements, lumbo-pelvic region, and lower extremities. This type of program conceptually minimizes mechanical stresses acting on spinal elements. For this reason, lumbar stabilization exercises are sometimes referred to as "core strengthening" programs. They are often the beginning elements of a spinal rehabilitation program, from which more dynamic, resistance and flexibility training is built.

A multitude of exercises and approaches exist to achieve these measures. Most produce a training effect by simulating basic functional movements of the lower abdomen, lumbar spine, pelvis, hip girdle, and gluteals. Movements involve direct isolation of specific muscles and more advanced, complex multimuscle patterns. They typically involve manual or body weight resistance of the trunk, limited to short arcs of motion. Exercises look to create a synergy between force coupled muscles, acting in concert to restore more natural biomechanics and a stable base. Efficiency and comfort of more complex movements can then be achieved by training the individual to operate from a more stable neutral spine position. A series of examples is presented, emphasizing this type of approach. Similar to more traditional strength training movements, stabilization programs can be divided into cervical, lumbar, spinal flexor, extensor, and accessory muscle exercises. Examples of basic and advanced movements targeting spinal flexors, extensors, and accessory musculature are demonstrated in Figures 1.2–1.13.

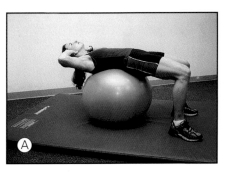
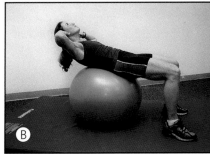

Figure 1.2
Basic abdominal stabilization movement targeting rectus abdominis.
A. Starting position, with slight hyperextension.
B. Finishing position, with maximal contraction of abdominals at end of movement.

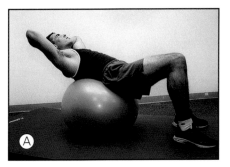
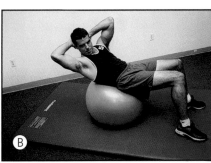

Figure 1.3
Basic abdominal stabilization movement targeting rectus abdominis and abdominal obliques.
A. Starting position.
B. Finishing position with maximal contraction of abdominals at end of movement.

Figure 1.4
Basic lumbar stabilization movement targeting abdominals, lumbar flexors, and lumbar extensors.
A. "Angry Cat" (starting position), emphasizing lumbar hyperextension.
B. "Camel" (finishing position), emphasizing lumbar flexion and pelvic rotation.

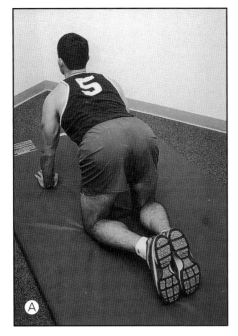

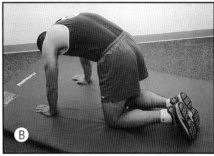

Figure 1.5
Lumbar stabilization movement.
A. Starting position.
B. "Bridging" (second position), emphasizing neutral spine position.
C. Single leg extension while holding bridge and neutral spine position.

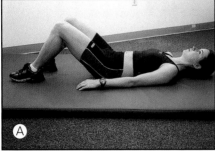

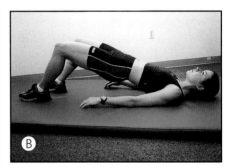

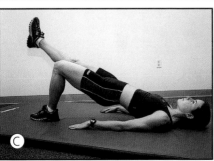

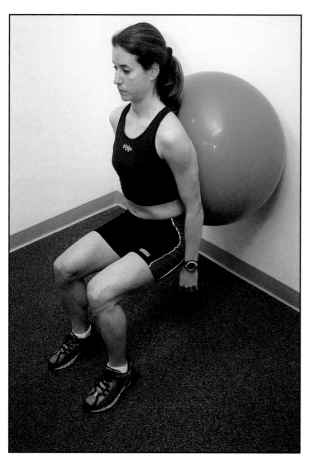

Figure 1.6
Isometric squat using physioball and maintaining neutral spine position. Feet are maintained parallel and tibio-femoral angle is maintained at 90 degrees.

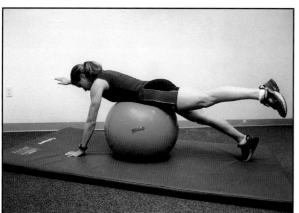

Figure 1.7
Advanced spinal stabilization movement targeting upper and lower spinal extensors, along with deltoids and gluteal accessory muscles.

Figure 1.8
Accessory muscle spinal stabilization movement, emphasizing spinal rotators, abdominal obliques, adductors, and hip flexors.
A. Finishing position 1.
B. Starting position.
C. Finishing position 2.

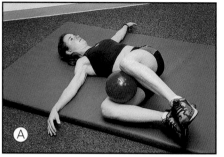

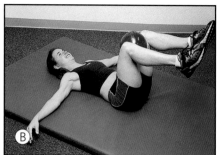

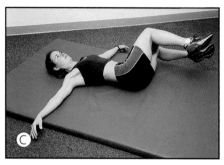

Figure 1.9
Upper spinal extensor stabilization movement targeting cervico-thoracic extensors, rear deltoids, lower traps, and rhomboids.
A. Starting position.
B. Finishing position with maximal contraction of rear deltoids and rhomboids at the end of the movement.

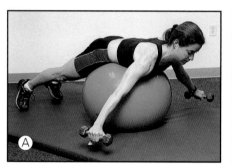

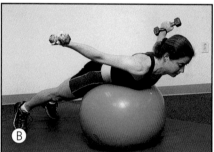

Figure 1.10
Upper spinal extensor stabilization movement, emphasizing cervico-thoracic paraspinals, middle/rear deltoids, rhomboids, and latissimus dorsi muscles.

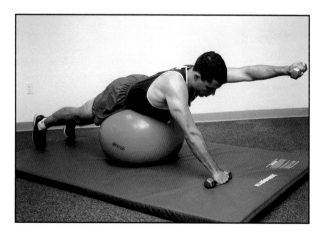

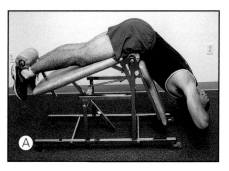

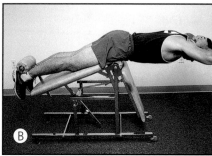

Figure 1.11
Roman Chair dynamic lumbar spinal extensor stabilization movement.
A. Starting position.
B. Finishing position, stopping at neutral spine, without hyperextension.

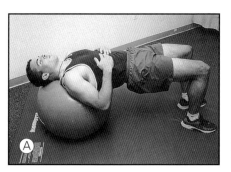

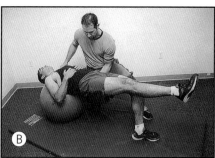

Figure 1.12
Advanced lumbar flexor spinal stabilization movement.
A. Starting position maintaining neutral spine, targeting abdominals, gluteals, quads, and hamstrings.
B. Second position – achieved by extending unilateral extremity, activating hip flexors, lower abdominals, quads, and abdominal obliques. Partial assist by examiner demonstrated to maintain neutral spine position.

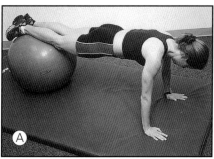

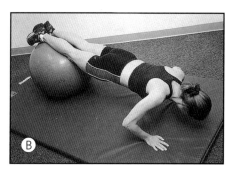

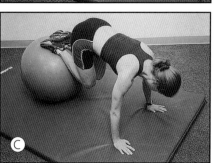

Figure 1.13
Advanced dynamic spinal stabilization movement targeting multiple muscle groups.
A. Starting position, maintaining neutral spine.
B. Position 2: pushup while maintaining neutral spine.
C. Position 3: lower extremity flexion, while maintaining neutral spine of thoraco-lumbar regions.

Conditioning and cross training

In addition to flexibility and strength training, the benefits of aerobic conditioning as part of a comprehensive exercise program have been well established. A detailed analysis of the physiology behind aerobic conditioning is beyond the scope of this chapter. As mentioned previously, training goals need to be clearly identified to maximize gains. It must be recognized, however, that maximal gains in strength and aerobic capacity cannot be obtained at the same time. Focused strength training requires an intense, focused progressive resistance program. Cardiovascular conditioning requires more aerobic, high-repetition, long-duration training. Athletes can often use periodization of training to enhance multiple aspects of their overall fitness. Under this premise, training can take on a different focus through scheduled intervals, with time spent on aerobic conditioning, strength, and power training. This is similar to *cross training*, where athletes balance participation in their primary sport, with crossover training in types of exercise that are atypical for the primary sport. These principles help to maintain overall fitness, allow for recovery time, and prevent overtraining.

Fitness is a global measure of cardiovascular functioning, muscle tissue performance, and general well-being. It is often quantified as a function of maximum oxygen consumption or maximum aerobic capacity ($VO_{2\,max}$). $VO_{2\,max}$ is defined as the maximum volume of oxygen consumed by the body per minute. This capacity can be increased with an aerobic or endurance training program. An increase in $VO_{2\,max}$ suggests an increase in the efficiency of the cardiovascular system and working muscle, which has a higher capacity to resist fatigue. These principles of peripheral adaptation apply to all skeletal muscle within the body, including those tissues closely associated with the spine.

Basic physiologic changes that occur in response to aerobic training involve the heart and peripheral cardiovascular system, respiratory system, and metabolism. A reduction in the resting and exercise driven pulse rate occurs, along with a decrease in resting and overall blood pressure. An increase in blood volume and blood hemoglobin levels occurs, as well as increased stroke volume and cardiac output. At the same time, enzymatic and biochemical changes occur in muscle tissue to increase oxygen extraction from circulating red blood cells. This increase in extraction leads to an increased utilization of available oxygen, and a decreased blood flow per kg of working muscle. Respiratory changes include larger lung volumes and greater alveolar-capillary surface area. This leads to increased ventilatory efficiency, but no change in maximal ventilation capacity. Metabolic adaptations include increased number and size of mitochondria, and increased muscle myoglobin concentration. With exercise, muscle glycogen is depleted at a slower rate and blood lactate levels are lower at submaximal workloads. Finally, there is an increased capacity to oxidize carbohydrate, or mobilize energy.

The adaptations presented involve complex physiologic mechanisms that were not reviewed. Most athletic endeavors involve some degree of endurance and aerobic activity. The manifestations of aerobic training augment and enhance performance, irregardless of the sport.

ASSESSMENT

Baseline health-related physical fitness testing

Introduction

As part of a thoughtful and comprehensive approach to athletic participation, baseline health-related fitness evaluation is recommended. The American College of Sports Medicine (ACSM) describes "health-related physical fitness" as typically including body composition, cardiorespiratory endurance, muscular strength and endurance, and flexibility.[42] The authors recognize that persons engaging in various sports cover a spectrum of ability and level of participation. At one end of the spectrum are gymnasts who are groomed from childhood for Olympic competition. At the other end of the spectrum is the "weekend warrior," recreating college grudge matches on the neighborhood basketball court. The skill and motivation levels of the particular athlete as well as access to training resources will determine the depth of a health-related fitness evaluation.

Baseline physical fitness testing, in addition to a medical evaluation, provides the foundation for identifying athletes at risk for illness and injury, for educating the athlete about general fitness and sports-specific injury prevention, and for achieving fitness or athletic goals. In addition to the baseline health-related fitness evaluation, assessment parameters relevant to "spine fitness" are also discussed.

The tests presented in this chapter are based on the wealth of information reviewed by the ACSM. The majority of tests described have proven to be valid and accurate, and are inexpensive and straightforward to administer. The reader is referred to the ACSM publication on exercise testing for detailed testing protocols. This chapter will briefly describe body composition determination, submaximal exercise testing for cardiorespiratory fitness, Borg's rating of perceived exertion (RPE), dynamic strength testing of 1-repetition maximum (1-RM), muscular endurance testing with the push-up and curl-up tests, and, finally, flexibility testing of the low back and hip girdle.

Body composition

A relative increase in percentage body fat versus lean body mass takes place in individuals at increased risk for type II diabetes, hypertension, and hyperlipidemia. The gold standard methods for determining body composition are hydrostatic (underwater) weighing and plethysmography, which measure body volume based on water and air displacement, respectively. The next best choice for determining body composition is to use the anthropometric method of skinfold measurement. This test requires a skilled technician. Skinfold measurement has a high correlation coefficient when compared to hydrostatic weighing ($r = 0.70–0.90$). The margin of error of skinfold measurement is $\pm$ 3.5%.

Calculation of the body mass index (BMI) and waist-hip circumference (WHR) are much less cumbersome methods; however, they are not as accurate. The BMI is the body weight (kg) divided by height (meters squared). The Expert Panel on the identification, evaluation, and treatment of overweight and obesity in adults[43] defined overweight as a BMI of 25.0–29.9 kg/m^2; obesity is defined as a BMI greater than or equal to 30.0 kg/m^2. Research has shown that health risks due to obesity increase with a BMI greater than 25.0 kg/m^2. Due to the large standard error ($\pm$ 5%), however, the ACSM does not recommend this test for fitness assessment.[44]

The WHR reflects the pattern of body fat distribution, being the ratio of waist-to-hip circumference. Increased fat distribution on the trunk, especially around the abdomen, is linked with a significantly greater risk of hypertension, type 2 diabetes, hyperlipidemia, coronary artery disease, and premature death. This correlation holds true in individuals with the same percentage of body fat. In the evaluation of abdominal obesity, waist circumference can also be used alone.[43] Studies have also shown that increased waist circumference is a marker for adverse health outcomes in persons of normal weight.

Cardiorespiratory fitness

Cardiorespiratory fitness depends on the heart, lungs, and skeletal muscle systems and is defined as the ability to perform large muscle, dynamic, moderate-to-high intensity exercise for prolonged periods.[42] The better an individual's cardiorespiratory fitness, the less likely he is to die from all causes. Individuals with poor cardiorespiratory fitness have a significant risk of premature death.[45–47] The gold standard for measuring cardiorespiratory fitness is the maximal oxygen uptake ($VO_{2\ max}$). The $VO_{2\ max}$ is the maximal cardiac output (L/min) multiplied by the arterial–venous difference (ml O_2/L). Maximal exercise testing requires technician expertise, time, and special equipment. An acceptable alternative is submaximal exercise testing. In these tests the heart rate response to submaximal work rates is used to predict $VO_{2\ max}$. The ACSM manual describes field tests such as the Cooper 12-minute test for distance, the 1.5 mile test for time and the Rockport one-mile fitness walking test (heart rate is measured during the last quarter mile). The other tests are more complex and use a motor-driven treadmill, mechanically braked cycle ergometers, or step testing. The treadmill, cycle, and step tests should include monitoring of the subject's heart rate, blood pressure, and rating of perceived exertion (RPE). Borg's RPE scale is a subjective assessment of individual exercise tolerance. Either the Borg category scale (6–20) or the category-ratio scale (0–10) can be used. Interestingly, on the scale a rating of "somewhat hard" to "hard" (12–16) or "moderate" to "strong" (4–5) is reliably correlated with the threshold for blood lactate accumulation and a cardiorespiratory training effect.

Muscular fitness

Muscular fitness is a term that includes both muscular strength (maximal force a muscle can generate at a given velocity in newtons or kilograms) and muscular endurance (ability of a muscle to make repeated contractions or to resist muscular fatigue).[48,49] The gold standard of evaluating muscular strength is to test dynamic strength with the 1-RM, which is the heaviest weight that a subject can lift while maintaining optimal technique. For upper body strength, either the bench press or military press are evaluated; for lower body strength, the leg press or leg extension are used. Other tests, using cable tensiometers or handgrip dynamometers, test static or isometric strength and allow determination of maximal voluntary contraction. These methods only test a specific muscle group, as opposed to the 1-RM, which better evaluates overall muscular strength.

Muscular endurance evaluates a muscle group's ability to perform repeated contractions over a period of time sufficient to cause muscular fatigue or maintain a specific percentage of maximal voluntary contraction for a prolonged period of time.[42] The standardized tests to evaluate are simple and inexpensive to administer and include the curl-up (crunch) test[50,51] for abdominal endurance and the push-up test for upper body endurance.[52] Another popular test is the YMCA test, which uses the bench press to measure muscular endurance by setting a submaximal resistance and counting the number of repetitions to fatigue. Using the YMCA test, the subject lifts at a rate of 30 lifts/min. Women use a 35 lb barbell and men use an 80 lb barbell. The score is the total number of repetitions until the muscles fatigue.

Flexibility

Flexibility is defined as the ability to move a joint through a complete range of motion. The American Academy of Orthopaedic Surgeons[9] has established normal values for all the joints in the body. Flexibility is affected by many intrinsic factors, including age, gender, genetic predisposition, and so forth. Extrinsic factors are also important, including level of fitness, type of athletic participation, etc. Moreover, the level of optimal flexibility depends on the individual's goal, whether that be simply to perform the activities of daily living or to become an Olympic gymnast. Flexibility can be measured through visual estimation, tape measures, goniometers, inclinometers, and so on. In terms of standards for health-related fitness testing, the sit-and-reach test has been used to grossly assess low-back and hip-girdle flexibility. For the purposes of spine fitness, the components of flexibility assessment should include the neck, shoulder girdle, trunk lateral bending, trunk forward flexion, trunk extension; hip girdle (including IR/ER and the Ely and Thomas tests); and straight leg-raise (also assess for neural tension signs).

Functional movement screen

In addition to the more standardized approaches to fitness evaluation, a new approach is being taken to baseline fitness testing which moves beyond the usual one-dimensional, traditional spine assessment. The typical spine examination includes measuring gross range of motion and a neurologic examination for sensation, strength, reflexes, and neural tension signs. Rehabilitation focuses on symptomatic-relief, achieving optimal flexibility, strengthening, conditioning, and ergonomic correction. In the occupational medicine literature, an important theoretical and simply practical leap was the introduction of "work hardening" to the rehabilitation. This method takes a functional approach to rehabilitation and has been successful in returning more injured workers to their jobs. From this research it follows that our rehabilitation should ideally include more functional assessment and functional rehabilitation. Bronner[53] notes that in rehabilitation we often neglect the most important link, the "return to functional movement with its multiple degrees of freedom and richness of expression." Specifically, Bronner states that "the crucial and often missing key is to provide the necessary neuromuscular learning experiences and feedback to achieve optimal safe motor control of the lumbopelvic area." The lumbopelvis is recognized by these authors as the key point of control for the optimal spine fitness. This approach to functional rehabilitation is also mirrored in the focus on core rehabilitation. The lumbopelvis is referred to the "hub" for weight-bearing and functional kinetic chain movement.[54]

Interestingly, a functional movement approach to rehabilitation can also be much more motivating for the patient/athlete than traditional rehabilitation strategies and thereby elicit greater compliance with the treatment regimens. The successful introduction of such practices as yoga and Pilates to training football players is a perfect example of this shift in prehabilitation and rehabilitation strategies. Of course, this strategy can only go so far, in that the athletic trainer may not be able to actually tell the football players that they are doing "dance" exercises.

One of the most compelling assessment tools born of this paradigm shift is the Functional Movement Screen™ created by Gray Cook, MPT.[55] The FMS™ consists of seven simple tests to assess functional movement quality. Each of the seven tests is scored on a three-point scale for a total score of 21. The tests were developed from observing the mobility and stability milestones of human development: stepping, reaching, striding or kicking, squatting, and lunging, as well as two additional movements that require anterior–posterior stress (pushing) and rotatory spine stabilization.[55] Also included are screening tests for shoulder impingement and back pain. The reader is referred to the original reference for a complete discussion of the seven tests and their significance.

This method is being adopted by athletic trainers in the NFL, NHL, and NBA. Data is limited so far, but early results are promising. There are times in science when looking only at the parts in a relatively static, quantitative, single-variable approach limits our understanding of the whole, dynamic, functional person. This approach to evaluating an athlete's fitness is appealing because it looks at a set of movement patterns that integrate multiple elements at one time, including optimal flexibility, strength, endurance, and core stability. This approach may be akin to mastering yoga postures or Pilates exercises, which draw from the whole of the body's physical (and mental) resources.

Gray Cook, MPT, challenges sports enthusiasts to look first at the quality of a movement. Instead of the foundation being a quantitative variable such as strength, the foundations of performance are "functional movement patterns and motor control."[55] Athletic movement is comprehensively assessed in the following three ways: [55]

1. Functional movement quality: basic fundamental movements that demonstrate full range of motion, body control, balance, and body stability.
2. Functional performance quantity: general, nonspecific performance demonstrating gross power, speed, endurance, and agility. This element is assessed by time or distance trials such as the 40-yard dash or vertical leap.
3. Sports-specific skills: skills that demonstrate sports-specific movement patterns.

In this brief introduction to Gray Cook's work, the discussion is focused on functional movement quality, as opposed to functional performance quantity or sports-specific skills, because this is a truly novel concept in our reinventing baseline fitness testing. The "building blocks"[55] of functional movement are mobility and stability coordinated by the neuromuscular system. In terms of the spine, we have only recently appreciated how the core muscles such as the transversus abdominus and multifidus muscles function to stabilize spinal segments so that an athlete can efficiently transfer power through the lumbopelvis to the extremities in motion.

Cook recommends assessing mobility of the lumbar spine and hip/pelvic girdle using functional movements such as performing an overhead squat with a bar or an in-line lunge. Stability is defined as a "representation of body control through strength, coordination, balance and efficiency of movement."[55] Stability is divided into static and dynamic types, where static stability involves maintenance of posture and balance and dynamic stability involves production and control of movement. Dynamic stability is further broken down into five components that must function optimally: mobility and flexibility, strength, coordination, local muscular endurance, and cardiovascular fitness.[55] For example, a sweep rower who has not optimized these building blocks may have a fast 2000 meter *stationary* rowing ergonometer time, representing strength and endurance, but then is not able to transfer that level of performance to a fast time in a boat, which requires greater coordination on the water and coordination with other rowers.

According to Cook,[55] the new paradigms in optimizing athletic potential can be drawn from observing the developmental patterns in infants. The healthy infant is born with more mobility than stability. During the infant's development, the core is selectively stabilized before the extremities. Specifically, the infant first learns head control, then sitting, then crawling, then cruising, then walking, and so forth. This pattern is also observed in motor recovery after a stroke. Whether in the setting of motor recovery or motor learning, motor control and stability proceed in a predictable pattern from head to toe and from proximal to distal.

In translating these concepts to the pre-rehabilitation or rehabilitation of athletes, the bottom line is that proper technique, mobility, and stability are emphasized before strengthening, conditioning, and sports-specific skills training. Cook emphasizes that "the most common mistake in sports conditioning today is training a movement pattern before achieving full range of motion and control of that movement."[55] Coaches, trainers and sports medicine experts have only recently dissuaded athletes from focusing only on the "mirror muscles" instead of the core. Unless the focus is on a foundation of mobility, stability, and neuromuscular control first, athletes risk hard-wiring movement patterns that may place them at greater risk for injury, as well as limiting athletic potential.

EXERCISE PRESCRIPTION

Comparisons between recreational and competitive athletes will reveal varying levels of training assistance and supervision. Levels of commitment and lifestyle factors will also affect preparedness for athletic participation with respect to training, nutrition, and recovery. With these factors in mind, developing and implementing an exercise program relies on clarity of communication between the physician and multiple potential parties: therapists, trainers, exercise physiologists, coaches, parents, and most often the athlete directly. A fundamental objective of the exercise prescription is to implement changes in personal health and training behavior. For the athlete, this change may lead to enhanced performance, injury prevention, or injury rehabilitation.

Traditional exercise prescription builds upon the training principle termed *specific adaptation to imposed demand* (SAID).[56] This principle anticipates predictable response of human tissues to a given demand. Tissues such as muscle that are subject to repetitive high-level training will respond with physiologic adaptation to function more efficiently at that higher level. Under this premise, workload can be varied to target a particular training goal. For example, low-resistance, high-repetition training will lead to improved endurance, whereas high-resistance, low-repetition training will build strength.

Identification of a targeted training goal is important to direct the progression of a proposed exercise program. It also allows for a selection of exercises that will maximize the potential that the desired training effect will be achieved. Traditional elements of the exercise prescription involve four basic elements (Box 1.9).

Box 1.9 Components of an exercise prescription

1. Mode of exercise
2. Intensity
3. Frequency
4. Duration

Mode of exercise

Specifics of the desired training activities should be outlined based on the goals of the program. Suggested components of the program should be identified and differentiated. General details for strength training, aerobic conditioning, or flexibility training should be specified. This includes the type of resistance exercise (isometric, isotonic, plyometric, etc.), details of flexibility training, and muscle groupings or tissues to be isolated. Free weights, variable resistance equipment, theraband, or other training equipment are some options to the practitioner. Mode of aerobic activity (bike, treadmill, elliptical, aquatic, etc, ...) should also be identified.

Intensity

Parameters on the intensity of both strength and aerobic training should be defined. Ranges for aerobic training vary based on $VO_{2\,max}$ or percent maximal heart rate. Typically, 40–85% $VO_{2\,max}$ or 55–90% max heart rate are the respective target ranges.[22] For lower level athletes, utilization of a rate of perceived exertion (RPE) scale can also be helpful. For strength training, a percentage of a one or ten repetition maximum is often identified to focus, define, and guide training and training progression.

Frequency

Frequency of exercise defines parameters on how often exercise or elements of exercise are performed. Typical programs suggest 3–5 days per week, depending on the intensity. Competitive athletes may have varying training schedules, depending on time of year, and how that applies to in and off season. Preseason workouts may be daily, sometimes multiple sessions, while in-season programs will often look to maintain general strength and fitness, with focused sport specific work, and injury rehab if needed. Practitioners must respect the need for scheduled rest intervals to allow for tissue recovery in response to intense training.

Duration

This parameter defines the length of individual training sessions. It is usually quantified by a proposed number of minutes at a given intensity. For power or strength training, sessions are typically of short duration, with target parameters defining a set number of repetitions per set, and a total number of sets per session. For aerobic training, longer, sustained sessions, at a specified percent max heart rate is needed to achieve an appreciable training effect. For both strength and aerobic training, exercise intensity typically has an inverse relationship with sustainable time of effort. Variable factors include continuous versus interrupted training, rest between sets, supersets, pyramid sets and isolation versus muscle group exercises.

To ensure a worthwhile and appropriate exercise program, practitioners must understand movement, energy contributions, and physical requirements in a sports-specific manner. Elements of strength, power, endurance, dexterity, and flexibility must all be considered based on their relative importance to enhance performance in a given athletic activity. Well-balanced training cannot be underemphasized, along with cross-training to augment more specific and focused approaches. Pre-participation warm-up and post training rest intervals are also vital elements that should be emphasized and stressed in a well-rounded program. Over-training occurs when sustained, intense exercise is not complemented by appropriate rest intervals and nutritional support to allow tissue regeneration and repair. This all too common scenario can be manifest as subtle, maladaptive symptoms of mild fatigue, poor sleep patterns, mood alterations, diffuse myalgias, and decreased performance. If uncorrected, this syndrome can lead to physiologic changes in hormonal, cardiovascular, and musculoskeletal systems. It can also lead to tissue breakdown and increase the risk of acute injury.

REFERENCES

1. Panjabi MM: The stabilizing system of the spine. Part I: function, dysfunction, adaptation and enhancement. J Spinal Disord 5(4):383–389, 1992.
2. Frymoyer JW, Pope MH: Risk factors in low back pain: an epidemiologic survey. J Bone Joint Surg (Am) 65A: 213–218, 1983.
3. Tall RL, DeVault W: Spinal injury in sport: epidemiologic considerations. Clin Sport Med 12(3):441–448, 1993.
4. Cole AJ, Herring S, Stratton, SA: The lumbar spine and sports. In: Cole AJ, Herring S, eds. The low back pain handbook: a practical guide for the primary care clinician. Philadelphia: Hanley & Belfus; 1997:309–321.
5. Gerbino PG, Micheli LJ: Back injuries in the young athlete. Clin Sports Med 14(3):571–590, 1995.
6. Panjabi MM, White AA: Clinical biomechanics of the spine, 2nd edn. Philadelphia: JB Lippincott; 1990:23–45.

7. Gleim GW, McHugh MP: Flexibility and its effects on sports injury and performance. Sports Med 24(5):289–299, 1997.

8. Luebbers P: Enhancing your flexibility. Fit: A quarterly publication of the American College of Sports Medicine, 2002:5 and 8.

9. Protas EJ: Flexibility. ACSM resource manual for guidelines for exercise testing and prescription, 3rd edn. Baltimore, MD: Williams and Wilkins; 1998:368–377.

10. Alter MJ: The science of flexibility, 2nd edn. Champaign, IL: Human Kinetics; 1996.

11. Blanke D: Flexibility. In: Mellion MB, ed. Sports medicine secrets, 2nd edn. Philadelphia, PA: Hanley and Belfus; 1999:70–75.

12. Krivickas LS: Training flexibility. In: Frontera WR, Dawson DM, Slonk DM, eds. Exercise in rehabilitation medicine. Champaign, IL: Human Kinetics; 1999:83–102.

13. Kendall HO, Kendall FP: Normal flexibility according to age groups. J Bone Joint Surg 30A(3):690–694, 1948.

14. Micheli LJ: Overuse injuries in children's sports: the growth factor. Orthop Clin N Am 14:337–360, 1983.

15. Barnekow-Bergkvist M, Hedberg G, Janlert U, Jansson E: Development of muscular endurance and strength from adolescence to adulthood and level of physical activity in men and women at the age of 34 years. Scand J Med Sci Sports 6:145–155, 1996.

16. Pratt M: Strength, flexibility, and maturity in adolescent athletes. Am J Dis Child 143(5):560–563, 1989.

17. Leibesman JL, Cafarelli E: Physiology of range of motion in human joints: a critical review. Crit Rev Phys Rehab Med 6:131–160, 1994.

18. Munns K: Effects of exercise on the range of joint motion in elderly subjects. In: Smith E, Serfass RC, eds. Exercise and aging: the scientific basis. Hillsdale, NJ: Enslow; 1981:167–178.

19. Rabb DM, Agre JC, McAdam M, Smith EL: Light resistance and stretching exercise in elderly women: effect upon flexibility. Arch Phys Med Rehabil 69(4):268–272, 1988.

20. Corbin CB, Noble, L: Flexibility: a major component of physical fitness. J Phys Ed Recreation 51(6):23–24, 57–60, 1980.

21. Mense S: Effect of temperature on the discharges of muscle spindles and tendon organs. Pflugers Arch 374:159–166, 1978.

22. Pollack ML, Wilmore JH: Exercise in health and disease. Evaluation and prescription for prevention and rehabilitation. Philadelphia: WB Saunders; 1990.

23. Jami L: Golgi tendon organs in mammalian skeletal muscle: functional properties and central actions. Physiol Rev 72(3):623–666, 1992.

24. Milne RA, Mierau DR: Hamstring distensibility in the general population: relationship to pelvic and low back stresses. J Manipul Physiol Therap 2(1):146–150, 1979.

25. Pheasant S: Bodyspace: anthropometry, ergonomics and design. London: Taylor & Francis; 1986.

26. Pheasant S: Ergonomics, work and health. Gaithersburg, MD: Aspen; 1991.

27. Lewitt K: Manipulative therapy in rehabilitation of the locomotor system, 2nd edn. Oxford: Butterworth-Heinemann; 1991.

28. Safran MR, Garrett WE, Seaber AV: The role of warm up in muscular injury prevention. Am J Sports Med 16(1):123–129, 1988.

29. Mair SD, Seaber AV, Glisson RL: The role of fatigue in susceptibility in acute muscle strain injury. Am J Sports Med 24:137–143, 1996.

30. Smith AD, Stroud L, McQueen C: Flexibility and anterior knee pain in adolescent elite figure skaters. J Pediatr Orthop 11:77–82, 1991.

31. Craib MW, Mitchell VA, Fields KB: The association between flexibility and running economy in sub-elite male distance runners. Med Sci Sports Exerc 28(6):737–743, 1996.

32. Harris BA, Watkins MP: Adaptations to strength conditioning. In: Frontera WR, Dawson DM, Slonk DM, eds. Exercise in rehabilitation medicine. Champaign, IL: Human Kinetics; 1999:71–81.

33. Frontera WR, Hughes VA, Lutz KJ, et al: A cross sectional study of muscle strength and mass in 45 to 78 year old men and women. J Appl Physiol 71:644–650, 1991.

34. Booth SW: Time course of muscular atrophy during immobilization of hind limbs of rats. J Appl Physiol 43:656–661, 1977.

35. Deschenes MR, Maresh JF, Crivello IE, et al: The effects of exercise training of different intensities on neuromuscular junction morphology. J Neurocytol 22:603–615, 1993.

36. Stone MH: Implications for connective tissue and bone alterations resulting from resistance exercise training. Med Sci Sports Exerc 20(Suppl):162–168, 1998.

37. Smith R, Rutherford OM: Spine and total body bone mineral density and serum testosterone levels in male athletes. Eur J Appl Physiol 67:330–334, 1993.

38. DeLorme T, Watkins A: Techniques of progressive resistance exercise. Arch Phys Med Rehab 29:263, 1948.

39. Kisner C, Colby AC: Therapeutic exercise: foundations and techniques, 2nd edn. Philadelphia: FA Davis; 1990.

40. O'Sullivan PB, Phyty GD, Twomey LT: Evaluation of specific stabilizing exercise in the treatment of chronic low back pain with radiologic diagnosis of spondylolysis or spondylolisthesis. Spine 22(24):2959–2967, 1997.

41. Hartigan C, Miller L, Liewehr SC: Rehabilitation of acute and subacute low back and neck pain in the work injured patient. Orth Clin N Am 27(4):841–860, 1996.

42. American College of Sports Medicine: Physical fitness testing and interpretation. In: Franklin BA, Whaley MH, Howley ET, eds. ACSMs guidelines for exercise testing and prescription, 6th edn. Philadelphia: Lippincott, Williams and Wilkins; 2000:57–90.

43. Expert Panel: Executive summary of the clinical guidelines on the identification, evaluation, and treatment of overweight and obesity in adults. Arch Intern Med 158:1855–1867, 1998.

44. Lohman TG: Dual energy X-ray absorptiometry. In: Roche AF, Heymsfield SB, Lohman TG, eds. Human body composition. Champaign, IL: Human Kinetics; 1996:63–78.

45. Blair SN, Kohl HW III, Barlow CE, et al: Changes in physical fitness and all-cause mortality: a prospective study of healthy and unhealthy men. JAMA 273:1093–1098, 1995.

46. Blair SN, Kohl HW III, Paffenbarger RS Jr, et al: Physical fitness and all-cause mortality: a prospective study of healthy men and women. JAMA 262:2395–2401, 1989.

47. Paffenbarger RS Jr, Hyde RT, Wing AL, et al: The association of changes in physical-activity level and other lifestyle characteristics with mortality among men. N Engl J Med 328:538–545, 1991.

48. Kramer WJ, Fry AC: Strength testing: developing and evaluation of methodology. In: Maud PJ, Foster C, eds. Physiological assessment of human fitness. Champaign, IL: Human Kinetics; 1995:115–138.

49. Graves JE, Pollack ML, Bryant CX: Assessment of muscular strength and endurance. In: Roitman JL, ed. ACSM's resource manual for guidelines for exercise testing and prescription, 3rd edn. Baltimore, MD: Williams and Wilkins; 1998:363–367.

50. Diener MH, Golding LA, Diener D: Validity and reliability of a one-minute half sit-up test of abdominal muscle strength and endurance. Sports Med Training Rehab 6:105–119, 1995.

51. Faulkner RA, Springings ES, McQuarrie A, et al: A partial curl-up protocol for adults based on an analysis of two procedures. Can J Sport Sci 14:135–141, 1989.

52. Canadian Standardized Test of Fitness Operations Manual, 3rd edn. Ottawa, Canada: Fitness and Amateur Sport Canada; 1986.

53. Bronner S: Functional rehabilitation of the spine: the lumbopelvis as the key point of control. In: Brownstein B, Bronner S, eds. Functional movement in orthopaedic and sports physical therapy: Evaluation, treatment, and outcomes. New York: Churchill Livingstone; 1997:141–190.

54. Porterfield JA, DeRosa C: Mechanical low back pain: perspectives in functional anatomy. Philadelphia: WB Saunders; 1991.

55. Cook G: Baseline sports-fitness testing. In: Foran B, ed. High-performance sports conditioning. Champaign, IL: Human Kinetics; 2001:19–55.
56. Young J, Press JM: Rehabilitation of lumbar spine injuries. In: Kibler WB, Herring SA, Press JM, eds. Functional rehabilitation of sports and musculoskeletal injuries. Gaithersburg, MD: Aspen; 1998:9–15.

FURTHER READING

Anderson B, Burke ER: Scientific, medical and practical aspects of stretching. Clin Sports Med 10(1):63–86, 1991.

Bandy WD, Irion JM, Briggler M: The effect of time and frequency of static stretching on flexibility of the hamstring muscles. Phys Ther 77:1090–1096, 1997.

Cole AJ, Farrell JP, Stratton SA: Functional rehabilitation of cervical spine athletic injuries. In: Kibler WB, Herring SA, Press JM, eds. Functional rehabilitation of sports and musculoskeletal injuries. Gaithersburg, MD: Aspen Inc.; 1998:127–144.

Congeni J, McCulloch J, Swanson K: Lumbar spondylosis: a study of natural progression in athletes. Am J Sports Med 25(2):248–253, 1997.

George SZ, Delitto A: Management of the athlete with low back pain. Clin Sports Med 21(1):105–132, 2002.

Geraci MC: Rehabilitation of hip, pelvis and thigh. In: Kibler WB, Herring SA, Press JM, eds. Functional rehabilitation of sports and musculoskeletal injuries. Gaithersburg, MD: Aspen Inc.; 1998:216–226.

Haher TR, O'Brian M, Kauffman C, et al: Biomechanics of the spine in sports. Clin Sport Med 12(3):449-464, 1993.

Hooker D: Back rehabilitation. In: Prentice WE, ed. Rehabilitation techniques in sports medicine, 2nd edn. St. Louis: Mosby; 1994:277–302.

Kaul M, Herring SA: Rehabilitation of lumbar spine injuries. In: Kibler WB, Herring SA, Press JM, eds. Functional rehabilitation of sports and musculoskeletal injuries. Gaithersburg, MD: Aspen Inc.; 1998:188–215.

Kraus D, Shapiro D: The symptomatic lumbar spine in the athlete. Clin Sports Med 8(1):59–69, 1989.

Krivickas LS: Anatomical factors associated with overuse sports injuries. Sports Med 2:132–146, 1997.

MacDougal JD, Wenger HA, Green HJ: Physiological testing of the high performance athlete, 2nd edn. Champaign, IL: Human Kinetics Books; 1991.

Pollock ML, Gaesser GA, Butcher JD, et al: The recommended quality and quantity of exercise for developing and maintaining cardiorespiratory and muscular fitness, and flexibility in healthy adults. Med Sci Sports Exerc 30(6):975–991, 1998.

Pu CT, Nelson ME: Aging, function, and exercise. In: Frontera WR, Silver JK, eds. Essentials of PM&R. Philadelphia: Hanley & Belfus; 2002:391–424.

Scherping SC: Cervical disc disease in the athlete. Clin Sports Med 21(1):37–47, 2002.

Schneck CD: Functional and clinical anatomy of the spine. Physical medicine and rehabilitation: state of the art reviews. Philadelphia: Hanley & Belfus; 9(3):571–604, 1995.

Stanish W: Low back pain in athletes: an overuse syndrome. Clin Sports Med 6(2):321–344, 1987.

Sward L: The thoracolumbar spine in young elite athletes: current concepts on the effects of physical training. Sports Med 13(5):357–364, 1992.

Trainor TJ, Wiesel SW: Epidemiology of back pain in the athlete. Clin Sports Med 21(1):93–99, 2002.

Watkins RG: Lumbar disc injury in the athlete. Clin Sports Med 21(1):147–165, 2002.

Wimberly RL, Lauerman WC: Spondylolisthesis in the athlete. Clin Sports Med 21(1):133, 2002.

Wood KB: Spinal deformity in the adolescent athlete. Clin Sports Med 21(1):77–91, 2002.

Section Two

Age-related changes of the spine in the athlete

CHAPTER

2

Common Spinal Disorders in the Young Athlete

Julian Lin
Frederick Boop

There is no doubt that over the past 20 years sports have played a major role in the daily life of American youth. More than 30 million children and adolescents (<18 years old) participate in some sort of organized sports, while many others are involved in non-organized recreational sports.[1] Approximately one-half of the boys and one-quarter of the girls between the ages of 14 and 17 in the US participate in some sort of organized sports.[2] The popularity in youth sports seen in this country is mainly due to health reasons and popular trends. This popular trend explains why sport is a multibillion dollar industry, and why some professional athletes attract almost cult-like followings, particularly from adolescents. With increasing participation and involvement in sports, sport injuries have become an important entity in pediatrics. Sports-related spinal injury in children is the third most common cause after motor vehicle accidents and falls.[3] Approximately 10–15% of all sports injuries are related to the spine.[4]

Sports can be organized into recreational nonsupervised or supervised categories.[5] Recreational nonsupervised sports that are frequently associated with spine injuries include diving, surfing, and trampoline. Supervised organized sports can be divided into five different types:

1. collision sports such as football and hockey
2. contact sports such as lacrosse or basketball
3. noncontact, high-velocity sports such as skiing or gymnastics
4. noncontact, repetitive load sports such as running
5. noncontact, low-impact sports such as golf and bowling.[6]

In regard to sports injuries, there are several important differences between adults and young athletes that are worth mentioning. First of all, an adolescent is in a dynamic growth process which can cause back pain by itself.[4] Developmentally, the paraspinal muscles and soft tissues do not grow at the same rate as the bone, so some of the paraspinal soft tissues may become excessively tight and cause additional mechanical stress on the growing spine. In the adolescent, the cartilaginous end plate of the intervertebral disc is weaker than the nucleus pulposis; therefore, excessive compressive forces can cause the end plate to fracture.[4] Increased flexibility in young children predisposes them to spinal cord injury without radiographic abnormality (SCIWORA), and increased stress on the bony structures, especially with hyperextension, may lead to spondylolysis, commonly seen between the ages of 6 and 10.

There are also important differences seen in athletes when compared to the nonathletic population. By definition, athletes are participants involved at the highest levels of competition in a physically demanding sport.[7] Strict criteria apply to the adolescent who is dedicated to intense year-round training and who competes to win. There are several physical factors that make athletes different in their response to illness and injuries. The elite athletes have the advantage of having inherent natural talents such as flexibility, strength, and coordination. Constant and disciplined training enhances and strengthens paraspinal soft tissues, which offer additional protection from injuries. Top-level athletes are extremely competitive and are motivated for several reasons, such as potential scholarships and lucrative professional careers.[7] It is not uncommon for talented high school students to advance directly to professional sports careers, completely bypassing higher education. For these reasons, athletes have different motivation to return to play after injury than industrial workers with back pain.

ACUTE SPINAL INJURIES IN YOUNG ATHLETES

Often, young athletes are injured acutely with an identifiable event. Fortunately, most of these injuries are self-limited as a result of muscle strain and ligamentous sprain. Most feared injuries are those involving the cervical spine, which may result in quadriplegia. Most if not all of the fractures occur in the cervical spine; it is extremely rare for sports-related thoracolumbar fractures to occur, with the exception of downhill skating or skiing. It is beyond the scope of this chapter to describe the various types of spinal fractures and their management. Therefore, we will limit our discussion to the most common acute injuries sustained by young athletes and some of the commonly associated sports.

Sprain and strain

Muscle strain and ligamentous sprain are soft tissue injuries to the musculotendinous structures of the cervical, thoracic, and lumbar spine commonly seen in athletic activities.[5] This is a direct result of mechanical overload that exceeds paraspinal soft tissue capacity. Response of the injured soft tissue may include localized pain, tenderness, weakness, swelling, and limited range of motion. The associated pain is nonradicular and without sensory disturbances. The ligamentous supporting structures of the spine may be damaged by repeated insults, leading to chronic tears, calcification, and fibrosis.[5] A cumulative effect of ligamentous injury may lead to fibrosis and chronic pain. In both strain and sprain syndromes, fractures, instability, and neurological injury must be excluded. In a series conducted with college athletes, 59.5% of all back injuries are related to either strain or sprain.[8] These self-limited injuries are treated with ice, rest, nonsteroidal anti-inflammatory drugs (NSAIDs), or occasional trigger point injections, and are prevented by stretching and/or strengthening.

Specific sports related to devastating spinal injuries in young athletes

In the US, there are approximately 1.5 million athletes participating in junior and senior high school football.[9–11] Statistics show that the incidence of quadriplegic injury ranges from 1/7000 to 1/58 000.[12–14] The vast majority of these injuries are sustained by high school players.[15] Preadolescent and early adolescent disabling football injuries are almost nonexistent, due to their small size and lack of high-speed collision.[12,16] In high school, there is a discrepancy in player size, age, maturity, and speed, accounting for devastating cervical spine injuries. Defensive players account for most of the injuries.[15] Injuries usually occur when a tackler strikes an opponent with his head vertex and straight neck (Fig. 2.1). This is called spearing, and was outlawed in 1976 following rule changes that also disallowed all use of the top of the helmet in tackling.[17,18] Following this rule change, Torg et al reported that the incidence of permanent cervical quadriplegia in high school and college players decreased from 34 in 1976 to 5 in 1984.[19]

Most severe injuries in ice hockey are reported from Canada. They are almost exclusively seen in males with a mean age 20 years.[20,21] The usual mechanism of injury is a push or check from behind, with the player striking his head with a vertex axial load against the ice or boards around rink.[22] For these reasons, the American Academy of Pediatrics (AAP) recommended in March 2000 that body checking not be allowed in youth hockey for children aged 15 years or younger.[23]

Figure 2.1
A defensive player "spear tackling" an offensive player running with the ball; injuries usually occur when a tackler strikes an opponent with his head vertex and straight neck.

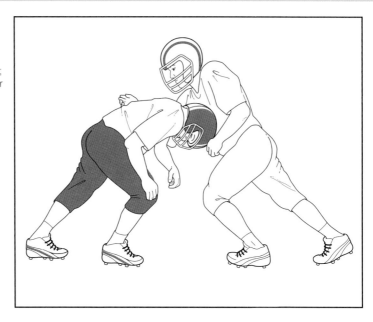

Diving is a recreational sport that is frequently associated with quadriplegic injuries. Diving injuries tend to occur in teenage males involved in recreational unsupervised activities in the summer.[24,25] According to the University of Pittsburgh's series, diving accounts for approximately 10% of all spinal injuries, with 55% occurring lakeside, 28% in a swimming pool, and 11% in rivers. Many diving injuries occur in swimming pools as young, athletic male divers leave the diving board and jump far enough out that they strike their head on the upslope of the pool (Fig. 2.2); C5 is the most commonly injured level. Neurologic involvement is seen in 70%, with 50% of these injuries being complete spinal cord injuries.[5,26]

Trampoline-related spinal injuries are the leading cause of serious spinal injuries in gymnastics. Torg and Das in 1984 identified 114 trampoline-related quadriplegias.[27] They found that injuries were

Figure 2.2
Many diving injuries occur in swimming pools as young, athletic male divers leave the diving board and jump far enough out that they strike their head on the upslope of the pool.

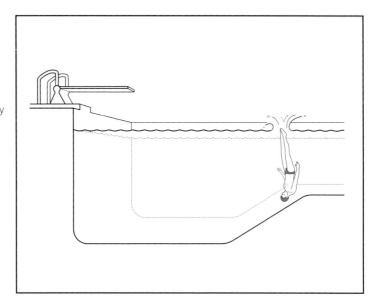

independent of the environment in which the trampoline was used, occurred despite mats and spotters, and were independent of the jumper's experience. Transient blackout may precede the accident. The AAP in 1977 issued a policy statement recommending that "trampolines be banned from use as part of physical education programs ... and also be abolished as a competitive sport."[28] Due to a decline in injuries in recent years, the AAP revised its position 4 years later to support trampoline use under certain conditions.[29]

Stingers, burners, burning hand syndromes, and transient cervical cord symptoms

Stingers and burners are named for dysesthetic burning pain in the shoulder radiating unilaterally into the hand usually in the C5 and C6 distribution. These are commonly seen among football players, with up to 50% of collegiate players reporting these symptoms during the course of a season.[30–32] The mechanism is believed to be due to traction of the upper brachial plexus, occurring when a force is applied that depresses the ipsilateral shoulder while the neck is laterally bent to the contralateral side. These injuries are usually self-limited but are commonly recurrent. Radiologic studies may show plexus injury without any evidence of spinal cord involvement. Electromyography may be helpful several weeks after the injury in confirming brachial plexus involvement by showing denervation potentials. Stingers and burners should be distinguished from the burning hand syndrome, which is a mild form of central spinal cord syndrome (Fig. 2.3). In the burning hand syndrome, there are usually bilateral transient paresthesias and dysesthesias in the upper limbs, most notably in the hands as a result of hyperextension occurring during collisions. There may be associated weakness, particularly in the distal upper extremities. In addition to the burning hand syndrome, other names for transient cervical cord symptoms include cervical cord neurapraxia, contusio cervicalis, cord concussion, and hysteria.[5,30–32]

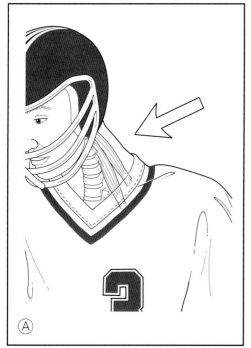

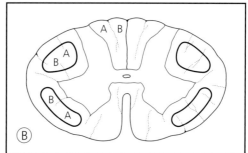

Figure 2.3
Anatomical differences between stingers and burning hand syndrome.
A. A stinger originating from brachial plexus traction injury.
B. The anatomy of the burning hand syndrome, which is a mild form of central cord syndrome usually affecting the upper distal extremities. Letter A corresponds to upper extremities, B to distal extremities.

For the most part, transient cervical cord symptoms are mostly an adult clinical entity associated with cervical stenosis and considered to be at high risk for recurrent injury. Other associated factors accounting for transient cervical symptoms include ligamentous instability, intervertebral disc disease, and congenital cervical anomalies. In children, transient cervical cord symptoms could be a mild form of SCIWORA rather than congenital cervical stenosis. Boockvar et al looked at 13 young athletes with a mean age of 11.5 years who sustained cervical cord neurapraxia.[33] Using sagittal canal diameter and Torg ratio, the authors did not find evidence of congenital cervical stenosis in this group of children with sports-related cervical cord neurapraxia.

Cervical stenosis

Congenital stenosis of the cervical spine is believed by many authorities to predispose athletes to injury.[34] What constitute stenosis or narrowing of the cervical spine canal is debatable. The range in normal adults is 10–17 mm for the C3–C7 levels. Most consider congenital cervical stenois to be present when the anteroposterior (AP) diameter is less than 13 mm. However, direct measurement of the canal width is sometimes difficult due to variations in X-ray magnification and measurement landmarks. In order to attempt to standardize the measurements of canal diameter to allow for, Torg proposed utilizing the canal-to-body ratio (Fig. 2.4). In this method, the distance of the anteroposterior width of the middle of the vertebral body compared with the corresponding level spinal canal measurement is measured. This canal-to-body, or Torg, ratio is considered abnormal, or indicative of significant cervical stenosis if the value is less than 0.8.[35] The main drawback to this method is that it tends to overestimate the degree of narrowing in athletes with large vertebral bodies. In a study of 80 professional football players, Herzog et al found that 49% had abnormal Torg ratios at one or more cervical canal levels.[36] The determining factor in their athletes was that the ratio was lowered by a larger value for the body width, not an abnormally small canal. The other pitfall of this ratio is that it does not consider the relationship between the spinal canal and spinal cord, which is often clarified by sagittal magnetic resonance imaging (MRI). Therefore, the Torg ratio should be used as a screening tool for stenosis, but abnormal values require further radiographic assessment.

Figure 2.4
Canal-to-body ratio; the distance of the anteroposterior width of the middle of the vertebral body is compared with the corresponding level spinal canal. This canal-to-body ratio, *A/B*, is considered abnormal if the value is less than 0.8.

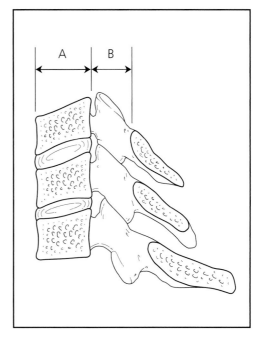

Cervical canal stenosis, when associated with high-velocity impact and combined with hyperextension, is considered dangerous by many. During hyperextension, the cervical canal is narrowed due to indentation of the ligamentum flavum and interspinous ligaments, and also by relaxation of the posterior longitudinal ligaments.[5] Reports have shown a frequency of recurrence of symptoms of up to 17%.[37,38] In a report of 10 patients with transient spinal cord symptoms for whom the authors had assessed the width of the cervical spinal canal, the authors found that 4 had canal diameters of less than 14 mm.[5] Interestingly, Torg et al did not find that football players with narrowed cervical canals were necessarily predisposed to subsequent injury if they returned to participate in contact sports after an episode of transient sensory symptoms of spinal cord origin.[35] However, these football players probably had a low Torg ratio due to large vertebral bodies and not true cervical stenosis. In our opinion, young athletes with symptomatic congenital cervical stenosis should avoid collision sports.

One other important clinical entity that can cause functional cervical spinal stenosis is the Chiari I hindbrain malformation. Cantu has proposed that obliteration of the subarachnoid space on MRI should be primary radiologic evidence of functional spinal stenosis.[39] Chiari malformation is a condition in which the cerebellar tonsils are caudally displaced (Fig. 2.5); it does satisfy Cantu's definition of functional stenosis. Callaway et al reported a case of transient quadriparesis in an 8-year-old football player after sustaining an axial blow to the head causing flexion of the neck during a tackle.[40] The patient was advised not to return to contact sports despite successful posterior fossa decompression. Syringomyelia is a fluid-filled cavity often found in the center of the spinal cord in conjunction with a Chiari malformation. Chiari I with syringomyelia is well described as a predisposition to spinal cord injury. Frogameni et al reported a 20-year-old college football player who sustained 10 minutes of left-sided hemiparesis after weightlifting.[41] MRI showed Chiari I with a C3–C7 syrinx. The patient was not treated but was advised to forgo sports.

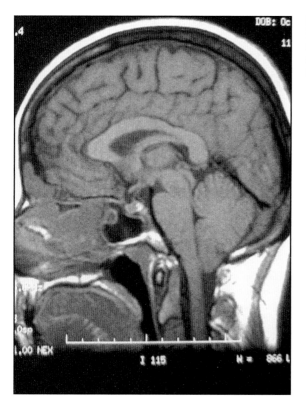

Figure 2.5
MRI findings of type I Chiari malformation with caudally displaced cerebellar tonsils causing functional stenosis.

Spinal cord injury without radiographic abnormality

In 1982, Pang and Wilberger described SCIWORA in 24 children.[42] Negative radiologic examinations are limited to plain films and computed tomography (CT). SCIWORA is seen primarily in children and is attributed to hypermobility of the spine related to ligamentous laxity, open ossification centers, a more horizontal orientation of the facets, wedge-shaped vertebral bodies, and a relatively larger head with underdeveloped musculature. Younger children are at higher risk of severe injury, but the overall prognosis for neurologic recovery is good. SCIWORA was described in the pre-MRI era. Therefore one would suspect that with the advent of MRI, fewer spinal cord injuries would remain undetected because of the high sensitivity of MRI for detecting mild spinal cord and ligamentous injuries. In a recent series of SCIWORA that correlated with MRI findings, most injuries (60%) were sports related, and each of these patients suffered a mild partial deficit. MRIs were all normal in these patients.[43] All these children with sports-related injuries made a good recovery. Two patients with more severe injuries had abnormal MRI findings and poor outcomes. In the current era, whether a child with transient cervical cord symptoms and negative MRI has SCIWORA or cervical cord neurapraxia is debatable and is significant only in the academic sense. However, MRI does prove its importance in the evaluation of SCIWORA as a method to exclude injuries undetected by plain films and CT. It also serves as a prognosticator for neurologic recovery.[33,43]

Criteria for return to play after cervical spine injuries

The decision to allow young athletes to return to play, especially to collision or contact sports, following spinal injury is a difficult one for the physician, the player, and his family. Risk assessment differs depending on the value system and biases of the physician. Difference in opinions exist for each scenario and are related to personal bias, clinical experience, clinical training, regional differences, and the medicolegal environment. Morganti et al surveyed a group of orthopedics and sports medicine physicians regarding their decision-making in terms of guidelines for return to play after sports-related cervical spine injuries.[6] Their results showed that respondents with a spine subspecialty interest recommended return to a higher level of play, whereas more senior physicians tended to recommend lower level of play. Torg and Watkins have independently derived general schemata to assist physicians in making these difficult decisions.[44,45]

Box 2.1 categorizes criteria for return to contact sports into low-, moderate-, and high-risk groups. The low-risk group includes conditions or injuries that are essentially benign, where the chance of further neurologic injury is minimal. There is a potential for permanent neurologic injury in the moderate risk group; decisions here of whether to allow an athlete to return to contact sport should be made on an individual basis. The high-risk category consists of conditions and injuries that are basically absolute contraindication to return to contact. One example of a high-risk athlete seen in our practice is a 13-year-old girl who developed neck and back pain while playing soccer. Plain films of the cervical spine showed a Klippel–Feil anomaly (see Fig. 2.6). A subsequent MRI showed a large cervical syrinx. A tethered spinal cord was found at surgery. Although postoperatively the patient remained neurologically intact, our recommendation to the patient, based on the criteria set by Torg and Watkins, was not to return to contact.[44,45] Controversy remains in the decision-making process for athletes with a history of cervical cord neurapraxia. Based on Box 2.1 criteria, a previous episode of neurapraxia is a relative contraindication for return to

---

Box 2.1 Risk assessment for return to play after cervical spine injury

Low risk or no contraindication

Congenital:
- spina bifida occulta
- type II Klippel–Feil at C3 and below without other anomalies

Developmental:
- Torg ratio <0.8
- nondisplaced stable healed fx of end plate
- one-level fusion
- asymptomatic bone spurs
- nondisplaced healed facet fractures
- brachial plexus neurapraxia
- healed disc herniations
- healed lamina fractures
- spinous process fractures

Box continued on following page

contact or collisions sports. Cervical cord neurapraxia with abnormal radiologic findings is an absolute contraindication. At the high school level, the decision for further participation of athletes with neurapraxia or transient quadriplegia is often made in conjunction with the parents. Frequently, the decision is to retire from collision or high-velocity sports.[6] In conclusion, there appears to be a difference of opinions regarding return to play after sports-related cervical spine injuries despite availability of several guidelines.

LOW BACK PAIN IN YOUNG ATHLETES

Low back pain is commonly seen in young athletes involved in either contact or noncontact sports. Some of the more common culprits include tennis, weightlifting, running, gymnastics, diving, basketball, soccer, wrestling, hockey, and football.[46] The constant twisting motion of racquet sports, such as tennis, predispose these athletes to back pain. The incidence of back pain in racquet sports is reported to be 12% in one series.[47] Biomechanical studies have shown that weightlifting places tremendous force on the lumbar spine, causing disc failure at 220 kg and often resulting in an accelerated rate of spondylosis.[48] Sports associated with hyperextension types of activities, such as gymnastics and diving, are often associated with back injuries.[46] Garrick reported 12.2% of injuries in gymnasts were of the spine.[49]

The prevalence of low back pain in 11–17 year olds is 30.4%.[2,50] This may be either acute or chronic, and caused by overuse, mechanical factors, developmental factors or a combination of all three.[51] Acute muscle strain is the most common diagnosis, followed by disc injury.[8] Predisposing factors to low back pain in young athletes should be investigated at the initial encounter with the athlete. These factors include a recent change in the training regimen, beginning of a new season, try-outs, and big games or events. Poor conditioning can predispose the athlete to back injury and pain. Often overlooked reasons include improper techniques such as football lineman blocking in erect position, and poor equipment such as improperly fitted gear or footwear.[4]

There is also an important distinction to make regarding the growing spine in young athletes. During the rapid adolescent growth phase, the skeleton is more vulnerable to overuse injury than the adult spine.[52] The repeated trauma to the discs, end plates, or ring apophyses may accelerate to the degenerative process.[49,53] The area between the vertebral body and the ring apophyses may be the weakest link in the vertebra–disc–vertebra

complex, which is very vulnerable to injury just prior to the fusion of apophyseal rings and the vertebral body at the age of 17–20 years old.[54] Multiple different forces such as traction to the ring apophysis by the annulus, ligaments, and paraspinous muscles as well as compression between the vertebral body and ring apophysis can injure the ring apophysis.[53,55] In one study, severe low back pain occurred only during the growth spurt, whereas none had occurred before the study begun.[52]

The most important factor in the initial evaluation of the young athletes with low back pain is a detailed history and physical examination. Since 80–90% of back problems will resolve within 4–6 weeks,

---

Box 2.1 Risk assessment for return to play after cervical spine injury *Continued*

Moderate risk or relative contraindication

- Torg ratio <0.8, with motor and/or sensory neurapraxia
- previous episodes of neurapraxia
- two- or three-level fusions
- healed but stable compression or posterior ring fx
- instability < 3.5 mm/11 degrees facet fractures
- lateral mass fractures
- nondisplaced healed odontoid fractures
- nondisplaced healed ring of C1 fx
- acute lateral disc herniations
- cervical radiculopathy due to foramen spurs

High risk or absolute contraindication

Congenital:
- odontoid agenesis
- odontoid hypoplasia
- os odontoideum
- C1–C2 anomaly or fusion
- type I Klippel–Feil anomaly
- type II Klippel–Feil anomaly with other anomalies

Developmental:
- spear tackler spine
- residual pain or limited range of motion
- acute fracture or central HNP
- recurrent cervical cord neurapraxia or with abnormal imaging studies
- C1–C2 fx or ligament injury
- C1–C2 fusion
- instability > 3.5 mm/11 degrees
- body fx with sagittal compression, arch fx, ligament injury, fragmentation at canal
- lateral mass fx with facet incongruity > three level fusion
- occipitocervical dislocation
- unstable fx–dislocation or ligamentous injury
- unstable Jefferson fx
- cervical cord anomaly
- symptomatic hard disc

fx, fracture.
Source: derived from Watkins' risk categories and Torg's criteria.

Figure 2.6
Example of a high-risk athlete with Klippel–Feil anomaly showed by X-ray on the left associated with a large cervical syrinx, depicted by MRI on the right.

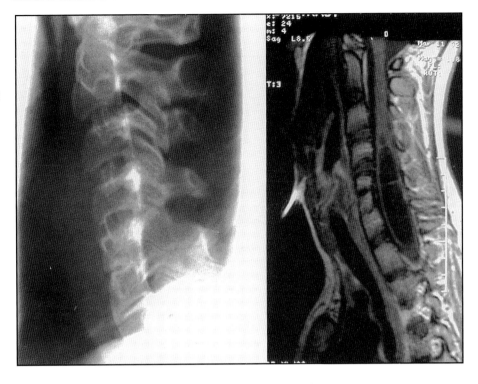

an extensive work up is not warranted initially.[4] Neurologic and orthopedic deficits must be excluded. Radiologic studies are ordered for specific scenarios. Patients with neurologic compromise will need plain films to exclude spinal instability in acute traumatic events. A bone scan may be helpful if one suspects acute spondylolysis. MRI is more helpful if disc or soft tissue injury is suspected.

The treatment principle for back pain in young athletes is to avoid prolonged periods of bedrest that will promote deconditioning (24–36 hours); to encourage walking; to treat muscle spasm with ice; and to prescribe NSAIDs and avoid narcotics, except for sleep.[4] Physical therapy should be started as soon as muscle spasms and pain subside. Exercises for back pain include Williams flexion and McKenzie extension exercises.[56] These should be focused on strengthening flexors' and extensors' musculature. However, extension should be avoided in spondylolysis, spondylolisthesis, and facet disorders, whereas flexion is contraindicated in acute disc disease.[4]

Lumbar disc herniations

There are three types of disc herniations:
- protruded disc, in which the annulus remains intact;
- extruded disc, in which posterior longitudinal ligament is intact but the annulus is disrupted;
- sequestered disc, in which there are free disc fragments in the canal and both the posterior longitudinal ligament and the annulus have been disrupted.[4,57]

Lumbar disc herniations are very rare in children and even rarer in young athletes. In a series of collegiate athletes with low back pain, only 7% had disc diseases.[8,56] Clinical presentations in children with lumbar disc disease are different than adults. First, radicular leg pain is usually absent, and physical limitation is far more prominent than focal sensory, motor, or reflex findings. Children are also less likely to admit to severity of pain. On examination, one often finds limitation of motion, positive straight leg raising, muscle spasms, and mild lumbar scoliosis. Most of the disc diseases in children and adolescents are self-limited and respond to conservative management. If discectomy is indicated after failed conservative management or progressive neurologic or bladder involvement, one will not find degenerated disc materials at surgery. Instead, disc materials in children and adolescents will be tough, fibrous, and difficult to remove. Oftentimes, the end plate has slipped with the disc. The overall outcome after discectomy in children or adolescents is excellent. In a surgical series of lumbar disc disease in the adolescent population, sports accounted for the mechanism of injury in 32% of patients.[58] The mean age of the patients was 15 years old with a fairly long-term follow-up of 8.5 years. The authors concluded that lumbar disc disease in the adolescent population did not appear to cause chronic back pain, and it did not appear to have a negative impact on overall health or quality of life.

Spondylolysis and spondylolisthesis

Spondylolysis is an acquired defect in the pars interarticularis that accounts for approximately 13–47% of referral for athletic back pain.[2] On the other hand, spondylolisthesis is defined as slippage of the superior vertebral body on the one below (Fig. 2.7). The degree of displacement of the vertebral body is graded I–IV by Myerding in increments of 25%. Gymnasts reportedly have a four-fold increased risk of developing spondylolysis due to repetitive hyperflexion–hyperextension maneuvers such as flipping, vaulting, dismounting, and backbending exercises.[59–61] Spondylolysis can be either hereditary or acquired and has been associated with spina bifida occulta.[62,63] The true cause is most likely multifactorial. Excessive lumbar lordosis with repetitive stress from overuse has been implicated in some cases. There is also a higher incidence in first-degree relatives. Approximately 90% of spondylolysis occur at L5, and the risk of slippage is at L5–S1.[2]

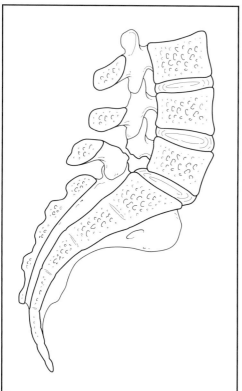

Figure 2.7
Spondylolisthesis, which is defined as slippage of the superior vertebral body on the one below. The degree of displacement of the vertebral body is graded I–IV by Myerding in increments of 25%. This L5–S1 slip is caused by a L5 pars defect.

Athletes with spondylolysis often present with dull, aching pain in the lumbosacral area that is exacerbated or reproduced by hyperextension.[2] In one study, up to 98% of adolescent patients with spondylolysis had pain with extension and rotation of the lumbar spine.[64] On examination, one often finds local tenderness, especially during single-leg hyperextension. The patient/athlete is frequently noted to have paraspinal muscle spasms, which causes splinting. Hamstring tightness is common and is found in up to 70% of patients.[62,65] Radicular pain is uncommon. The diagnosis of spondylolysis is made with the classical finding of the broken neck in the "Scottie Dog" on an oblique X-ray of the lumbar and sacral spine (Fig. 2.8).

Spondylolysis can be missed in up to 20% of all cases if good oblique views are not obtained.[66] Pierce has reported the anteroposterior view of lumbosacral X-ray in diagnosing spondylolysis to have a sensitivity of 32%, the lateral view 75%, and the oblique view 77%.[67] X-rays may be normal in the acute setting; therefore, a bone scan or SPECT (single-photon emission computerized tomography) scan will be required to make the diagnosis of spondylolysis (Fig. 2.9).

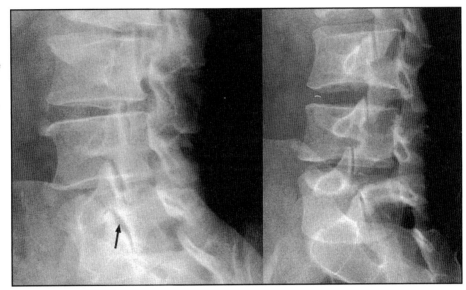

Figure 2.8
The diagnosis of spondylolysis is made with the classical finding of the broken neck in the "Scottie Dog" on an oblique X-ray of the lumbar and sacral spine. Left, the arrow indicates the normal neck of "Scottie Dog." Right, L5 pars defect.

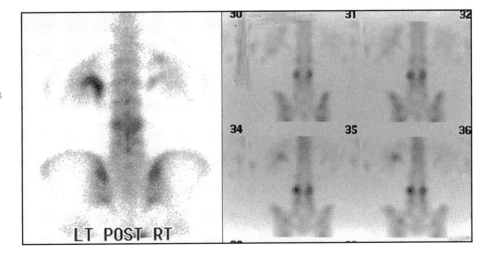

Figure 2.9
Bone scan on the left shows diffuse uptake at L4 pedicles, which is better seen with SPECT scan on the right, confirming the diagnosis of bilateral L4 spondylolysis.

The timely diagnosis of an early spondylolysis will lead to an improved outcome. Some authors have reported that the longer the symptoms were present before treatment, the more likely that surgical intervention will be needed.[59,64] If the diagnosis is made prior to the development of a frank fracture, then conservative treatment is more likely to be successful.[59] The goals of treatment are to provide pain relief, healing of the defect, and prevention of further injury. This is usually done by means of activity restriction and physical therapy. Bracing of spondylolysis depends on the presence of a stress fracture or a true fracture, need for pain control, and compliance.[2] The advantage of bracing is that it limits motion, thereby reducing stress. The results of bracing vary from complete healing, with resolution of back pain, to nonunion, persistence of pain, or progression to spondylolisthesis.[62,64,68] Using return to sports as an endpoint, success of bracing ranged widely from 7% to 84%.[69–72] Bracing mainly provides pain control through the limitation of movement and reduction in stress on the injured segment. The lumbosacral orthosis should be worn a minimum of 2 months, particularly if the former interventions do not provide adequate pain relief, or if the patient is noncompliant with the prescribed activity restriction.[69,71,73] It has been recommended that individuals with normal X-rays but a positive bone scan can be treated without bracing, although some do recommend bracing acute spondylolysis and spondylolisthesis to optimize healing.[6,74] A unilateral spondylolysis with normal X-rays probably does not require bracing. Surgery may be indicated in failed conservative management with persistent pain for more than 6 months, progression of slippage, slippage >50% in growth spurt, or neurologic compromise.[62]

By itself, spondylolisthesis is not a contraindication to competitive or contact sports even though the progression of symptomatic displacement has been reported in young athletes. Muschik et al reported that 43% of observed athletes involved in competitive sports had an increase in displacement of only 5%; 13% of athletes had an increase in displacement of >10%.[75] Seitsalo et al observed a greater than 10% displacement in 62 of 272 subjects with spondylolisthesis with clinical symptoms.[76] Blackburne and Velikas found such a progression in 15% of their patients.[77] McPhee et al reported 24% progressive spondylolisthesis.[78] An increase of 20% progression was seen by Danielson et al.[70] Given that despite intensive training, most athletes with spondylolisthesis remain asymptomatic and the progression of vertebral displacement is minimal, it is not appropriate to advise young athletes with asymptomatic spondylolisthesis to avoid sports completely unless acute instability can be demonstrated.

SPINAL DEFORMITIES IN YOUNG ATHLETES

The most common spinal deformity seen in the adolescent population is idiopathic scoliosis. The etiology of idiopathic scoliosis is unknown although a multifactorial origin is commonly accepted.[79] The risks of athletic activities of developmental spine is well known and is strongly influenced by external forces acting upon them.[80] Sports can provide such forces from muscular exertion and body motions. Immature bone is much more sensitive to cyclic loading than mature bone, and multiple repeated loading cycles could increase the chance of a spinal deformity. As the normal spine growth in girls stops at an average age of 14–15 years old, and between ages 16 and 17 years old in boys, this would be considered prime time for the development of any growth-related deformity.[81]

Certain sports have been associated with scoliosis, whether directly or indirectly. These include gymnastics, swimming, and volleyball, in which asymmetrical loading of the spine is often seen.[80,82] Tanchev et al recently described a distinct entity of "sports scoliosis" seen in rhythmic gymnastics.[83] Rhythmic gymnastics is very popular in Bulgaria; almost every school has training groups. Training usually starts at the age of 5 years old, 6 days weekly, and 5 hours a day. Athletes tend to be thin with flat backs and manifest an obvious delay in growth and maturation. The dangerous triad of generalized laxity, delayed maturity, and asymmetric spinal loading predispose these athletes to "sports scoliosis," with a 10-fold higher incidence of scoliosis than the general population (Fig. 2.10).[83] Ballet dancers, tennis players, and javelin throwers are also at risk, with girls being at higher risk than boys. Hypoestrogenism, a complication of weight loss, dieting, and physical training in girls, is a contributing factor.[84] Estrogen has an essential effect on bone; it stimulates epiphyseal closure. Delayed growth and maturity cause prolongation of "vulnerable growing years," which exposes growth plates to unfavorable mechanical factors longer than usual.[85] These factors also explain why idiopathic scoliosis is seen more commonly in girls.

Figure 2.10
Photograph of a rhythmic gymnast with generalized laxity.

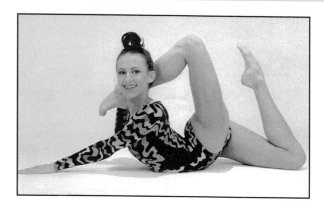

The prevalence of idiopathic scoliosis in the general population is 2–3%.[86] It is a painless condition and is more common among girls. Kyphosis, also known as Scheuermann's disease, is a developmental roundback deformity of the thoracic spine caused by abnormal growth of vertebral end plates, Schmorl's nodes, and occasional apophyseal ring fractures.[87] The incidence is estimated at between 2 and 8%.[88] There appears to be an increase in the incidence of scoliosis among swimmers and kyphosis among water skiers. This is attributed to drag and inertial forces producing sufficient load to cause changes in the paraspinal musculature, with resultant spine deformity.[89] The inability of the musculature to keep up with the demand can lead to an increase in sagittal deformity such as kyphosis.[90] Several opinions exist regarding sports participation in athletes with spinal deformity. In the past, restrictions have been placed on swimming, and professional volleyball was not recommended.[91,92] Currently, however, most physicians feel there are no contraindications to swimming or contact sports in patients with scoliosis.[92,93] One should not expect sports to reverse scoliosis but participation has other therapeutic and psychological benefits. In children who are treated with a brace, participation in sports is encouraged during hours out of the brace. Some sports allow in-brace participation, such as bicycling, horseback riding, or cheerleading. Swimming during the hours out of brace is encouraged with the rationale being that swimming would remove the deforming effects of gravity on the spinal curvature while enhancing muscular conditioning, improving vital capacity, and increasing overall fitness. The butterfly stroke, however, continues to be discouraged by some for fear that overdevelopment of the pectoral muscles might worsen a kyphotic deformity.[93] Contact sports were initially discouraged with or without a brace; however, recent advancement in brace technology has allowed athletes with spinal deformity to compete in these sports with or without the brace.

Athletic activity after fusion with segmental instrumentation

Resuming athletic activity after fusion with segmental instrumentation is often a difficult recommendation for the surgeon to make. There are no generally accepted guidelines for surgeons regarding appropriate sport activities or appropriate time to resume athletic activities. One author suggested that for patients treated with fusion and instrumentation, recreational sports such as swimming, biking, and hiking is allowed at 2 months; light physical activity such as tennis and shooting basketball is allowed at 4 months; and contact and twisting sports are allowed at 6 months if fusion is solid. If fusion is below L3, heavy twisting and contact sports should be avoided. However, a more conservative approach has been advocated by other individuals for fear of catastrophic injuries. There have been reports of spinal fracture–dislocation in the adjacent nonfused segments of the spine in young patients after spinal fusion for scoliosis.[94] Most of these injuries are due to motor vehicle accidents.[95,96] It is postulated that the loss of spine mobility due to segmental spinal fusion creates a rigid lever arm and an increased stress concentration at the adjacent mobile segment, resulting in vulnerability. The ability of the fused thoracic spine to evenly distribute force upon impact is lost.[94] For these reasons, some recommend that patients who have undergone posterior spinal fusion for idiopathic scoliosis should not participate in high-impact sports such as football, or in activities in which spinal mobility is critical, such as cheerleading and gymnastics.

In a survey of the members of the Scoliosis Research Society, clinicians demonstrated great variation with regard to recommendations about resuming sports after scoliosis surgery.[97] The most popular time to resume low-impact, noncontact sports was 6 months. Contact sports were most frequently allowed at 12 months, although 13% of respondents thought that they should never be resumed. Sixty percent of respondents recommended against collision sports. There were also varied recommendations after fusion for spondylolisthesis. Surgeons seemed to suggest very similar timing for patients, regardless of whether they were fused for high- or low-grade slips. Six months was the preferred time for resuming low-impact/noncontact and noncontact sports. Contact sports were most often permitted at 1 year; however, 14% of respondents who treated low-grade slips and 21% of those who treated high-grade slips believed that those sports should not be resumed. Between 49% and 58% of respondents believed that collision sports should never be resumed. If permitted, they were usually withheld for 1 year. Factors that influenced the decision included time from surgery, use of instrumentation, and chosen sport. This survey demonstrated a broad variation of opinion with regard to timing, safety, and types of athletic activity that are appropriate after spinal surgery in children and adolescents.

REFERENCES

1. Metzl JD: Sports medicine in pediatric practice: keeping pace with the changing times. Ped Annals 29:146–148, 2000.

2. Garry JP, McShane J: Lumbar spondylolysis in adolescent athletes. J Fam Pract 47:145–149, 1998.

3. Tall RL: Spinal injury in sports: epidemiologic considerations. Clin Sport Med 12:441, 1993.

4. Trainor TJ, Weisel SW: Epidemiology of back pain in the athlete. Spine Sports 21:93–103, 2002.

5. Bailes JE: Spinal injuries in athletes. In: Menezes AH, Sonntag VK, eds. Principles of spinal surgery. New York: McGraw-Hill; 1996:465–491.

6. Morganti C, Sweeney CA, Albanese SA, et al: Return to play after cervical spine injury. Spine 26:1131–1136, 2001.

7. Day A, Chandler HC: Herniated nucleus pulposus in the athlete. In: Menezes AH, Sonntag VK, eds. Principles of spinal surgery. New York: McGraw-Hill; 1996: 411–421.

8. Keene JS, Albert MJ, Springer SL, et al: Back injuries in college athletes. J Spinal Disord: 2:190–195, 1989.

9. Hill SA, Miller CA, Kosnik EJ, et al: Pediatric neck injuries. A clinical study. J Neurosurg 60:700–706, 1984.

10. Mueller FO, Cantu RC: The annual survey of catastrophic football injuries: 1977–1989. Exerc Sport Sci Rev 19:261–312, 1991.

11. Mueller FO, Schindler RD: Annual survey of football injury research 1931–1987; Mission, KS: National Collegiate Athletic Association and American Football Coaches Association, 1987.

12. Maroon JC: Catastrophic neck injuries from football in western Pennsylvania. Physician Sports Med 9:83–86, 1981.

13. Maroon JC, Steele PB, Berlin R: Football head and neck injuries – an update. Clin Neurosurg 27:414–429, 1980.

14. Mueller FO, Blythe CS: Catastrophic head and neck injuries. Physician Sports Med 7:71–76, 1979.

15. Cantu RC, Mueller FO: Catastrophic spine injuries in football. J Spinal Disord 3:227–231, 1990.

16. Burstein AH, Otis JC, Torg JS: Mechanisms and pathomechanics of athletic injuries to the cervical spine. In: Torg JS, ed. Athletic injuries to the head, neck and face. Philadelphia: Lea & Febiger; 1982:139–142.

17. Poindexter DP, Johnson EW: Football shoulder and neck injury: a study of the "stinger." Arch Phys Med Rehab 65:601–602, 1984.

18. Torg JS, Sennett B, Pavlov H, et al: Spear tackler's spine: an entity precluding participation in tackle football and collision activities that expose the cervical spine to axial energy inputs. Am J Sports Med 21:640–649, 1993.

19. Torg JS, Vegso JJ, Sennett B, et al: The national football head and neck injury registry: 14 year report on cervical quadriplegia, 1971–1984. JAMA 254:3439–3443, 1985.

20. Tator CH: Neck injuries in ice hockey. Clin Sports Med 6:101–114, 1987.

21. Tator CH, Edmonds VE: National survey of spinal injuries in hockey players. Can Med Assoc J 130:875–880, 1984.

22. Tator CH, Ekong CEU, Rowed CA, et al: Spinal injuries due to hockey. Can J Neurol Sci 11:34–41, 1984.

23. American Academy of Pediatrics. Committee on Sports Medicine and Fitness: safety in youth ice hockey: the effects of body checking. Pediatrics 105:657–658, 2000.

24. Albrand OW, Corkill G: Broken necks from diving accidents: a summer epidemic in young men. Am J Sports Med 4:107–110, 1976.

25. Raymond CA: Summer's drought reinforces diving's dangers. JAMA 260:1199–2000, 1988.

26. Bailes JE, Herman JM, Quigley MR, et al: Diving injuries of the cervical spine. Surg Neurol 34:155–158, 1990.

27. Torg JS, Das M: Trampoline-related quadriplegia: review of the literature and reflections on the American Academy of Pediatrics' position statement. Pediatrics 74:804–812, 1984.

28. American Academy of Pediatrics. Committee on Accident and Poison Prevention: policy statement. Trampolines. Evanston, IL: American Academy of Pediatrics; September 1977.

29. American Academy of Pediatrics. Trampolines II. Pediatrics 67:438, 1981.

30. Maroon JC: "Burning hands" in football spinal cord injuries. JAMA 238:2049–2051, 1977.

31. Shannon B, Klimkiewicz JJ: Cervical burners in the athlete. Spine Sports 21:29–35, 2002.

32. Wilberger JE, Abla A, Maroon JC: Burning hands syndrome revisited. Neurosurgery 19:1038–1040, 1986.

33. Boockvar JA, Durham SR, Sun PP: Cervical spinal stenosis and sports-related cervical cord neurapraxia in children. Spine 26:2709–2713, 2001.

34. Hashimoto I, Tak YK: The true sagittal diameter of the cervical spinal canal and its diagnostic significance in cervical myelopathy. J Neurosurg 47:912–916, 1977.

35. Torg JS, Pavlov H, Genuario SE, et al: Neurapraxia of the cervical spinal cord with transient quadriplegia. J Bone Joint Surg Am 68A:1354–1370, 1986.

36. Herzog RJ, Wiens JJ, Dillingham MF, et al: Normal cervical spine morphometry and cervical spinal stenosis in asymptomatic professional football players. Spine 16:5178–5186, 1991.

37. Albright JP, Moses JM, Feldick HG, et al: Nonfatal cervical spine injuries in interscholastic football. JAMA 236:1243–1245, 1976.

38. Ladd AL, Scranton PE: Congenital cervical stenosis presenting as transient quadriplegia in athletes. J Bone Joint Surg Am 68A:1371–1374, 1986.

39. Cantu RC: Functional cervical spinal stenosis: a contraindication to participation in contact sports. Med Sci Sports Exer 25:316–317, 1993.

40. Callaway GH, O'Brien SJ, Tehrany AM: Chiari I malformation and spinal cord injury: cause for concern in contact athletes. Med Sci Sports Exer 28:1218–1220, 1996.

41. Frogameni A, Widoff B, Jackson D: Syringomyelia causing acute hemiparesis in a college football player. Orthopedics 17:552–553, 1994.

42. Pang D, Wilberger JE: Spinal cord injury without radiographic abnormality in children. J Neurosurg 57:114–129, 1982.

43. Dare AO, Dias MS, Li V: Magnetic resonance imaging correlation in pediatric spinal cord injury without radiographic abnormality. J Neurosurg (Spine 1) 97:33–39, 2002.

44. Torg JS, Glasgow SG: Criteria for return to contact activities following cervical spine injuries. Clin J Sports Med 1:12–26, 1991.

45. Watkins R: Neck injuries in football players. Clin Sports Med 4:215–246, 1986.

46. Goldsetin JD, Berger PE, Windler GE, et al: Spine injuries in gymnasts and swimmers: an epidemiologic investigation. Am J Sports Med 19:463–468, 1991.

47. Chard MD, Lachmann MA: Racquet sports – patterns of injury presenting to a sports injury clinic. BR Sports 21:150, 1987.

48. Gatt CJ, Hosea TM, Palumbo RC, et al: Impact loading of the lumbar spine during football blocking. Am J Sports Med 25:317–321, 1997.

49. Garrick JG, Requa PK: Epidemiology of women gymnast injuries. Am J Sports Med 8:261, 1980.

50. Bernhardt DT, Landry GL: Sports injuries in young athletes. Advan Ped 42:465–500, 1995.

51. King HA: Back pain in children. Pediatr Clin N Am 31:1083-1095, 1984.

52. Kujala UM, Taimela S, Erkintalo M, et al: Low-back pain in adolescent athletes. Med Sci Sports Exer 28:165–170, 1996.

53. Sward L, Hellstrom M, Jacobson R, et al: Acute injury of the vertebral ring apophysis and intervertebral disc in adolescent gymnasts. Spine 15:144–148, 1990.

54. Epstein NE, Epstein JA: Limbus lumbar vertebral fractures in 27 adolescents and adults. Spine 16:962–966, 1991.

55. Sward L: The toracolumbar spine in young elite athletes. Current concepts on the effects of physical training. Sports Med 13:357–364, 1992.

56. Keene JS, Drummond DS: Mechanical back pain in the athlete. Compr Ther 11:1–14, 1985.

57. Kraus DR, Shapiro D: The symptomatic lumbar spine in the athlete. Clin Sports Med 8:59–69, 1998.

58. Durham SR, Sun PP, Sutton LN: Surgically treated lumbar disc disease in the pediatric population: an outcome study. J Neurosurg (Spine 1) 92:1–6, 2000.

59. Ciullo JV, Jackson DW: Pars interarticularis stress reaction, spondylolysis and spondylolisthesis in gymnasts. Clin Sports Med 4:95–110, 1985.

60. Jackson DW, Wiltse LL, Cirinsione RJ: Spondylolysis in the female gymnast. Clin Orthop 117:68–73, 1976.

61. Jackson DW, Wiltse LL, Dingeman RD, et al: Stress reactions involving the pars interarticularis in young athletes. Am J Sports Med 9:304–312, 1981.

62. Hensinger RN: Spondylolysis and spondylolisthesis in children and adolescents. J Bone Joint Surg 71A:1098–1107, 1989.

63. Rossi F: Spondylolysis, spondylolisthesis and sports. J Sports Med Phys Fitness 18:317–340, 1988.

64. Blanda J, Bethem D, Moats W, et al: Defects of pars interarticularis in athletes: a protocol for nonoperative treatment. J Spinal Disord 6:406–411, 1993.

65. Bell DF, Ehrlich MG, Zaleske DJ: Brace treatment for symptomatic spondylolisthesis. Clin Orthop 236:192–198, 1988.

66. Libson E, Bloom RA, Dinari G, et al: Oblique lumbar spine radiographs: importance in young patients. Radiology 151:89–90, 1984.

67. Pierce ME: Spondylolysis: what does it mean? Australas Radiol 31:391–394, 1987.

68. Hensinger RN, Lang JR, MacEwin GD: Surgical management of spondylolisthesis in children and adolescents. Spine 1:207–216, 1976.

69. Daniel JN, Polly DW, Van Dam BE: A study of the efficacy of nonoperative treatment of presumed traumatic spondylolysis in a young patient population. Mil Med 160:553–555, 1995.

70. Danielson BI, Frennered AK, Irstam LKH: Radiologic progression of isthmic lumbar spondylolisthesis in young patients. Spine 16:422–425, 1991.

71. Micheli LJ, Hall JE, Miller ME: Use of modified Boston brace for back injuries in athletes. Am J Sports Med 8:351–356, 1980.

72. Pizzutillo PD, Hummer CD: Nonoperative treatment for painful adolescent spondylolysis or spondylolisthesis. J Pediatr Orthop 9:538–540, 1989.

73. Micheli LJ: Back injuries in gymnastics. Clin Sports Med 4:85–93, 1985.

74. Stinson JT: Spondylolysis and spondylolisthesis in the athlete. Clin Sports Med 12:517–528, 1993.

75. Muschik M, Hahnel H, Robinson PN, et al: Competitive sports and the progression of spondylolisthesis. J Pediatr Orthop: 16:364–369, 1996.

76. Seitsalo S, Osterman K, Hyvarinen H, et al: Progression of spondylolisthesis in children and adolescents: a long term follow-up of 272 patients. Spine 16:417–421, 1991.

77. Blackburne BJS, Velikas EP: Spondylolisthesis in children and adolescents. J Bone Surg B59:490–494, 1977.

78. McPhee IB, O'Brien JP, McCall IW, et al: Progression of lumbosacral spondylolisthesis. Aust Radiol 25:91–94, 1981.

79. Harrington PR: The etiology of idiopathic scoliosis. Clin Orthop 126:17–25, 1977.

80. Becker TJ: Scoliosis in swimmers. Clin Sports Med 5:149, 1986.

81. Hou JC, Salem GJ, Zernicke RF: Structural and mechanical adaptations of immature trabecular bone to strenuous exercise. J Appl Physiol 63:1309, 1990.

82. Omey ML, Micheli LJ, Gerbino PG: Idiopathic scoliosis and spondylolysis in the female athlete: tips for treatment. Clin Orthop Rel Res 372:74, 2000.

83. Tanchev PI, Dzherov AD, Parushev AD, et al: Scoliosis in rhythmic gymnasts. Spine 25:1367–1372, 2000.

84. Underwood LE, Van Wyk JJ: Hormones in normal and aberrant growth. In: Williams RH, ed. Textbook of endocrinology, 6th edn. Philadelphia: WB Saunders; 1981: 1149–1191.

85. Warren MP, Brook-Gunn J, Hamilton LH, et al: The effects of exercise on pubertal progression and reproductive function in girls. J Clin Endocrinol Metab 51:1150–1157, 1980.

86. Weinstein SL: Idiopathic scoliosis: natural history. Spine 11:780, 1986.

87. Lowe TG: Scheuermann disease. J Bone Joint Surg 72A:940, 1990.

88. Scoles PV, Latimer BM, DiGiovanni BF, et al: Vertebral alterations in Scheuermann's kyphosis. Spine 16:509, 1991.

89. Jensen RK, Bellow DG: Upper extremity contraction moments and their relationship to swimming training. J Biomechanics 9:219, 1976.

90. Ohlen G, Wredmark T, Spangfort E: Spinal sagittal configuration and mobility related to low-back pain in the female gymnast. Spine 14:847, 1989.

91. Williams L: Volleyball. In: Watkins RG, ed. The spine in sports. St. Louis: Mosby-Year Book; 1996:522.

92. Wilson FD, Lindseth RE: The adolescent "swimmer's back." Am J Sports Med 10:174, 1982.

93. Wood KB: Spinal deformity in the adolescent athlete. Spine Sports 21:77–92, 2002.

94. Fuchs PD, Bertrand S, Iwinski H, et al: Traumatic C6–C7 dislocation in a 14 year old with posterior spinal fusion for idiopathic scoliosis. J Trauma 51:1004–1007, 2001.

95. Drennan JD, King EW: Cervical dislocation following fusion of the upper thoracic spine for scoliosis. J Bone Joint Surg 60A:1003–1005, 1978.

96. Neyt JG, Wienstein SL: Fracture–dislocation of the lumbar spine after arthrodesis with instrumentation for idiopathic scoliosis. J Bone Joint Surg 81A:111–114, 1999.

97. Rubery PT, Bradford DS: Athletic activity after spine surgery in children and adolescents: results of a survey. Spine 27:423–427, 2002.

FURTHER READING

Grant TT, Puffer J: Cervical stenosis: a developmental anomaly with quadriparesis during football. Am J Sports Med 4:219–221, 1976.

Nagib MG, Maxwell RE, Chou SN: Identification and management of high-risk patients with Klippel–Feil syndrome. J Neurosurg 61:523–530, 1984.

Taylor AR: The mechanism of injury to the spinal cord in the neck without damage to the vertebral column. J Bone Joint Surg Br 33B:543–547, 1951.

CHAPTER

3

Spine Problems in the Older Athlete

Thomas D Fulbright

SPINE PROBLEMS

Spinal difficulties that plague the older athlete are of interest to athletes, clinicians, and to those who aspire to a higher than average level of physical activity. The cardiovascular benefits of regular aerobic exercise are generally established and accepted. Reduced musculoskeletal disability and mortality have been demonstrated in runners by longitudinal study.[1] Degenerative changes as assessed by roentgenographic evaluation may be accelerated in certain sporting activities. A significant number of athletic endeavors are associated with spondylolysis and spondylolisthesis. Whether there is a spinal price to be paid, or a benefit to the spine of various athletic endeavors is examined in this chapter.

Low back pain

The incidence and prevalence of low back pain in retired wrestlers and weight lifters has been examined in comparison to historical controls.[2] Wrestlers were noted to have a higher incidence (79% vs 61%) and prevalence (59% vs 31%) of low back pain than controls. Despite this difference, wrestlers reported less interference with work than controls and enjoyed substantial continued participation in sporting activity. No significant difference in the prevalence or incidence of low back pain from the control group was noted among weight lifters. Evaluation of previously elite Finnish athletes demonstrated a decreased prevalence of low back pain across a broad cross section of sportsmen. This was noted despite the finding of increased degenerative change in weight lifters and soccer players by magnetic resonance (MR) evaluation.[3]

Radiographic features

Little argument is likely to arise regarding the poor correlation of spinal symptoms and radiographic abnormalities; however, an increased incidence of degenerative change in athletes would at least imply a physiologic cost of sporting activity. Currently active elite athletes of young age demonstrate an increased frequency of multiple radiographic abnormalities in the lumbar and thoracic spine compared to the nonathletic individual of comparable age. This is particularly true of gymnasts and weight lifters.[4] Healy et al[5] reviewed MR scans of 19 asymptomatic athletes over 40 years old who were actively engaged in regular vigorous triathlon training or handball. They found a similar incidence of lumbar degenerative change and a somewhat greater incidence of cervical degenerative change than that observed in other, less-active asymptomatic populations.

Osteoporosis

Lumbar bone mass has been shown to be increased with exercise under certain circumstances;[6] however, athletes, particularly those involved in endurance sports, may actually be at risk for osteoporosis. Diminished levels of sex hormones have been found in endurance athletes and to a lesser extent in strength-training athletes.[7] The association of diminished hormone levels and decreased lumbar bone mineralization is established (Fig. 3.1). Vertebral mineral content has been found to be diminished by as much as 27% in women with exercise-induced amenorrhea.[8] Irregular menses may be present in up to two-thirds of female athletes. Amenorrhea persisting for more than 3 years leads to decreased bone mineral density that is not reversible with calcium supplementation.[9]

Elite male runners have been demonstrated to have a decreased lumbar bone mineral content of up to 19%.[10] The significance of hormonal factors is less apparent in the male athletic population.

Spondylolysis and spondylolisthesis

A high incidence of spondylolysis has been reported in various sports, particularly those that involve lumbar hyperextension and rotation such as gymnastics,[11] weightlifting, and wrestling.[2] It has been suggested that spondylolysis in the athlete is distinct from the "silent" pars defect commonly found incidentally in youth in that it is said to occur later in life and in association with vigorous extension and rotation stresses and is generally symptomatic.[12] What specifically differentiates incidental and athletic spondylolysis is unclear. The incidental spondylolytic defect is not found in infants[13] and is uncommon before 5 years of age, after which the incidence rises precipitously to about 80% of its eventual adult level

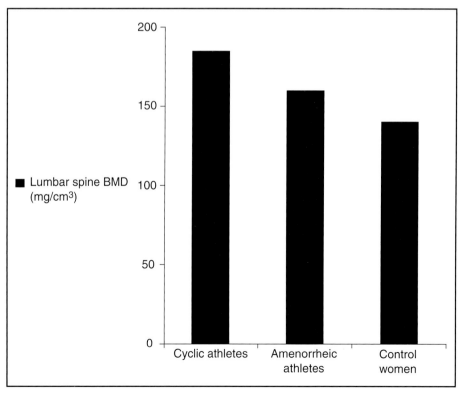

Figure 3.1
Lumbar bone mineralization in athletes. BMD = bone mineral density. (Reproduced from Snow-Harter with permission.[9])

before age 7. Spondylolisthesis is present in two-thirds of patients when initially diagnosed with incidental spondylolysis and is present in about 80% by adulthood. Progression of spondylolisthesis after age 16 is rare.[14] A genetic predisposition to spondylolysis has been well documented.[15] A 5.8% incidence in the US white population and a 1.95% incidence in the US Afro-American population have been reported. Pre-European Inuit populations have shown a frequency of over 50%; however, the defect appeared most commonly in adult life and would therefore be more consistent with athletic or traumatic spondylolysis rather than the silent variety.[16] Fatigue fracture is thought to be the basic lesion of isthmic spondylolisthesis, with genetic factors playing some role in how much stress is required to generate the lesion.[17]

Spondylolysis and spondylolisthesis are commonly found in athletes, with about half reporting the existence of back pain. Soler and Calderon have reviewed the prevalence of spondylolysis in the Spanish athletic elite and have taken an incidence of greater than 9% as more than two standard deviations above the upper limit for spondylolysis in the general population (Table 3.1). They concluded that rotation and

Table 3-1 The prevalence of spondylolysis among athletes

Sport	Number of athletes	Prevalence N (%)	Athletes with spondylolysis who were symptomatic N (%)
Track and field:	685	69 (8.9)	32 (52.5)
Races	512	37 (7.3)	19 (51.3)
Throwing	45	12 (26.7)	8 (6.7)
Heptathlon/decathlon	31	4 (12.9)	1 (25.0)
Bobsledding	15	3 (20.0)	0 (0.0)
Canoeing	47	4 (8.5)	2 (50.0)
Combat sports:	207	23 (11.1)	9 (39.1)
Boxing	21	3 (14.3)	2 (66.7)
Judo/wrestling	143	16 (11.2)	6 (37.5)
Karate	43	4 (9.3)	1 (25.0)
Fencing	56	6 (10.7)	4 (66.7)
Gymnastics:	235	33 (14.0)	19 (57.6)
Artistic	112	19 (17.0)	10 (52.6)
Rhythmic	92	9 (9.8)	6 (66.7)
Trampoline	31	5 (16.1)	3 (60.0)
Paddleball	20	2 (10.0)	1 (50.0)
Rowing	77	13 (16.9)	8 (61.5)
Swimming	176	18 (10.2)	6 (33.3)
Volleyball	70	7 (10.0)	4 (57.1)
Weightlifting	85	11 (12.9)	6 (54.5)

Source: adapted from Soler and Calderon[18] with permission of the American Journal of Sports Medicine.

torsion against resistance should be included, with lumbar hyperextension and rotation as precipitating factors.[18]

Conservative management will lead to symptomatic relief in the majority of patients, although only one-third will experience healing.[19] Temporary restriction of activity, external support, or no alterations of training routine have all been employed with success.

DIAGNOSIS AND TREATMENT

As with any patient, evaluation of spinal ailments in athletes should begin with a careful history and physical as the first and most important step in creating a proper plan for diagnosis and treatment. Given the ubiquity of this axiom, it is curious that responsibility is so soon delegated and so often found in the hands of various physician extenders. It would appear that the axiom and the practice are at odds with each other.

As with all symptom evaluations, the patient should be queried regarding the character, time of onset, precipitating factors, and exacerbating and relieving features of their complaint. A review of current and past training activity should be obtained as well as a dietary history. Physical examination should include a complete motor and sensory examination in addition to evaluation of spinal mechanics. A rectal examination should be completed in men. Given the currently held views of gynecologic evaluations, women are asked if they have had a normal pelvic examination within the last 6 months. If they have not, it is recommended that they do so.

Given that patients have sought medical evaluation for their spinal complaints, they should be subjected to sufficient radiologic imaging to rule out pain-producing pathology that could be potentially dangerous if not diagnosed before empiric conservative treatment is prescribed. Generally, a spinal MR scan, supplemented by other studies as indicated by history and physical examination, is appropriate.

Osteoporosis

Female athletes and male endurance athletes should undergo screening with DEXA (dual energy X-ray absorptiometry) evaluation for osteoporosis. If osteoporosis is found, evaluation of a training regimen and diet should be undertaken. Calcium intake should be increased to 1500 mg per day and proper caloric and protein intake should be insured. Reduction in training regimen is advisable but difficult to achieve. Estrogen replacement in the postmenopausal athlete or oral contraceptives in the younger athlete should be considered. The use of bisphosphonates and calcitonin can be considered.

Low back pain

The patient with low back pain without radicular symptoms or focal neurologic findings, who has a magnetic scan remarkable only for degenerative changes such as disc dehydration and collapse and facet arthropathy, should undergo flexion–extension lumbar spine films to rule out overt instability and oblique views to evaluate the pars interarticularis. Bone scanning can be useful to demonstrate acuity of such defects and determine the metabolic activity of morphologically apparent arthropathy. Diagnostic injections, guided by bone scanning, may be useful and can be followed by focal steroid administration. Neuroablative interventions, such as facet rhizotomy, carry the risk of allowing persistent engagement in injurious activity. Active modes of physical therapy for strengthening of spinal supporting musculature and proper stretching techniques may be beneficial. Pharmacologic options include anti-inflammatory agents, analgesics, muscle relaxants, and pain modifiers. Narcotic analgesics and narcotic analogs are generally to be avoided in the treatment of chronic pain despite their newfound benignity made possible by narrow definitions of addiction. Muscle relaxants may be particularly useful in the presence of spasm. Pain modifiers useful in the active population include nonsedative antidepressants such as Zoloft (sertraline), Prozac (fluoxetine), and Paxil (paroxetine), and anticonvulsants such as gabapentin.

Spondylolysis and spondylolisthesis

Following a diagnostic workup consisting of a magnetic scan, bone scan, and plain films, with flexion–extension views, the same conservative measures may be employed for spondylolysis as for low back pain. An acute spondylolytic defect is unlikely in the older athlete and should be effectively ruled out by bone scanning. Patients with radicular pain with minimal low back pain may be effectively treated with decompression alone via the Gill procedure.[20] If back pain is equal to or more significant than radicular pain, fusion can be considered. Discography is sometimes performed, although its utility is highly suspect. A trial of bracing might be considered. The older athlete should be advised to make lifestyle alterations rather than undergo fusion with the expectation that such an intervention will return him to premorbid activity.

Cervical disc herniation

Conservative measures for treatment of cervical disc herniation do not differ significantly in the older athlete in comparison to the general population. With failure of conservative management, surgical intervention is reasonable. If radiculopathy is accompanied by substantial mechanical pain, if significant stenosis is present, or if the anatomy of the herniation would require significant cord manipulation during discectomy, the anterior approach is selected. In the absence of the aforementioned conditions, a posterior approach may avoid restriction of range of motion and the potential of induction of junctional degeneration.

Lumbar disc herniation

As in cervical disc herniation, treatment of lumbar disc herniation does not differ significantly in the older athlete in comparison to the general population. Failure of conservation management can be followed by discectomy, utilizing general principles of surgical management. Matsunaga et al reported on a small series of athletes undergoing simple disc excision or percutaneous discectomy: three-fourths of these patients returned to some sporting activity, although only one-third of these were described as enjoying a complete return.[21]

Lumbar stenosis

In cases of lumbar stenosis, the most conservative surgical option that will adequately address the problem is in order. Preservation of posterior supporting structures is to be encouraged in any case, particularly so in the active individual. The presence of subluxation or sagittally oriented facet joints, especially when associated with well-preserved disc height, should raise concern about inducing instability. If fusion is contemplated, it should be emphasized that it is questionable that such intervention will return the patient to vigorous physical activity.

CONCLUSION

In general, it appears that there is an eventual cost to the spine attributable to engagement in sporting activity. Proper training and nutrition are likely to reduce this cost. The benefits to general health and well-being may outweigh the consequences of the traumatic, degenerative, or metabolic effects. These effects should not be ignored, but rather considered among the effects of vigorous physical exercise.

REFERENCES

1. Fries JF, Singh G, Morfeld, D, et al: Relationship of running to musculoskeletal pain with age. Arthritis and Rheumatism 39(1):64–72, 1996.

2. Granhed H, Morelli B: Low back pain among retired wrestlers and weightlifters. Am J Sports Med 16:530–533, 1988.

3. Videman T, Sarna S, Battie MC, et al: The long-term effects of physical loading and exercise lifestyles on back-related symptoms, disability, and spinal pathology among men. Spine 20:699–709, 1995.

4. Hellstrom M, Jacobbson B, Sward L, et al: Radiological abnormalities of the thoraco-lumbar spine in athletes. Acta Radiol 31:127–132b, 1990.

5. Healy JF, Healy BB, Wong WHM, et al: Cervical and lumbar MRI in older male lifelong athletes: frequency of degenerative findings. J Comp Assist Tomog 20(1):107–112, 1996.

6. Michel BA, Lane NE, Bloch DA, et al: Effect of changes in weight-bearing exercise on lumbar bone mass after age fifty. Ann Med 23:397–401, 1991.

7. Voss LA, Fadale PD, Hulstyn MJ: Exercise-induced loss of bone density in athletes. J Am Acad Orthop Surg 6:349–357, 1998.

8. Cann CE, Martin MC, Genant HK, et al: Decreased spinal mineral content in amenorrheic women. JAMA 251:626–629, 1984.

9. Snow-Harter CM: Bone health and prevention of osteoporosis in active and athletic women. Clin Sports Med 13:389–404, 1994.

10. Hetland ML, Haarbo J, Christiansen C: Low bone mass and high bone turnover in male long distance runners. J Clin End Metab 77:770–775, 1993.

11. Jackson DW, Wiltse LL, Cirincione RJ: Spondylolysis in the female gymnast. Clin Orthop Rel Res 117:68–73, 1976.

12. Stinson JT: Spondylolysis and spondylolisthesis in the athlete. Clin Invest Sports Med: 12:517–528, 1993.

13. Rowe GG, Roche MB: The etiology of separate neural arch. JBJS 35-A:102–110, 1953.

14. Fredrickson BE, Baker D, McHolick WJ, et al: The natural history of spondylolysis and spondylolisthesis. JBJS 66-A:699–707, 1984.

15. Wiltse LL: The etiology of spondylolisthesis. JBJS 44-A:539–560, 1962.

16. Simper LB: Spondylolysis in eskimo skeletons. Acta Orthop Scand 57:78–80, 1986.

17. Wiltse LL, Widel EH, Jackson DW: Fatigue fracture: the basic lesion in isthmic spondylolisthesis. JBJS 57-A:17–22, 1975.

18. Soler T, Calderon C: The prevalence of spondylolysis in the Spanish elite athlete. Am J Sports Med 28:57–62, 2000.

19. Micheli, L: Back injuries in gymnasts. Clin Sports Med 4:85, 1985.

20. Gill GG, Manning JG, White HL: Surgical treatment of spondylolisthesis without spine fusion. JBJS 37-A:493–520, 1955.

21. Matsunaga S, Sakou T, Taketomi E, Iuiri K: Comparison of operative results of lumbar disc herniation in manual laborers and athletes. Spine 18:2222–2226, 1993.

Section Three

Sports-specific spine disorders and maintenance

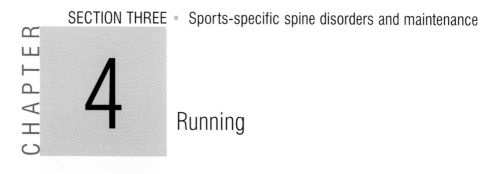

CHAPTER

4

Running

Jeffrey L Woodward

BIOMECHANICS

Running activities typically require that the spine, including the lumbar region, be moved through only a limited range of flexion/extension, rotation or lateral bending movements. Serious acute traumatic injuries to the spine directly related to running activities are relatively infrequent due to the limited motion of the spine from the neutral position. The most frequent and significant spine injuries directly related to running are due more to the repetitive axial or compressive loading of the spine that occurs during foot strike with each stride. It is common, however, for lumbar injuries and symptoms that have been caused by non-running injuries to be aggravated symptomatically by running, post-injury.

Casual observation of runners indicates that the lumbosacral spine angle typically ranges from mild flexion to mild extension alignment during routine running activities. The sagittal spine angle varies based on that runner's habitual spine posture, as well as the upward or downward slope of the ground being traversed at a given time. Complex scientific three-dimensional (3D) angular kynomatic patterns of the lumbar spine and pelvis that occur during running have been studied and documented in previous reports.[1] These studies have shown that there is a high correlation between the flexion–extension position of the lumbar spine during running motions and the corresponding anterior–posterior tilt of the pelvis. The lateral bending movements of the lumbar spine during running also correlate closely with pelvic obliquity or tilt throughout the running cycle. There has been no significant correlation found when comparing lumbar spine axial rotation with the corresponding axial rotation of the pelvis during running.

Schache et al[1] reported that, based on a study of 20 male runners, the average total flexion–extension motion during the running cycle was a total of 13.3° (SD 3.8°), about a mildly extended spine position (Fig. 4.1) and that the pelvis typically rotated through 7.6° (SD 2.0°) of total anterior–posterior tilt motion about an average anterior tilted position (Fig. 4.2). During running, the pelvis was routinely noted to tilt more anteriorly when the lumbar spine was extended and vice-versa. The average angular position of the lumbar spine during the running cycle was 22.9° (SD 6.2°) of extension from the vertical plane, as measured from the posterior superior iliac spine up to the T12 spinous process with the lumbar spine oscillating about this average angular position over the running cycle. The lumbar spine was noted to complete one phase of extension and flexion for each stride of the running cycle. The lumbar spine was reported to flex and the pelvis to tilt posteriorly slightly during the foot loading or heel strike response. By mid-stance, these lumbosacral movements reversed, so that the lumbar spine was extending and the pelvis had begun to tilt anteriorly. Maximum extension of the lumbar spine was noted immediately preceding the toe-off phase of the running cycle. The lumbar spine was reported to undergo lateral

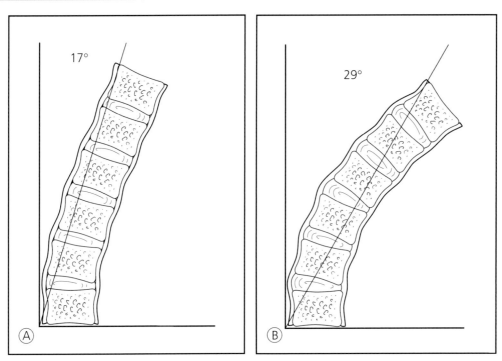

Figure 4.1
Lumbar spine diagrams showing the average maximum spine range of motion during the running cycle.

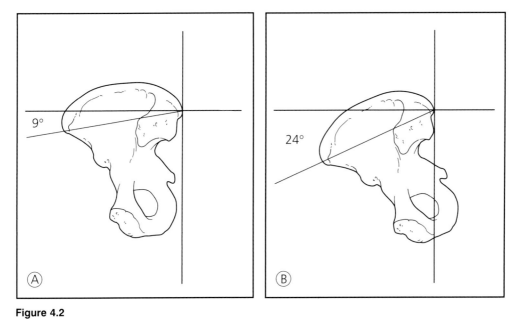

Figure 4.2
A. Pelvic diagram showing the average maximum posterior pelvic tilt during the running cycle.
B. Pelvic diagram showing the average maximum anterior pelvic tilt during the running cycle.

bending motion during running, with an average amplitude of total side-bending about 9° (SD 3.9°) to each side (Fig. 4.3), and the pelvic obliquity lateral motion, with an average of about 5° (SD 3.0°) to each side (Fig. 4.4). When the right foot was loaded with weight, the lumbar spine was noted to bend laterally to the right, with the pelvis then being lower on the left side. By the time of right toe-off, the lumbar spine had a maximum left lateral bend and the pelvis elevated on the left. Schache's study also showed that the greatest variability across test subjects of all measurements taken was in amount of total lumbar flexion–extension motion displayed, thought most likely to be due to differences in the natural lordotic posture of the lumbar spine between subjects.[1] Whittle[2] had also studied the lumbar spine extension motion during running and found an average lumbar spine extension position during running of 25.9°, which is similar to the 22.9° value found in the above study. Any prolonged running on unlevel ground could clearly increase the amount of lumbar motion, particularly the lumbar lateral bending required to maintain balance with side hill running.

While the size and shape of both the lumbar spinal canal and the neuroforamen are prone to change significantly with lumbar postural changes which could aggravate central or lateral spinal stenosis conditions, I could find no published reports indicating the degree of such spinal canal changes specifically during running activities.[3] Clinically, the most significant injurious affects from running appear to result from the highly repetitive axial compressive loads that occur at heel strike with each stride. A typical distance runner running about 130 km per week in training would subject his body to approximately 40 000 foot strikes per week.[4] Numerous measurements have been made of lumbar intradiscal compressive loads with various activities in the past. Increased intradiscal loads and pressures will occur during running from axial spine loading at heel strike and, to a lesser extent, the activation of lumbar spine extensor muscles during the running cycle. Cappozzo and Berme reported that during walking activity, the L3–L4 segment loading varied during the gait cycle from a minimum of 0.2–0.8 times body weight up to maximum of 2.7–5.7 times body weight during heel strike.[5] In comparison, loads up to eight times body weight have been demonstrated to occur in the hip joint during jogging.[6] Keller et al stated that

Figure 4.3

Lumbar spine diagrams showing the average lumbar lateral tilting, right (**A**) and left (**B**), respectively, occurring during the running cycle.

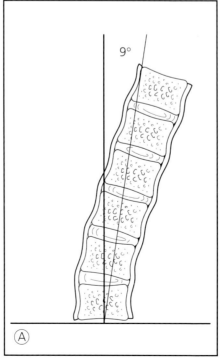

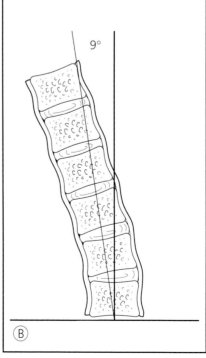

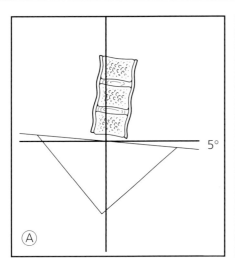 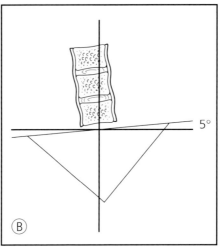

Figure 4.4
Pelvic diagram showing the average lateral pelvic obliquity motions, right (**A**) and left (**B**), respectively, during the running cycle.

the ground reaction and spine loading forces were proportional for female and male runners. Also, walking activity was associated with a maximum loading force up to 1.2 times body weight and running at 6.0 ms^{-1} caused spine loading forces of 2.5 times body weight.[7] No changes in ground reaction force loading of the spine were noted with increased running speeds or with more forward leaning during sprinting, including at higher speeds. Slow jogging at about 3.0 ms^{-1} was noted, with up to 50% higher ground reaction forces and loading in comparison to walking or fast running, which was stated to be due to a higher and more variable center of gravity during jogging, which increases impact forces. Wilke, in 1999, used newer technology to measure intradiscal pressures during activity in comparison with Nachemson's prior intradiscal studies. Wilke et al reported that a 45-year-old male with a non-degenerated L4–L5 disc had an intradiscal pressure with relaxed standing of 0.5 MPa and with standing in a forward flexed posture, the intradiscal pressure increased to 1.1 MPa. The study also reported that jogging with tennis shoes resulted in intradiscal pressures ranging from 0.35–0.85 MPa.[8] Rohlmann recorded a maximum intradiscal pressure while jogging on a treadmill of 0.85 MPa or 170% of the pressure noted in standing.[9] Spine extensor muscle contraction can also increase the intradiscal pressure to some extent. Thoracic and lumbar spine extensor muscles are known to have a burst of contraction activity at the time of ipsilateral toe off; however, the actual biomechanical effects and loading forces to the lumbar discs from this muscle activity is thought to be relatively small compared to postural effects.[5,10] Longitudinal lumbar spine shrinkage has been measured in marathon runners at different speeds running for a total testing time of 30 minutes.[11] The maximum amount of lumbar spine shrinkage occurred during the first 15 minutes of running, and faster running speed resulted in a greater amount of shrinkage.[11] The maximum shrinkage noted after 30 minutes of running at full marathon pace resulted in a 7.69 mm decrease in stature. There was no correlation noted between the presence of low back pain and the amount of spine shrinkage. The clinical effects of increased intradiscal pressure and increased spine loading with various speeds of running are not known.

The effects of spine posture and lower extremity biomechanical changes that occur during exhaustive running, as fatigue occurs, is not well known but has undergone preliminary evaluation. One study has shown prolonged running to exhaustion causes biomechanical changes in the legs that lead to a lower effective body mass during heel strike impact. This reduced impact loading to lower extremity joints results from better shock absorption with changes in leg movements and a change in the center of gravity which may change the spine-loading forces with fatigue.[12] Therefore, spine forces and disc pressure may actually vary during a run, depending on lower extremity activity and level of fatigue.

Another factor that may have some clinical effect on spine loading with running is the type of running shoe and insole materials utilized. Ogon et al. showed that certain running shoes and insoles slow the rate of shock transmission to the spine significantly, which may allow the lumbar spine muscles more time to activate and contract, to provide more effective spine-stabilizing forces around the lumbar spine during peak loads in the running cycle.[13] Running shoes that have a higher arch support, which maintains a greater medial longitudinal arch height while running, have been shown to be better shock absorbers with regard to the lumbar spine than shoes maintaining a lower arch height.[14] These biomechanical considerations regarding running shoes and insoles assume a relatively normal and symmetric lumbosacral and pelvic alignment. Prior studies have documented an increased incidence of low back pain associated with running on harder surfaces, which would also indicate that any variable causing increased shock and loading forces through the legs and spine may well increase the incidence of lumbar injury and pain.[15]

For years there has been discussion regarding the possible deleterious effects of a significant leg length discrepancy, including its contribution to low back pain and other lumbosacral/pelvis disorders. There continues to be some disagreement on the extent to which leg length discrepancy and its biomechanical effects actually contribute to the development of spinal osteoarthritis and lumbosacral pain and no clear evidence on the magnitude of length discrepancy is necessary to cause such problems.[16] Wen and associates did, however, find a direct and statistically significant correlation between leg length discrepancy and onset of lumbar pain within 12 months of running in a marathon training program.[15] The clinical importance of leg length discrepancies with running shorter distances is not clear.

COMMON DISORDERS

Overall, running activities are not associated with a significant incidence of spine injuries due to the absence of any heavy lifting or collision activity with this sport and the relatively limited spine motion required for running. Injuries specifically to the lumbar spine and pelvis account for only 11–13% of all running injuries that usually involve the lower extremities.[17] Most commonly, running aggravates spine pain that was originally caused by an injury resulting from a more strenuous activity.

In general, routine physical activity done for at least 3 hours per week reduces the risk of low back pain episodes over the course of the participant's lifetime.[18] However, while swimming seems to reduce the prevalence of low back pain significantly, there was no similar effect noted from running activities. A prospective study of women runners reported injuries at a rate of 2.44 per 100 hours of jogging and running for all injuries, including lower extremity muscle pain.[19] Spine injuries and pain are included in this injury rate and would constitute just a portion of this relatively small rate of running injury reports, supporting the low incidence of spine injuries caused by running activity. The majority of all injuries reported from the running group in this study were mild temporary injuries that were consistent with mild sprain/strain or delayed-onset muscle pain abnormalities. Former elite male runners have reported a decreased prevalence of monthly low back pain as compared to other elite athletes, which included soccer players and weight lifters.[20] Also, the average intensity of low back pain occurring during the study was clearly higher in weight lifters and soccer players than for the runners group in the study. However, the running athletes did report having more frequent and more severe episodes of hip pain over a prolonged period of time than the other athletes.[20] Middle-aged and elderly joggers (a total of 316 subjects) who ran regularly have been noted to have no report of serious lumbar injuries or pain from their jogging activities.[21] The elderly joggers were documented to report a significantly higher incidence of knee joint pain. Also, the number of joggers in this study reporting any illness was significantly lower than the non-running control group for both men and women, supporting the overall health benefits of a jogging or running program.

Raty et al reported that long-distance running, along with other sports activities that do not require extremes of spinal motion, does not cause lumbar flexion–extension immobility or decreased disc space height later in life.[22] In terms of the development of significant disability with advancing age, members of a running club were compared with non-running community controls and the runners had a rate of disability development over time that was several times lower than the controls, after adjusting for age, sex, body mass, smoking history, arthritis, and other premorbid conditions.[23] During this 8-year study, there were also significant differences in mortality recorded between the runners' club members (1.49%)

and the controls (7.09%) (p <0.001) noted after adjustments for age, sex, body mass, smoking history, and mean blood pressure.

Two studies have indicated that jogging and running may well have a protective effect on the development of both low back pain and the development of cervical or lumbar disc herniations.[24,25] Videman et al studied the long-term effects of both endurance running and sprinting versus sedentary controls, and the overall prevalence of back pain was noted to be less in runners than for controls. There were also no significant differences in the occurrence of sciatica, hospitalizations for back pain, or in back-related pensions between runners and controls. Also, lumbar magnetic resonance images (MRI) of 24 runners were noted to have no significant disc degeneration or disc bulging as compared to the sedentary control group and included no signs of accelerated disc degeneration found among competitive runners.[25]

With regard to lumbar radicular pain, joggers have been noted to have no increased risk of developing this pain condition with a routine running program.[25] However, for individuals developing sciatica symptoms from non-running lumbar injuries, the patients that continue to run or jog have a higher risk for persisting leg symptoms associated with their running activities.[26] Inoue et al described three patients who presented with sciatica occurring specifically with running: the sciatica alternated from one leg to the other with each stride, even while jogging. These patients were subsequently found to have either a lumbosacral spinal cord or cauda equina tumor, with the radicular pain during running presenting as an early symptom of the disease and with no mention of any disc pathology contributing to the sciatica symptoms.[27] These authors speculated that the inertial force induced while jogging, acting on the small mobile tumor in the intradural space, caused this alternating pain and reviewed the potential spinal tumor diagnosis associated with runners having these symptoms.

Based on my review of prior studies, hip and gluteal region pain from jogging or running is more commonly caused by focal hip joint pathology than from spine disorders. However, lumbosacral pain of spine origin can often be difficult to discern from similar pain of gluteal or hip joint origin. Gluteal pain in runners can occur from various conditions, with one report of confirmed piriformis syndrome as the pain generator.[28] In this patient, the chronic left gluteal pain limited the patient's ability to run, with focal examination indicating pain from the hip/gluteal region that resolved with treatments specifically to the gluteal musculature.

Running activities have been associated with the development of both spine and sacral stress fractures: these are not common, but should be included in the differential diagnosis for any running athlete presenting with lumbosacral pain. The repetitive axial weight and force loading on the lower lumbosacral vertebrae can potentially cause stress fractures to any part of the posterior bony vertebral structures, including the pedicle, pars, or lamina.[29] Lumbar pars interarticularis fractures have been reported in both sprinters and distance runners, although the prevalence of spine stress fractures in runners is much less than stress fractures in the tibia, fibular, and metatarsal regions.[30] Atypical sources of low back and sacral pain in athletes, including runners, that have been recently identified are fatigue-type stress fractures of the sacrum.[31] These stress fractures have often been associated with a prolonged period of low back pain after diagnosis before gradual resolution of symptoms, with an average of 6.6 months back pain during recovery. One recent article reported a literature review of 29 cases of sacral stress fractures occurring in athletes who were predominantly runners.[32] The stress fractures have been documented to involve both the sacral ala as well as stress reactions of the sacroiliac joint.[33] Sacral ala stress fractures have been reported both in adult and adolescent runners.[34] Several of these medical reports concerning sacral fractures in runners clearly document that the presenting symptoms can include low back pain with or without focal sacral or buttocks pain. The most common site of the sacral stress fracture was noted to be the superior aspect of the ala, with one patient's fracture line extending inferior to the S1 foramina.[35] Major and Helms report that while sacral stress fractures are rare, sacral stress fracture symptoms may mimic lumbosacral disc disease and sciatica, leading to a delay in diagnosis and treatment. One of their studies included 11 athletes with stress fractures; those were mostly male long-distance runners, with one patient having complaints of sciatica later found to have a sacral stress fracture. Several of the other athletes in that study were experiencing groin and sacral pain with running, with both pubic symphysis and sacroiliac joint bone stress reaction and fracture abnormalities identified on radiologic studies. They seemed to find a correlation between patients having radiologic abnormalities of the sacroiliac joint also having coexisting pubic symphysis bony abnormalities with concordant pain symptoms while running.[36]

The chronic effects of jogging and running on bone structure, including the lumbosacral spine, with respect to osteoarthritis and bone mineral density have been reviewed. I could find no studies indicating a direct relationship between jogging or running and spine osteoarthritis consistent with other previous review articles.[37] However, an increased incidence of symptomatic osteoarthritis among men under 50 years old who routinely run 20 or more miles per week was noted in the knee and hip joints, with no such increased extremity osteoarthritis for either young or elderly individuals performing recreational running of less than 20 miles per week.[38,39]

The relationship of walking and jogging/running physical activity on the bone mineral density of both adolescent and perimenopausal women has been studied in the past. A recent prospective study of adolescent female athletes did indicate that female runners had a significantly higher lumbar spine and femoral neck bone mineral density as compared to cyclists and control subjects.[40] Peri- and postmenopausal women have been studied for over a 5-year period, and those subjects performing regular jogging activity were shown to have a significantly reduced rate of bone mineral density loss in the lumbar vertebrae L2–L4 levels versus controls, which supports the beneficial effect of jogging on maintenance of spine bone density over time.[41] However, any benefits that routine running activity has on maintaining bone mineral density in postmenopausal women have been shown to reverse and revert to control base-line levels with cessation of the weight-bearing jogging or running exercise program.[42] While no studies assessing bone mineral density in the lumbar spine in men from jogging activity were found, prior studies have demonstrated a significant increase in femoral bone mineral density in men with jogging and significantly higher bone density occurring for those subjects jogging nine or more times per month. Based on a review of the beneficial effects of jogging and running activity on female lumbar and femoral bone mineral density, there would most probably also be a beneficial effect to lumbar bone density in men with jogging/running exercise.[43]

CLINICAL EXAMINATION

Owing to the relatively infrequent and non-traumatic lumbosacral spine injuries occurring from jogging and running activity, no atypical or specialized physical examination procedures are necessary when evaluating acute running low back pain patients. However, due to the possibility of a variety of conditions contributing to the onset of low back/gluteal region pain with running, including pelvic, hip and groin injuries, a thorough spine and lower extremity physical examination is warranted. In particular, patients presenting specifically with gluteal region pain must be carefully examined in an attempt to isolate the specific pain generator, which may range from lower lumbar ligament/disc abnormality to pelvic/sacral or thigh musculature or joint disorder.

Focused physical examination of not only the spine but also hip and lower extremities must be performed routinely in order to make an accurate diagnosis. Although the actual contribution of pelvic obliquity and leg length discrepancy in causation of lumbosacral injuries with running is clinically unclear, thorough evaluation of the patient's bony pelvic and lower extremity alignment, as well as careful physical examination for a functional leg length discrepancy should be performed. Routine leg length measurements using standard bony landmarks should be done, as well as functional examination in long sitting and standing positions to diagnose the presence and possible contribution of leg length discrepancy to a lumbosacral pain condition.

The most common pain complaints reported by joggers and runners involve primarily lower extremity symptoms. However, maintaining a clinical suspicion for referred pain patterns to the lower extremities due to lumbar radicular symptoms caused by lumbar bony/disc pathology should be pursued during the examination of every runner. As with any other patient presenting with lumbar radicular symptoms, a detailed history and examination will usually provide clinical information that allows the physician to identify the presence of an active lumbosacral pain generator.

Ideally, an evaluation of the patient's standing and jogging/running posture should be performed as part of the routine evaluation of spine pain associated with running activity. If abnormal lumbosacral postures such as significant lumbar hyperlordosis are identified, routine physical examination should include a thorough evaluation of not only the spine but also of pelvic and lower extremity motion to identify coexisting conditions such as hip flexor-rectus femoris or posterior thigh/calf inflexibility contributing to the hyperlordotic posture. As with any running injury, footwear should be examined for additional information regarding the patient's running biomechanics that may provide useful diagnostic information. Patients reporting a significant amount of lumbosacral pain with running activity may have injured their back performing some other lifting or sports activity, with running only an aggravating activity, and a thorough history should be obtained to explore this possibility to allow for accurate diagnosis.

Common spine pain complaints associated with jogging or running activity should be evaluated radiologically, as indicated for any spine condition. Persisting lumbar radicular pain should be examined with an MR scan after failure of appropriate conservative care, even with the relatively low incidence of significant disc abnormalities associated with running activities. The only unusual lumbosacral conditions known to be associated with jogging or running activities that may require more in-depth diagnostic testing would be the lumbar and sacral stress fractures reviewed previously. Many studies have reported the uncertainty in finding and diagnosing posterior vertebral and sacral stress fractures using only plain X-rays.[44] The most commonly recommended radiologic test after plain X-ray to diagnose these types of stress fractures is bone scintigraphy, particularly for acute and sub-acute pain onset.[35] The bone scan can also isolate the location of the stress fracture with abnormal uptake at the sacral ala or with a linear pattern that parallels the sacroiliac joint, indicating active bony stress abnormality along the sacroiliac joint. Computed tomography (CT) can also provide diagnostic images for either vertebral or sacral stress fractures and would be the imaging study of choice for a stress fracture condition with incomplete healing and persisting pain complaints to study the degree of bone recovery. Garces et al studied 33 athletes with low back pain of more than 1 month's duration, all having normal radiography of the lumbar spine, and subsequent bone scintigraphy showed increased uptake in 17 of 33 patients and single-photon emission computed tomography (SPECT) positive in 16 of 24 patients despite normal initial plain X-ray.[45]

TREATMENT AND REHABILITATION

For acute episodes of lumbosacral pain caused by running activity, the first treatment should involve cessation of jogging or running activities for at least several days, which will often provide significant recovery and pain relief from the most common mild lumbosacral injuries caused directly by running. Any other sports activities that involve significant lower extremity impact loading should also be temporarily suspended. Cold and heat modalities at home may also be helpful during the acute injury time, to provide pain relief. Early initiation of nonsteroidal anti-inflammatory medications that are not medically contraindicated for the patient should also be started as early as possible after the injury, to provide acute pain relief and reduce acute post-injury inflammation.

For patients sustaining running injuries to the lumbosacral region that do not recover quickly with rest, a standard spine clinical evaluation and treatment protocol should be followed. Since acute running lumbar injuries typically do not involve any serious structural damage to the lumbosacral region, a 4–6 weeks period of routine conservative treatments is reasonable and most commonly will result in excellent injury recovery. Longer recovery times are possible, however, with one patient who sustained a vertebral laminar stress fracture reporting pain with running almost 2 years after the initial injury, although the discomfort was not disabling.[29]

For patients having persisting lumbosacral pain following the initial conservative treatment, more aggressive diagnostic testing can then be pursued, including standard radiologic evaluation, which may include lumbosacral CT scanning and bone scan imaging to evaluate for possible stress fractures when clinically indicated.

Interventional treatment such as lumbosacral anesthetic and corticosteroid injections under fluoroscopy may be provided, following the established guidelines for these treatments that is well documented in the available spine literature. As pointed out previously, running injuries to the lumbar spine typically do not result in significant acute disc structural injuries such as disc herniations, and a need for surgical intervention for running injuries would be rare but still should be pursued whenever clinically indicated.

Initial rehabilitation treatments following running lumbosacral injuries should focus on relative rest from impact loading forces on the injured region. During the acute injury treatment phase, non-impact loading aerobic exercises can be substituted for running, including aquajogging (simulated running in deep water aided by flotation devices) and aerobic activities such as biking and the use of elliptical trainers. For patients who are identified as having significant lumbar, pelvic and lower extremity motion restrictions that may have contributed to the injury, an early progressive flexibility program should be started to normalize these abnormalities; this could often include lumbar flexion restriction, hip flexion contracture and gastrocnemius-soleus restriction. If a patient is diagnosed with even a mild leg length discrepancy, then it is reasonable to correct this discrepancy with appropriate foot orthotic prescription. With postinjury lumbar pain reduction and physical recovery, patients are usually able to slowly and gradually resume running and gradually progress back to the preinjury level. A return to running on a treadmill or the softest running surface available such as grass or a padded track could allow the patient to progress more aggressively without significant reinjury or reaggravation of pain.

The acute treatment of lumbosacral stress fractures from running should include a complete restriction from all painful sports and running activities. Patients having posterior vertebral arch stress fractures may require the use of a lumbar brace for approximately the first 3 months.[46] With regard to treatment and recovery from lumbosacral stress fractures related to running, Johnson et al reported a protracted clinical course of prolonged back pain for an average of 6.6 months for these injuries prior to resolution of symptoms. However, a sacral stress fracture diagnosis did not preclude the patient from returning to his previous level of sports participation once complete bone healing had occurred.[31] All patients sustaining running-related bone stress fractures should be screened for any metabolic abnormality that could predispose the patient to stress fractures, particularly in the postmenopausal female athlete, related to osteoporosis, and in younger female athletes, for the presence of the amenorrhea, anorexia, and osteoporosis triad.[35] Lumbosacral stress fractures caused by running are usually associated with an abrupt significant change in training regimen that usually involves significant increased mileage, a change of shoes or a change in the running surface.

TRAINING AND PREVENTION

One of the most important factors contributing to the onset of running overuse injuries in the lower extremities and the lumbosacral region is the total mileage run by the athlete. A reasonable limitation of the total miles run per week to moderate amounts would be a logical first step in reducing the risk of lumbosacral running injuries. Running every other day would also probably reduce the potential deleterious repetitive axial loading effects and injuries to the spine occurring while running by providing recovery time, especially following longer runs. Aerobic cross-training using aquatic/swimming exercise and non-impact lower extremity loading activities such as biking, ski machine, stair stepper and elliptical trainers could also be helpful in maintaining excellent cardiovascular fitness while reducing the overall risk of lumbosacral overuse injuries from long distance running. As with lower extremity running injuries, references reviewed for this chapter have indicated that the onset of acute lumbosacral injuries are usually associated with a significant change in the individual's running program, such as rapidly increasing running distance, change in footwear or running surface. A general rule of thumb for progressing running distances gradually to reduce the risk of overuse injuries is to increase total running distance no greater than 10% increase per week. Obtaining well-fitting footwear with adequate shock-absorbing capability can also potentially reduce the total amount of repetitive loading forces on the lumbar spine, although an accurate measure of the efficacy of good footwear in reducing the incidence of running spine injuries is not available.

Repetitive impact loading on the spine can also be reduced for lumbar pain relief as needed by locating more forgiving running surfaces than concrete, such as grass, mulched pathways, treadmill or a padded running track, which can allow athletes to progress total mileage more rapidly, with potentially less risk of injury. While correction of any significant leg length inequality is a reasonable preventive measure, even for less severe leg length discrepancies, there has been no rigorous testing of the efficacy of this preventive treatment.[47] A thorough lumbosacral, pelvic and lower extremity flexibility program is typically recommended for all athletes, including runners, for the prevention of sports injuries. However, Brier and Nyfield[48] found no significant correlation between hip and low back inflexibility and the incidence of low back pain or disability in runners with no history of pre-existing lumbar spine disorder. Biomechanically, it would seem that stretching, specifically of the lumbar spine in runners, would be less important with regard to injuries, since running activities do not require the lumbar spine to bend or rotate excessively. However, pelvic and lower extremity flexibility training would be more likely to have a positive effect in the reduction of lower extremity injuries with running. With regard to lumbar spine strengthening, one recent study has shown that participation in a core strengthening program had no significant effect on the incidence of low back pain in athletes.[49] These authors did, however, note a significant correlation between the presence of right and left hip strength asymmetry and low back pain requiring treatment, which may indicate the importance of maintaining adequate and symmetric pelvic/hip muscle strength as an important preventive measure for reducing incidents of low back pain.

Some patients may benefit from a lumbosacral strengthening and exercise program and may be able to jog without significant pain after treatment with a trunk stabilization program and develop the ability to find and maintain the spine in the neutral pain-free position while running. Patients with ongoing spine posterior element pain from facet joint syndrome or posterior stress fracture may return to running more successfully after learning to run with less spine extension. It has been recommended that patients recovering from lumbosacral injuries should avoid running hills until they recover adequately and gain enough spine strength to run on unlevel ground comfortably.[37]

REFERENCES

1. Schache AG, Blanch P, Rath D, et al: Three dimensional angular kinematics of the lumbar spine and pelvis during running. Human Movement Sci 21:273–293, 2002.

2. Whittle MW, Levine D, Pharo EC: Sagittal plane motion of the pelvis and lumbar spine during level, uphill and downhill walking and running. Gait and Posture 11:162, 2000.

3. Chung SS, Lee CF, Kim SH, et al: Effect of low back posture on the morphology of the spine canal. Skeletal Radiol 29:217–223, 2000.

4. Cavanagh PR, LaFortune MA: Ground reaction forces in distance running. J Biomech 13:397–406, 1980.

5. Cappozzo A, Berme N: Loads on the lumbar spine during running. In Winter DA, Normal RW, Wells RP, et al, eds: Biomechanics IX-B. Champaign, IL: Human Kinetics Publishers; 1985:97–100.

6. Anderson K, Strickland SM, Warren R: Hip and groin injuries in athletes. Am J Sports Med 29:521–533, 2001.

7. Keller TS, Weisberger AM, Ray JL, et al: Relationship between vertical ground reaction force and speed during walking, slow jogging, and running. Clin Biomech 11:253–259, 1996.

8. Wilke HJ, Neef P, Caimi M, et al: New in vivo measurements of pressures in the intervertebral disc in daily life. Spine 24:755–762, 1999.

9. Rohlmann A, Claes LE, Bergmann G, et al: Comparison of intradiscal pressures in spinal fixator loads for different body positions and exercises. Ergonomics 44:781–794, 2001.

10. Zander T, Rohlmann A, Calisse J, Bergmann G: Estimation of muscle forces in the lumbar spine during upper-body inclination. Clin Biomech 16 (Suppl 1):F73–80, 2001.

11. Garbutt G, Boocock MG, Reilly T, Troup, JD: Running speed and spinal shrinkage in runners with and without low back pain. Med Sci Sports Exerc 22:769–772, 1990.

12. Derrick TR, Dereu D, McLean SP: Impacts and kinematic adjustments during an exhaustive run. Med Sci Sports Exerc 34:998–1002, 2002.

13. Ogon M, Aleksiev AR, Spratt KF, et al: Footwear affects the behavior of low back muscles when jogging. Int J Sports Med 22:414–419, 2001.

14. Ogon M, Aleksiev AR, Pope MH, et al: Does arch height affect impact loading at the lower back level in running? Foot Ankle Int 20:263–266, 1999.

15. Wen DY, Puffer JC, Schmalzried TP: Lower extremity alignment and risk of overuse injuries in runners. Med Sci Sports Exerc 29:1291–1298, 1997.

16. Gurney B: Leg length discrepancy. Gait posture 15:195–206, 2002.

17. Bennell KL, Crossley K: Musculoskeletal injuries in track and field: incidents, distribution and risk factors. Australian J Sci Med Sport 28:69–75, 1996.

18. Harreby M, Hesselsoe G, Kjer J, Neergaard K: Low back pain and physical exercise in leisure time in 38-year-old men and women: a 25 year prospective cohort study of 640 school children. Eur Spine J 6:181–186, 1997.

19. Williford HN, Richards LA, Scharff-Olson M, et al: Bench stepping and running in women. Changes in fitness and injury status. J Sports Med Phys Fitness 38:221–226, 1998.

20. Raty HP, Kujala UM, Videman T, et al: Lifetime musculoskeletal symptoms and injuries among former elite male athletes. Int J Sports Med 18:625–632, 1997.

21. Komura T, Muraki S, Irizawa M, Yamasaki M: Characteristics of physical health conditions in middle-aged and elderly joggers. J Hum Ergol (Tokyo) 26:83–88, 1997.

22. Raty HP, Battie MC, Videman T, Sarna S: Lumbar mobility in former elite male weight-lifters, soccer players, long distance runners and shooters. Clin Biomech 12:325–330, 1997.

23. Fries JF, Singh G, Morfeld D, et al: Running and the development of disability with age. Ann Intern Med 121:502–509, 1994.

24. Mundt DJ, Kelsey JL, Golden AL, et al: An epidemiological study of sports and weight lifting as possible risk factors for herniated lumbar and cervical discs. The Northeast Collaborative Group on Low Back Pain. Am J Sports Med 21:854–860, 1993.

25. Videman T, Sarna S, Battie MC, et al: The long-term effects of physical loading and exercise lifestyles on back-related symptoms, disability, and spinal pathology among men. Spine 20:699–709, 1995.

26. Miranda H, Viikari-Juntura E, Martikainen R, et al: Individual factors, occupational loading, and physical exercise as predictors of sciatic pain. Spine 27:1102–1109, 2002.

27. Inoue K, Hukuda S, Katsuura A, Saruhashi Y: Alternating sciatica while jogging: an early symptom of cauda equina tumor. Clin Orthop 328:102–107, 1996.

28. Julsrud NE: Piriformis syndrome. J Am Podiatr Med Assoc 79:128–131, 1989.

29. Abel MS: Jogger's fracture and other stress fractures of the lumbo-sacral spine. Skeletal Radiol 13:221–227, 1985.

30. Brukner, P, Bradshaw C, Khan KM, White S, et al: Stress fractures: a review of 180 cases. Clin J Sports Med 6:85–89, 1996.

31. Johnson AW, Weiss CB Jr, Sento K, Wheeler DL: Stress fractures of the sacrum. An atypical cause of low back pain in the female athlete. Am J Sports Med 29:498–508, 2001.

32. Shah MK, Stewart GW: Sacral stress fractures: an unusual cause of low back pain in an athlete. Spine 27:E104–108, 2002.

33. Marymont JV, Aynch MA, Henning CE: Exercise-related stress reaction of the sacroiliac joint. An unusual cause of low back pain in athletes. Am J Sports Med 14:320–323, 1986.

34. Haasbeek JF, Green NE: Adolescent stress fractures of the sacrum: two case reports. J Pediatr Orthop 14:336–338, 1994.

35. Major NM, Helms CA: Sacral stress fractures in long-distance runners. Am J Roentgenol 174:727–729, 2000.

36. Major NM, Helms CA: Pelvic stress injuries. The relationship between osteitis pubis (synthesis pubis stress injury) and sacroiliac abnormalities in athletes. Skeletal Radiol 26:711–717, 1997.

37. Liemohn W: Exercise and arthritis. Exercise and the back. Rheum Dis Clin North Am 16:945–970, 1990.

38. Cheng Y, Macera CA, Davis DR, Ainsworth BE, et al: Physical activity and self-reported, physician-diagnosed osteoarthritis: is physical activity a risk factor? J Clin Epidemiol 53:315–322, 2000.

39. Conaghan PG: Update on osteoarthritis part 1: current concepts in the relation to exercise. Br J Sports Med 36:330–333, 2002.

40. Duncan CS, Blinkie CJ, Cowell CT, et al: Bone mineral density in adolescent female athletes: relationship of exercise type and muscle strength. Med Sci Sports Exerc 34:286–294, 2002.

41. Puntila E, Kroger H, Lakka T, et al: Leisure-time physical activity and rate of bone loss among peri- and postmenopausal women: a longitudinal study. Bone 29:442–446, 2001.

42. Dalsky GP, Stocke KS, Ehsani AA, et al: Weight-bearing exercise training and lumbar bone mineral content in postmenopausal women. Ann Intern Med 108:824–828, 1988.

43. Mussolino ME, Looker AC, Orwoll ES: Jogging and bone mineral density in men: results from NHANE III. Am J Public Health 91:1056–1059, 2001.

44. McFarland EG, Gingarra C: Sacral stress fractures in athletes. Clin Orthop 329:240–243, 1996.

45. Garces GL, Gonzolas-Montoro I, Rasines JL, Santonja F: Early diagnosis of stress fracture of the lumbar spine in athletes. Int Orthop 23:213–215, 1999.

46. Kujala UM, Kinnunen J, Helenius P: Prolonged low back pain in young athletes: a prospective case series study of findings and prognosis. Eur Spine J 8:480–484, 1999.

47. McCaw ST: Leg length and equality. Implications for running injury prevention. Sports Med 14:422–429, 1992.

48. Brier SR, Nyfield B: A comparison of hip and lumbopelvic inflexibility and low back pain in runners and cyclists. J Manipulative Physiol Ther 18:25–28, 1995.

49. Nadler SF, Malanga GA, Bartoli LA, et al: Hip muscle imbalance and low back pain in athletes: influence of core strengthening. Med Sci Sports Exerc 34:9–16, 2002.

CHAPTER

5

Spine Injuries in Racquet Sports

Scott F Nadler

Matthew Chalfin

Luke Rigolosi

INTRODUCTION

Racquet sports such as tennis, squash, racquetball, and badminton are a recreational pastime to millions of people as well as a competitive sport to thousands of professional, college and high school athletes. Injuries may occur throughout the lifetime of the competitive and recreational player, as they are sports that can be played from youth to senior citizen. Racquet sports require many different skills, including strength, flexibility, and coordination. Strength and flexibility are two factors that are well maintained in the athlete who does off-court conditioning.

Coordination encompasses two different entities: hand–eye coordination and quickness. Hand–eye coordination deteriorates at a slow rate and is well maintained in even senior tennis players, whereas quickness of the lower extremities may be more of an age-related problem.[1] Injuries may occur when a player who has lost quickness attempts to compensate and uses poor body mechanics in an attempt to maintain the same level of play. Acute injuries to the spine may thus occur secondary to poor body mechanics, resulting from insufficiency of strength, flexibility, and coordination, or as the result of repetitive strain/overuse secondary to the same factors.

Lumbar spine injuries are far less common in racquet sports than injuries to the lower extremities.[2,3] Despite the lower frequency of injuries, spine injuries can result in significant disability at all skill levels. Thirty-eight percent of male professional tennis players reported missing at least one tournament because of low back pain.[4] Swan showed that 50% of randomly selected elite tennis players had a history of low back pain of at least 1-week duration and 46.7% had received a medical evaluation. Muscular injuries to the paraspinals were the most commonly reported injuries in these athletes.[5] The other causes of low back pain described in tennis included intervertebral disc degeneration, disc herniation, facet impingement, and spondylolysis, although the frequencies of these injuries are not clearly known.[6]

BIOMECHANICS

Racquet sports require significant neuromuscular coordination between the lower extremities, spine, and upper extremities. There are many movements and reactions within the kinetic chain that must occur in order to insure a successful strike of the ball. In order to understand the possible injuries that may occur, we must first understand the biomechanics associated with the various swings in tennis.

The serve

The serve is arguably the most important shot in tennis. Each point starts with a serve and the player has complete control over how and where he strikes each serve. The serve requires synchronous coordination of both upper and lower limbs and the force that must be produced alone makes it the most likely stroke that will cause injury[7] (Fig. 5.1). The most susceptible areas to injury are the vertebral column, caused by the hyperextension and rotation necessary to initiate the serve and generate force, and the resultant lumbar flexion and rotation to decelerate the serve. These movements are part of every serve, which may occur several hundred times during the course of practice and match play.

The serve starts with the ball toss. Toss height should be to the sweet spot of the racquet and optimally should be contacted at the peak of the toss so that the velocity is zero.[8] After the toss, the racquet is brought behind the back in a loop. The mean minimum elbow angle is 63 degrees during the loop and is combined with rotation of the humerus in an abducted position to allow the racquet to travel behind the players back and be pointing towards the ground. The scapula must also rotate 165 degrees with the serve, producing a glenohumoral rotation of 65%.[9] These kinetics put a lot of stress on the systems that stabilize the shoulder joint. If too large a loop is used during the swing back, the medial side of the elbow will be stressed and place the athlete at risk for injury.[10] As the player prepares for the forward swing, the spine is rotated, sidebent and hyperextended and begins to be transferred posterior to anterior. The forward swing begins with downward rotation of the shoulder with an average velocity of 5.8 meters/second.[11] The internally rotating shoulder reaches velocities of up to 1715 degrees per second, with

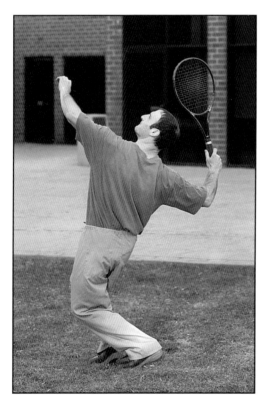

Figure 5.1
The serve.

extension velocity reaching 1000 degrees per second.[5] This is followed by medial rotation of the upper arm followed by pronation. Lastly, flexion of the hand and racquet occur at the wrist joint. All this occurs as the server's weight is transferred forward through impact. The service must be hit with forward rotation, so that it can land in front of the opponent's service line.

According to Elliot et al, a serve that travels straight must be impacted at 10 feet in the air in order for it to land within the opponent's service line.[11] It was shown that this is not the height where most professionals impact the ball on their serves. Thus, forward flexion and rotation of the spine along with gravity are needed to accomplish this. Therefore, to achieve forward ball rotation the racquet trajectory must be upwards and forwards.

The energy generated for the serve and other tennis shots is generated mainly in the legs and trunk. A total of 51% of the kinetic energy (KE) and 54% of the force is generated by the legs and trunk. The shoulder generates 13% of KE and 21% of force, but acts to aim the generated energy as opposed to creating it.[7] The concentric to eccentric contraction of the paraspinal and trunk musculature during the act of serving places these tissues at great risk for injury in the fatigued or poorly conditioned athlete.

The backhand

The kinematics of the one-handed backhand involves five body parts[12] (Fig. 5.2). It starts, as most strokes in tennis do, with a step toward the incoming ball. This is followed by a slight turn of the hips, opening to the projected path of return. As the hips turn, momentum is transferred to the trunk, which rotates in the same direction as the hips, which is open to the projected path of return. The upper limb, which had been moving away from the incoming ball prior to the initiating step towards the ball, begins to move forward toward the incoming ball as momentum and force is transferred to it.[13] This is followed by slight forearm movement, which will vary depending on the type of spin the player is trying to impart on the ball. We will cover the biomechanics specifically associated with backspin and topspin in a subsequent section. All of the previous movements bring the hand and racquet into position for impact. The shoulder velocity generated with the backhand may reach up to 895 degrees per second with a hand speed of 33 miles per hour.[5] Typically, the follow-through is a continuation of swing path that follows the same plane as was initiated prior to contact. There are differences encountered, depending on the spin that the player is attempting to impart, but basically the follow-through functions to insure maximum racquet velocity through impact and deceleration of the racquet. The two-handed backhand has much simpler biomechanics. A two-handed shot allows for less variation in position of the athlete's body and calls into

Figure 5.2
The backhand.

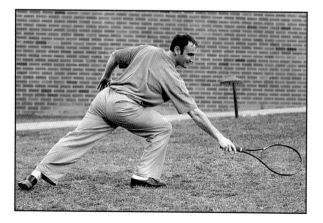

play less muscle groups. There are two body parts involved in the two-handed backhand.[13] The first initiating movement as with most ball strikes is a step toward the incoming ball. The hips then begin to open, rotating toward the projected path of the return. This is followed by trunk rotation in the same direction as the hips. However, the trunk rotates in unison with both upper limbs.[14] There is no movement of the elbows or wrists up to impact. The post-impact follow-through is similar to the one-handed backhand and functions in the same capacity. Again, there are variations in the swing plane, depending on the spin desired.

As with any sport, skill level plays a large role in the variations seen in biomechanics. The higher-skilled players will be more efficient at developing force via transferring the maximum amount of momentum to the racquet prior to impact. An obvious advantage to the two-handed backhand is that it requires less coordination of body parts. This means that there is less opportunity for deviation from proper form and more opportunity to generate as much force as needed to execute the desired shot velocity and placement. A disadvantage of the one-handed backhand, which is often encountered by less-skilled players, is improper ball strike. This means that a ball strike too far from the fulcrum, which in this instance is the shoulder, will cause excessive stress on the musculature of the shoulder and arm, which will need to absorb and stabilize the disorientating forces generated. In addition, the significant rotation and shear created at the spine may result in tissue damage and resultant injury.[15] Overall, the one-handed backhand allows for more opportunity for stress of the soft tissues of the spine.

The forehand

The forehand is a fundamental part of every tennis players' arsenal. It is most commonly used to impart force and spin to the ball with greater forces generated than during the backspin. The forehand shot begins with trunk rotation on a plane that is perpendicular to the net. The upper arm and trunk rotate with relatively stationary lower extremities, allowing for generation of the great forces generated during the forehand and the great shear and compressive forces generated at the spine. The shoulder velocity generated during the forehand can reach 387 degrees per second, with hand velocity up to 37 miles per hour.[5]

Topspin and backspin

Topspin is used to increase the ball's velocity and decrease the ball's height after it strikes the ground. Backspin is primarily used to decrease the ball's velocity and traveling distance after striking the ground on the opponent's side of the court. We will look at the biomechanics of the forehand in conjunction with topspin and backspin.

The upper arm is extended away from body but is flexed at the elbow with varying degrees of flexion. However, there is less flexion in the elbow with the topspin than is encountered with the backspin, where the upper arm is further away from the trunk.[16] The topspin back-swing involves greater hip and trunk rotation, allowing for a larger displacement of the racquet. The through-swing begins with a step forward with the anterior foot, creating a line through both feet that extends to the projected path of return. The topspin through-swing requires an upward racquet trajectory in order to impart the desired spin on the ball.[16] This requires that the racquet and upper arm start at a lower position relative to the shoulder as compared to the backspin start point. In addition, there is less flexion at the elbow with a topspin forehand. This increases the velocity at the wrist and allows for wrist flexion at impact. In contrast, the backspin forehand starts higher relative to the shoulder and follows a downward swing path. Elbow joint angle and wrist joint angle are maintained through impact. Typically, impact occurs in front of the body and approximately 0.05 meters in front of the front ankle for backspin and 0.26 meters in front of the ankle for topspin.[16] The follow-through for both shots continues on pre-impact trajectory.

EVALUATION OF THE INJURED ATHLETE

History

The basic history should include a temporal account of the patient's symptoms as well as a complete description of his complaint. If the chief complaint is pain, the primary location, intensity, and radiation should be noted. A pain diagram can be helpful in visually demonstrating the location and quality of the patient's complaint. A history oriented towards those participating in racquet sports should be performed, including questions regarding the mechanism of injury if known, the amount of practice and competition time, off-court conditioning, psychosocial issues, and success during play.

In addition to questions pertaining to the racquet sport, a comprehensive history should be undertaken. Physicians should be aware that true "sciatica" is a pain which radiates from the back, down below the knee, as it is the first indication of nerve root compression. The patient should be specifically questioned regarding provocative or relieving maneuvers or postures. The detailed history should also include a description of those activities which provoke pain and their previous medical treatment. This inquiry should include information pertaining to any office visits, diagnostic testing, as well the success of therapeutic interventions including medications.

Patients should also be questioned regarding previous participation in a physical therapy program. If this was included in previous treatment efforts, it is important to make an attempt to understand the specific therapeutic exercises and modalities employed. This information can be obtained from the patient or from the therapist's documentation. If, according to the patient, previous therapy failed, questions should be included regarding the type of therapy, the utilization of modalities, and the inclusion and compliance with a home exercise program. This approach will help the evaluating physician appreciate the extent and comprehensiveness of previous treatment strategies and allow a valid assumption as to whether a particular mode of treatment was successful or not.

Physical examination

A comprehensive physical examination of a patient with acute low back pain should include an in-depth evaluation of the neurologic and musculoskeletal systems. The neurologic examination should always include an evaluation of lower body sensation, strength, and reflexes. This portion of the examination will allow the examiner to detect sensory or motor deficits which may be consistent with an associated radiculopathy or cauda equina syndrome. Provocative maneuvers, such as straight leg raising, may provide evidence of increased dural tension, indicating underlying nerve root pathology.[17,18] Attempts at pain centralization through postural changes, i.e., lumbar extension, may suggest a discogenic etiology for pain and may also assist in determining the success of future treatment strategies.[19] Local pain reproduced with extension of the spine, especially when combined with rotation and sidebending, may support a mechanical etiology to athlete's pain, such as is noted with facet pathology or spondylolysis.

The musculoskeletal evaluation should include an assessment of the lower extremity joints and flexibility, as pain referral patterns may be confused with underlying nerve root pathology. By evaluating lower extremity flexibility, muscular balance, and ligamentous stability, the evaluating physician might be alerted to the patient's predisposition towards an acute low back pain episode.[20] In addition, the comprehensive evaluation should include an assessment of the thoracic spine and trunk, inspecting for signs of scoliosis or increased kyphosis brought on by inflexibility of the latissimus dorsi and pectoralis muscle groups, which may also result in compensatory lumbar spine difficulty. Combining the findings of the history and physical examination findings will increase the overall predictive value of the evaluation process.[21] Only upon completion of a thorough history and physical examination, as outlined above, and the establishment of a differential diagnosis, should further diagnostic studies, including X-ray, bone scan, magnetic resonance imaging (MRI), or electrodiagnostic testing, be undertaken.

DIFFERENTIAL DIAGNOSIS

Lumbar strain

Lumbar strain is one of the most common back injuries among tennis players. The erector spinae and multifidus muscles are most at risk due to the repetitive trunk extension and rotation performed during tennis play.[22] The mechanism of injury is one of repetitive contraction, causing muscle exhaustion and ischemia. The resultant lactic acid accumulation causes reflex spasm and pain.[23]

Presenting symptoms are unilateral or bilateral low back pain with paraspinal muscle spasm. Patients will often present with a history of a change in technique, intensity, or duration of play.[23] The patient may or may not complain of any pain radiation. On physical examination, there will be pain with back extension and flexion and tenderness over the paraspinal muscles. The patient will display negative straight leg raising and other provocative maneuvers, indicating adverse neural tension, but will have tenderness on palpation and restricted range of motion.

The initial treatment (Box 5.1) will consist of relative rest, avoidance of play, ice, and nonsteroidal anti-inflammatory drugs (NSAIDs). The addition of soft tissue myofascial technique and other osteopathic manipulative techniques including muscle energy may additionally be appropriate at this early stage. High-velocity, low-amplitude manipulation should be performed with caution immediately after injury and may be better utilized several days later when acute muscle spasm has resolved. When the acute pain subsides, a progressive program of flexibility and strengthening regimen of the back, upper and lower limb should begin (Figs 5.3 and 5.4). Incorporating the entire kinetic chain into functional balance and reaching activities along with more sport-specific conditioning may better prepare the athlete for return to play.

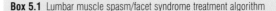

Box 5.1 Lumbar muscle spasm/facet syndrome treatment algorithm

Initial phase (pain control):
Activity modification
Anti-inflammatory medication with muscle relaxants
Therapeutic modalities
Soft tissue mobilization
Muscle energy techniques
High-velocity, low-amplitude manipulation
Consider intra-articular steroid injection of refractory pain in facet syndrome

Reactivation phase (correct postural, flexibility, and strength imbalance):
Active modalities
Spinal stabilization – progressive
Stretching hamstrings, hip flexors, quadriceps
Core strengthening, including quadratus lumborum, hip extensors, abductors
Address remaining issues pertaining to the entire kinetic chain
Sport-specific training

Maintenance phase (functional adaptations):
Continue with maintenance core stabilization
Upgraded sport-specific training with return to play
Comprehensive independent exercise program

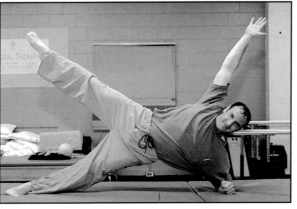

Figure 5.3
Strengthening of the quadratus lumborum as part of a core conditioning program.

Figure 5.4
Spine stabilization program –
quadruped position.

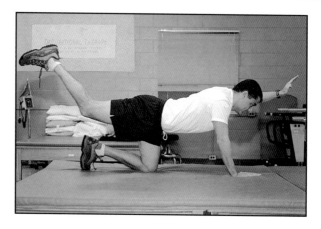

Facet syndrome

Facet joint syndrome and arthropathy may be the result of sudden flexion or extension combined with rotation, such as may occur with hitting a serve or an off-balanced shot. Facet syndrome may also occur in the presence of acute lumbar strain, where muscle spasm of the multifidi or rotatores results in restricted facet mobility, or as the result of degenerative disc disease, where loss of disc height results in increased compressive load on the posterior elements.[23,24] The latter would be more likely to occur in the more senior tennis player with degenerative disc and joint changes.

The presenting symptoms may vary, but often include movement-related low back pain with or without pain referral into the buttocks. Pain is often worsened with standing and extension, although flexion may also be painful secondary to compensatory muscle spasm. These patients may also present with a history of episodic back pain. On physical examination, there will be an exacerbation of pain with extension, local muscle fullness on inspection, and tenderness with palpation along with a negative neurologic examination and provocative maneuvers of adverse neural tension. Diagnostic testing is often not necessary, although this may be confused with spondylolysis, which should be carefully ruled out with appropriate diagnostic testing, which may include plain X-rays, bone scan with single-photon emission computed tomography (SPECT), and/or CT scan. The treatment plan would be the same as that for lumbar strain (see Box 5.1)

Disc herniation/radiculopathy

Lumbar disc herniation is one of the more serious problems encountered by the tennis enthusiast. There are many etiologies described to explain the occurrence in tennis players. Overuse of the paraspinal and trunk musculature may result in the loss of the dynamic stability of the lumbar spine, placing greater stress on the static structures such as the ligaments and intervertebral discs.[25,26] The significant rotational requirements and shear created during all the major tennis shots, including forehand, backhand, and serve, may also result in increased shear and compressive loads on the intervertebral disc, leading to tearing of the annulus fibrosus.[22,23] The least understood may be result of genetic predisposition to disc degeneration and tearing, which has been described in studies of identical twins.[27] In young tennis players, disc herniation may be on the continuum of disc degeneration or secondary to acute traumatic load caused by acute flexion and rotation maneuvering such as may occur in the follow-through from a serve or reaching forward and off balance for a net shot.[23] Isolated lumbar radiculopathy without disc pathology may be the result of traction injury secondary to a tethering of the lumbar nerve roots. Radiculopathy is most commonly encountered in the player with concomitant disc degeneration with loss of disc height and resultant spondylolysis, resulting in lateral recess stenosis.

The injured player may present with complaints of low back, leg pain, or a combination of the two. The patient can usually recall the onset of symptoms and may have had a long history of intermittent episodes of low back pain. They will be most uncomfortable with sitting or bending forward, whereas lying supine or quiet standing may be the most comfortable position. In the older athlete with stenosis, the converse may be true, with flexion relieving the symptoms whereas standing and/or extending back-wards worsen the symptoms. True radiculopathy is defined by pain extending down the back of the leg, below the calf. On physical examination, athletes with disc herniation will display pain-limited forward trunk flexion, occasionally with reproduction of leg symptoms. Back extension may improve their radicular symptoms, with centralization of pain.[19] Straight leg raising may cause ipsilateral pain when performed in the range of 30–70 degrees and may be exacerbated with ankle dorsi-flexion and/or neck flexion. Contralateral straight leg raising, where elevation of the non-painful extremity causes a repro-duction of symptoms into the painful extremity, is a rare finding but is highly sensitive for lumbar disc injury.[28] The results of provocative testing must be correlated with history, and most especially with the remainder of the neurologic examination, especially strength, sensation, and reflexes.[29] The high lumbar radiculopathy is a much rarer finding, but can present with a confusing clinical picture, with pain radiating down the front of the leg or groin; symptoms worsen while standing and often improve while sitting.[30] A careful physical examination will help to exclude this confusing diagnosis. Diagnostic testing, including MRI and/or electrodiagnostic testing, may be appro-priate in the case of a tennis player with radicular symptoms who has patchy objective findings that may be consistent with other diagnoses.

Initial treatment may consist of relative rest and NSAIDs (Box 5.2). An epidural corticosteroid injection may be considered in athletes who remain in pain despite analgesics and are having difficulty centralizing their pain with a McKenzie program.[31] Physical therapy should be initiated, with emphasis on flexibility and strengthening of the trunk and abdominal muscles initially in the context of a spine stabilization program and later progress-ing towards a more comprehensive core-strengthening program. Surgery is considered for those refractory to conservative care who demonstrate progressive neurologic loss or unremitting pain despite treatment.

> **Box 5.2** Lumbar disc herniation/radiculopathy treatment algorithm
>
> *Initial phase (pain control)*:
> Activity modification
> Anti-inflammatory medication with muscle relaxants
> Therapeutic modalities
> Soft tissue mobilization
> Epidural steroids
> McKenzie program
>
> *Reactivation phase (correct postural, flexibility, and strength imbalance)*:
> Continue McKenzie program
> Active modalities – Continuous low-level heatwrap therapy
> Spinal stabilization – progressive
> Nerve gliding techniques
> Stretching hamstrings
> Squat program
> Address remaining issues pertaining to the entire kinetic chain
> Advance to overall core strengthening
> Sport-specific training
>
> *Maintenance phase (functional adaptations)*:
> Continue with maintenance core stabilization
> Upgraded sport-specific training with return to play
> Comprehensive independent exercise program

Spondylolysis

Spondylolysis or fracture of the pars interarticularis can be related to an acute traumatic event or an overuse phenomenon causing stress fracture. Up to 4–6% of adults without a history of back pain will show this abnormality on X-ray. Seventy percent of these fractures occur at the L5 level, 25% at L4, and 4% at higher levels. Athletes presenting with these fractures will complain of various symptoms, including localized lower back pain, worsening of pain with back extension, pain with standing, walking, or lying prone, with pain relieved with sitting, bending, or lying supine. On physical assessment, athletes may

Box 5.3 Spondylolysis treatment algorithm

Initial phase (pain control):
Activity modification – avoid extension activities
Analgesics if necessary
Therapeutic modalities for local muscle spasm
Utilize soft lumbosacral support for protection and proprioception

Reactivation phase (correct postural, flexibility, and strength imbalance):
Stretch hamstrings, hip flexors, quadriceps
Strengthen abdominal musculature
Spinal stabilization – progressive
Address remaining issues pertaining to the entire kinetic chain
Sport-specific training – modify technique

Maintenance phase (functional adaptations):
Continue with maintenance core stabilization
Upgraded sport-specific training with return to play
Comprehensive independent exercise program

present with a hyperlordotic posture, tight hip flexors or hamstrings, weak abdominal muscles, pain, tenderness, and muscle spasm of the lower back. Spondylolysis is diagnosed with information noted in the history and physical examination along with X-ray and/or specialized bone scan studies (SPECT) and/or thin-section CT scan to evaluate the status of the fracture. Treatment is somewhat controversial, with some physicians advocating bracing for up to 23 hours per day.[32]

Newer approaches (Box 5.3) utilize activity modification (avoidance of extension activities) in combination with stretching that involves lower extremity musculature and core muscle strengthening in neutral position while the fracture heals. No research has been performed to demonstrate the advantage of bracing over functional rehabilitation at this time. It is important to diagnose these fractures as early as possible and initiate treatment, as significant delay may impact upon outcome. Morita et al demonstrated that a significant percentage of early fractures will heal and that bone healing is less likely as the fracture becomes older.[33] The ultimate goal of treatment is to return the athlete back to their sport pain-free and to prevent the likelihood of recurrence.

CONCLUSION

Spine injuries in racquet sports are a significant source of disability in the competitive athlete. They need to be carefully evaluated and aggressively treated. A comprehensive program addressing the entire kinetic chain with ultimate focus on core strengthening and sports-specific conditioning are key to returning these individuals to play.

REFERENCES

1. Leach RE, Abramowitz A: The senior tennis player. Clin Sports Med 10(2):283–290, 1991.

2. Jorgensen U, Winge S: Epidemiology of badminton injuries. Int J Sports Med 8:379–382, 1987.

3. Hutchinson MR, Laprade RF, Burnett QM: Injury surveillance at the USTA Boys' Tennis Championships: a 6-year study. Med Sci Sports Exerc 7:826–830, 1995.

4. Marks MR, Haas SS, Weisel SW: Low back pain in competitive tennis players. Clin Sports Med 7:277–287, 1988.

5. Kibler WB, Chandler TJ: Raquet sports. In: Fu FH, Stone D, eds. Sports injuries – mechanism, prevention, and treatment. Baltimore: Williams & Wilkins; 1994:278–292.

6. Hainline B: Low back injury. Clin Sports Med 14:241–265, 1995.

7. Kibler BW: Biomechanical analysis of the shoulder during tennis activities. Clin Sports Med 14(1):79–85, 1995.

8. Beerman J, Sher L: Improve tennis service through mathematics. J Health Phys Educ Recr September: 55, 1981.

9. Elliot BC: Biomechanics of the serve in tennis. A biomechanical perspective. Sports Med 6(5):285–294, 1988.

10. Allman FL, Nirschl RP: Tennis elbow: who's most likely to get it and how? Phys Sports Med 3:43–58, 1975.

11. Elliot B, Marsh A, Blanksby B: A three dimensional cinematographic analysis of the tennis serve. Int J Sports Biomech 2(4):260–270, 1986.

12. Groppel JL: Teaching one-handed and two-handed backhand drives. J Phys Educ Recr Dance May: 23–25, 1983.

13. Roetert EP, Brody H: The biomechanics of tennis elbow. Clin Sports Med 14(1):47–57, 1995.

14. Groppel JL: Control versus power – which is more important? Champaign, IL: High Tech Tennis Leisure Press, 1992: 81.

15. Blackwell JR, Cahalan T: Wrist positions for skilled and unskilled tennis players at ball racquet impact: implications for the onset of lateral epicondylitis. First World Congress of Biomechanics, 1990.

16. Elliot B, Marsh T: A biomechanical comparison of topspin and backspin forehand approach shots in tennis. J Sports Sci 7(3):215–227, 1989.

17. Cram RH: A sign of sciatic nerve root pressure. J Bone Joint Surg 35B:192–194, 1953.

18. Kortelainen P, Puranen J, Karvisto E, Lahde S: Symptoms and signs of sciatica and their relation to the location of the lumbar disc herniation. Spine 10:88–92, 1985.

19. Donelson R, Aprill C, Medcalf PT, Grant W: A prospective study of centralization of lumbar and referred pain. A predictor of symptomatic discs and anular competence. Spine 22(10):1115–1122, 1997.

20. Nadler SF, Wu KD, Galski T, Feinberg JH: Low back pain in college athletes: a prospective study correlating lower extremity overuse or acquired ligamentous laxity with low back pain. Spine 23(7):828–833, 1998.

21. Andersson GBJ, Deyo RA: History and physical examination in patients with herniated lumbar discs. Spine 21(24S):10–18, 1996.

22. Cailliet R: Low back pain syndrome. Philadelphia: FA Davis; 1981.

23. Hainline B: Low back injury. Clin Sports Med 14(1):241–265, 1995.

24. Haher T, Felmly W, Baruch H: The contribution of the three columns of the spine to rotational stability: a biomechanical model. Paraplegia 27:432, 1989.

25. Cochran GA: Primer of orthopedic biomechanics. New York: Churchill Livingstone; 1982:226.

26. Radin E, Simon S, Paul I: Practical biomechanics for the orthopedic surgeon. New York: John Wiley and Sons; 1979:8.

27. Battie MC, Videman T, Gibbons LE, et al: 1995 Volvo Award in Clinical Sciences. Determinants of lumbar disc degeneration. A study relating lifetime exposures and magnetic resonance imaging findings in identical twins. Spine 20(24):2601–2612, 1995.

28. Hudgins WR: The crossed straight leg raising test: a diagnostic sign of herniated disc. J Occup Med 21(6):407–408, 1979.

29. Malanga GA, Nadler SF: Nonoperative treatment of low back pain. Mayo Clinic Proc 74:1135–1148, 1999.

30. Nadler SF, Campagnolo DI, Tomaio A, Stitik TP: The high lumbar disc: a diagnostic and treatment dilemma. Am J Phys Med Rehab 77(6):538–544, 1998.

31. Benzon HT: Epidural steroid injections for low back pain and lumbosacral radiculopathy. Pain 24:277, 1986.

32. Micheli LJ, Wood R: Back pain in young athletes: significant differences from adults in causes and patterns. Arch Pediatr Adolesc Med 149:115–118, 1995.

33. Morita T, Ikata T, Katoh S, et al: Lumbar spondylolysis in children and adolescents. J Bone Joint Surg (Br) 77-B:620–625, 1995.

CHAPTER

6

Spine Injuries in Volleyball

Scott F. Nadler
Peter Yonclas
Luke Rigolosi

Volleyball was invented in 1895 by William Morgan as a training sport for track and field. Over the last century it has evolved into one of the most popular sports in the world, with millions of participants worldwide. It is played recreationally at all levels, from the local gym classes to the adult recreational leagues. Competitively, teams are found at all levels, from the junior and high school level to collegiate, national, and professional levels. Over the last decade, in part from the success of world competition in both beach and indoor volleyball, the sport has continued to grow. Volleyball is now one of the top five international sports, and with its 218 affiliated national federations, it is the largest international sporting federation in the world.

Although volleyball is often viewed as a limited contact team sport, it is not without frequent injuries. Studies of Scandinavian athletes have found that the incidence of injury in elite volleyball players was similar to or slightly lower than that in basketball players, but significantly higher than the incidence found in soccer, handball, and ice hockey, making volleyball a high-injury risk sport.[1] The very explosive nature of the game creates a number of opportunities for acute activity-related injuries, while the repetitive jumping, moving, and hitting required as part of sport-specific skills contribute to overuse injuries commonly encountered. Injuries to the spine in volleyball are not uncommon, with the incidence of low back pain estimated to be between 10 and 14% of all volleyball-related injuries, making it the fourth most common injury in volleyball.[2,3] Other factors which may contribute to spine injuries in the volleyball player include the different ages and skill levels of its participants and the variety of surfaces on which the sport is played; they all increase the potential for injury to volleyball participants. Solgard et al found that injury patterns depend on the age of the participants, their skill level, and their gender.[4] As the sport has grown in popularity, so has our knowledge grown regarding the etiology and biomechanics of injury.

BIOMECHANICS OF THE SPORT

Volleyball is a complex game of simple skills. It is a limited contact sport that requires a combination of fitness and technical skills. Players must be able to master various skills, including serving, passing, setting, hitting (or spiking), blocking, and digging while also having the strength and endurance to repeat these same skills numerous times in the course of a match. Because volleyball is a rebound sport (the ball cannot come to rest during play), it is a game of constant motion, requiring skill, quick decision-making, teamwork, and anticipation for success. In the course of a match, a team can touch the ball only three times on its side of the net. A typical sequence is begun with a pass or dig, a set (an overhead pass made with the hands), and a spike (the overhead attacking shot). Teams can also try to block the opponent's spike as it crosses the net.

Serving

A serve begins each point. A player must hit the ball with his or her hand over the net and within the lines of an opponent's court. Serving can be done several ways. At the recreational level, an underhand or overhand serve is used to place the ball in play. At more competitive levels, a jump serve is often used to add increased speed and spin on the ball to make the first pass more difficult. The overhand serve is typically accomplished by following a motion analogous to drawing back a bow and arrow to place the trunk and contact hand in a position to generate force required to put a ball into play (Fig. 6.1). Players will typically toss the ball with the non-contact hand while rotating and extending their trunk, abducting and extending a flexed arm while keeping their palm either face down or in a neutral position, before externally rotating their upper arm and extending their wrist. Repeated hyperextension of the trunk places repetitive stress on the posterior elements of the spine, particularly the facet joints and the pars interarticularis, while the reversal of this positioning into a more flexed posture may subject the disc to injury. This rotation and flexion of the trunk requires great muscular endurance and may lead to fatigue overload of the dynamic, muscular stabilizers of the spine. In the course of the serve, the contact point between the ball and the hand can additionally be varied to alter the trajectory of the ball by creating "floater" or knuckle ball serve, topspin, or curves to make the first pass more difficult to receive. The jump serve is typically accomplished by following a two- or four-step spike approach, while self-tossing the ball to generate more speed, spin, and power in the serve (see below for spike technique).

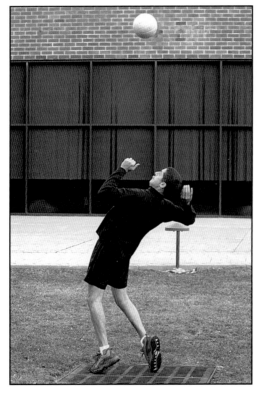

Figure 6.1
The serve.

Passing

Passing the ball is critical to initiating a team's offensive play. A pass is accomplished by contacting the ball on the volar aspect of a player's extended forearms while squatting at the knees and flexing at the waist to redirect the ball towards a setter at the net (Fig. 6.2). A "dig" is a defensive pass that is used to prevent an opponent's attack from hitting the floor. Because a spike can be coming at speeds of up to 90 mph, a receiver must assess the incoming angle, decide where to pass the ball, and control it in less than a second (Fig. 6.3). It requires anticipation, agility, and speed to get to the area of the court to pass it. Because of the speed at which a spiked ball is often hit, players sometimes must sprawl or dive on the floor to prevent it from touching the ground. The diving technique, which often involves hyperextension to cushion the dive, must be mastered to prevent injury to the knees, hips, back, wrist, elbow, and face.[5] This is why volleyball may be considered a contact sport, but in this case the contact is against a playing surface instead of an opposing player.

Setting

The set is typically an overhead pass used to alter the direction of the pass or dig and put the ball in a good position for the hitter to attack the ball. The set is usually the second contact and is generally

Figure 6.2
Passing.

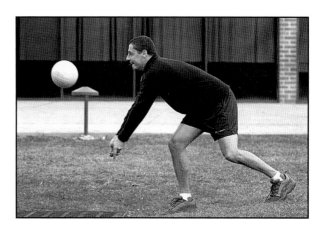

Figure 6.3
Digging.

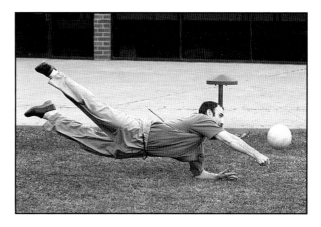

performed with open hands and fingers to place the ball in a prime hitting position. The setter is the tactical quarterback for a volleyball team, directing the attack to their team's best hitter or at an opponent's defensive weakness, often at shorter or slower blockers.

Spiking

The spike or hit is typically the third hit in a team's attack and often the most explosive. Hitters must adjust their approach, depending on the location and type of set being made by a team's setter. Hitters usually follow a four-step approach in which the first step is a small readying step and the last is a planting step that closes the gap before the player jumps.[5] The hitter often uses a preparatory countermovement between the third and fourth steps, which results in a coordinated flexion of the hips, knees, and ankles before a rapid extension at these joints while jumping. Simultaneously, most hitters will use a rapid extension of the elbows and arms between the third and fourth step, followed by an opposite rapid arm swing that results in extreme shoulder flexion and arm extension. This arm swing augments the ability of the hip and knee musculature to create extensor torque during the propulsive period of the jump and helps the hitter to jump higher.[6]

Once airborne, hitters will often follow a similar sequence as that employed by servers. Hitters will rotate and extend their trunk so that their torso is angled away from the net while simultaneously drawing back or extending their abducted and flexed arm, while their opposite arm will point towards the ball. Players will then cock their hitting arm by externally rotating their upper arm and extending their wrist. They will then uncoil and reverse these motions before contacting the ball. They will rotate and flex their trunk into a neutral position, while internally rotating and extending their arm before contacting the ball by snapping their wrist over the ball at a position approximately a foot in front of their torso. As with most overhead activities, the speed of the hitting hand comes primarily from the internal rotation of the arm and pronation of the forearm.[7] The contact point on the ball and the activity of the forearm and wrist movements will help to direct the ball towards a specific spot on the opponent's court.[8]

Blocking

Blocking is usually the first line of defense used in volleyball. The block is used to stop the spiked ball from crossing the net or to channel the spike to defenders who will dig the ball and redirect it towards the setter. In indoor volleyball the three frontcourt players share blocking, whereas in beach volleyball the responsibilities are generally performed by a single player. A vertical jump by one–three players is coordinated to prevent an opponent's attack from crossing the net. The blockers will spread their fingers and angle their hands to maximize the amount of area defended and to angle an attack towards the back row defenders. The key to blocking is penetration. The blockers will often "pike" or flex at the waist to help reach their hands over the net and into the opponent's court rather than reaching straight up, where they can be easily "tooled" or hit off of by the opposing team's hitter. If "tooled" or if the block is passed, the blocker will have to immediately land after the block and rotate towards the court to pick up the flight of the ball, a motion which may predispose a player to low back injury.

BIOMECHANICS OF VOLLEYBALL INJURIES

Although volleyball is a limited contact sport, a volleyball player's body and in particular the spine is subjected to various stresses throughout the course of a game and season. Because a volleyball player often has to jump countless times during a match, the player's spine is subjected to stress not only during the course of hitting approaches but also during landing from a spike or block. Nicholas et al described the link theory in which the ankle, knees, and hips act as a link system, making possible the transmission of forces into the pelvis and spine during running, jumping, kicking, and throwing.[9] Biomechanical studies have confirmed not only how the joints of the lower limb work together to transfer forces between limb segments during motion[10] but also how a compromised joint will lead to proximal and distal joint dysfunction.[10–12] Studies of ground reaction forces on jumping athletes demonstrate that their body must absorb a ground reaction force of up to 4.6 times their body weight.[13] Because hitters in volleyball will often rapidly move towards the point of take off during their approach and jump horizontally as well as vertically towards the ball, they will often land several feet in front of their contact point, forcing their spine to absorb not only vertical ground reaction force but also horizontal ground reaction forces. Repetitive jumping as well as poor technique in landing may lead to an increased risk of lumbar spine injury.

Because of the repetitive nature of the many specific skills of volleyball, volleyball players commonly experience lower extremity injuries that may increase the risk of low back pain. In addition to the transfer of power from the lower extremity to the spine via the kinetic chain, many physicians have proposed that any deficiency or alteration in the human link system will produce or aggravate disease either distal or proximal within the link.[10,11,14–18] Despite the common perception of the existence of the kinetic chain or link theory, there is limited research in the peer-reviewed literature regarding this entity.[11] As an exact biomechanical model has not been completely defined at this time, research has focused on individual issues related to the kinetic chain, such as flexibility, strength, and their relationship to injury, to define this phenomena. In a pilot study, Nadler et al demonstrated the association between a history of low back pain and the presence of hip flexor tightness, leg length discrepancy, and lower extremity instability or overuse.[19] In this same study, female volleyball players were found to have the highest incidence of reported low back pain (LBP) compared to all other men's and women's sports. In a prospective study on the same population, athletes with lower extremity overuse or acquired ligamentous injuries were significantly more likely to require treatment for low back pain during the ensuing year.[11] Nadler et al noted that clinically asymptomatic NCAA Division I athletes with a previous history of LBP were found to be significantly slower during performance of a timed 20-meter shuttle run compared to athletes without LBP history, suggesting that athletes with a previous history of LBP may have residual limitations within the lower extremity kinetic chain.[20] Because volleyball players are prone to both acute injuries at the ankle and overuse injuries at the knee, they may be prone to further back injury during the season.

In addition to the stresses that a volleyball player commonly encounters via the kinetic chain and alterations in normal mechanics, a volleyball player's spine is also subjected to stresses through the repetitive volleyball-specific motions required in the sport, in particular the spike. An attacker will often repeat the hitting motion hundreds of times a week during the season through practice, warm-up, and games. The rapid extension during the approach, combined with the hyper-rotation and oblique extension to cock the hitting arm followed by the rapid counter rotation and forced flexion, produce forces that will cause strains, sprains, and possibly overload of bone-causing stress fracture. Repetitive hitting in volleyball players has been associated with overuse injuries of the back, including lumbar strains, facet syndrome, pars fractures, and even disc herniations.[21]

Although there are limited studies on the mechanical factors specific to spine injuries in volleyball players to date, studies on other athletes who are subjected to similar stresses via repetitive counter-rotation throwing activities have shown an increased risk of low back injury depending on the angles used in the counter-rotation movement. For example, studies in cricket fast bowlers found that greater counter rotation of the shoulders and trunk rotation away from a batsman during bowling was associated with higher incidence of low back injury.[22] Volleyball players, in particular swing or outside hitters, who must hit at different set heights with different approaches and sometimes with varied trunk rotations in attempts to hit around blocks, will subject themselves to increased chance of low back injury. These repetitive motions as well as the occasional mistimed hitting, where a player gets under a ball and is forced to reach back in a hyperextended, torqued position, may result in acute muscular strains or overuse injuries.[21]

Because of the increase in specialization in volleyball today, the frequent substitutions from the bench made during a match may also contribute to the increased risk of spine injury. As with most other sports, volleyball players will often perform a warm-up period, including hitting followed by stretching. Because only six players start the match, the remaining players will sit on the bench for an indefinite time in positions that may increase the risk of injury before being called back into the match.[23] Green et al found that a warm-up followed by bench rest in varsity-level volleyball players was associated with increased spine stiffness, in particular with extension and side bending.[23] This increased stiffness may increase the risk of low back injury when subjected to the increased demands placed on the spine.

In regard to muscular influences as they relate to the kinetic chain, the hip musculature theoretically plays a significant role within the kinetic chain. Biomechanically, the hip extensors and abductors are important in all ambulatory activities, stabilizing the trunk and hip and helping to transfer force from the lower extremities to the pelvis.[24–26] The gluteus medius/minimus are the major stabilizers of the pelvis during single limb stance[24–26] Activation of these muscles prevents the Trendelenburg sign whereby the pelvis contralateral to the weight-bearing extremity tilts downward during the stance phase of gait. The hip musculature thus plays a significant role in transferring forces from the lower extremity up towards the spine during upright activities, and in particular transferring forces from the lower extremity as part of the approach in a hitter's take-off. Poor endurance and delayed firing of the hip extensor (gluteus maximus) and abductor (gluteus medius) muscles have previously been noted in individuals with lower extremity instability or LBP.[27–29] Beckman and Buchanan noted a significant delay in latency of gluteus medius muscle in those with chronic ankle instability as compared to normal controls.[29] Kankanaapa et al and Leinonen et al demonstrated poor endurance in the gluteus maximus in people suffering from chronic low back pain.[30,31] Nadler et al demonstrated a significant asymmetry in hip extensor strength in female athletes with reported low back pain and prospectively who developed low back pain.[32,33] Overall, the hip appears to play a significant role in transferring forces from the lower extremities to the pelvis and spine, and impaired or delayed firing in a volleyball player may contribute to the development of low back pain.

The four abdominal muscles may also influence the kinetic chain and low back pain development. The rectus abdominis flexes the trunk while compressing abdominal viscera, whereas the internal and external obliques flex and rotate the trunk. The transversus abdominis, the innermost of the four abdominal muscles, has fibers that run horizontally, except for the most inferior fibers, which run in line with the internal oblique muscle. The transverse orientation of its fibers contribute little to dynamic movement of the trunk throughout the range of motion of the trunk.[34] The transversus abdominis and the multifidus are considered to be stabilizing muscles that are continually modulated by the central nervous system and provide feedback regarding joint position, whereas the larger torque-producing muscles (e.g. gluteus maximus, hip flexors, and obliques) control acceleration and deceleration.[35] The transversus abdominis is one muscle that has been studied extensively in this regard. Hodges et al noted the transversus abdominis to be active 30 ms prior to movement of the shoulder and 110 ms prior to leg movement.[35] The neuromuscular stabilization provided by the deeper trunk musculature may be altered in individuals with impairment of the lower extremities or spine. A delay in activation of the transversus abdominis as compared to activation of the primary movers of the lower extremity has been noted in individuals with chronic LBP.[36] Volleyball players who generate large amounts of torque force for hitting via contraction of their rectus and oblique abdominal muscles may be at increased risk for low back injury if they have weakness or delay in firing of their tranversus abdominis.

DIFFERENTIAL DIAGNOSIS FOR LOW BACK PAIN IN VOLLEYBALL

Lumbar disc injury

The intervertebral disc is a hydrodynamic elastic structure which has two components: the annulus fibrosus and nucleus pulposus. In early life until the later 30s, blood vessels passing to the end plate are progressively obliterated, with most nutrition provided for via the process of imbibition, where compression and distraction force nutrients into the disc. The annulus fibrosus is composed of layered sheets of collagen fiber with the individual fibers enhancing overall mechanical efficiency. The nucleus pulposus is composed of a homogenous mucopolysaccharide matrix containing a network of fine protein-based fibrils. Biomechanically, intrinsic disc pressure functions to separate vertebral endplates and maintain tension within annular fibers. Flexion and extension forces are well tolerated by the annulus, whereas the addition of rotational forces causes excessive stress to the annulus, leading to failure.

Lumbar disc injury is a relatively uncommon injury in the young competitive athlete.[37] Micheli and Wood noted 11% of adolescents as compared to 48% of adults with low back pain had evidence for disc injury.[38] Although uncommon, there may be more significant changes to the structure of the disc in athletes as compared to non-athletes. Sward et al noted disc degeneration in 75% of male gymnasts as compared to 31% in an age-matched group of non-athletes.[39] Various sports have been evaluated in regards to the potential increased risk of disc herniation. Mundt et al found only a weak association between bowling and herniation of the lumbar disc, with no significant association found in other sports such as baseball, softball, golf, swimming, diving, weightlifting, or racquet sports.[40]

The individual suffering an acute herniated disc with radiculopathy may complain of both leg and back pain at the onset, with the pain noted to travel below the knee. On physical examination, sensory loss in a dermatomal distribution, myotomal strength loss, and decrease or absence of the muscle stretch reflexes may be noted. Provocative maneuvers such as the straight leg raising test are often positive between the ranges of 30 and 70 degrees, causing pain to be referred distally below the knee. Other provocative maneuvers include the use of neck flexion, ankle dorsiflexion, or compression in the popliteal fossa (i.e., "bowstring maneuver"), all of which should exacerbate symptoms of referred pain into the extremity. The femoral nerve stretch test must be performed in individuals with groin pain or symptoms in the anterior thigh, as a high lumbar radiculopathy may be difficult to diagnose.[41]

Diagnostic testing may include X-ray, computed tomography (CT) scan, magnetic resonance imaging (MRI), and electrodiagnosis (electromyography or EMG). An X-ray is of limited value in the diagnosis of a lumbar disc injury but may demonstrate evidence for disc space narrowing, osteophyte formation, or evidence for spondylolisthesis which may predispose to the development of a radiculopathy. A CT scan may be used to identify disc herniation, but has more limited use in this regard secondary to the superior anatomic picture provided by MRI. MRI provides for great anatomic detail, allowing the clinician to visualize disc herniation or focal stenosis predisposing to radiculopathy. The MRI is an adjunct to the history and physical examination, supporting information from the latter two diagnostic assessments.[42] Jensen et al demonstrated that in asymptomatic individuals, more than 27% of those less than 50 years of age and 67% of those greater than 50 years of age had multiple abnormalities on MRI.[43] Therefore, clinicians must cautiously evaluate the results of MRI in conjunction with the history and physical examination. Electrodiagnosis gives a dynamic picture of any pathologic process affecting the lumbar nerve root. It can be used at the onset of injury, with pathologic changes noted in recording of the H-reflex and motor unit recruitment. It is best used 3 weeks or more after injury, at which time spontaneous (abnormal) activity may be noted throughout the axial and peripheral musculature.

Treatment should be dictated by the presentation of the disc herniation and whether the player has axial alone or with radicular features (Box 6.1). The initial strategy should focus on pain reduction through the use of pharmacologic and non-pharmacologic means, including the use of the McKenzie evaluation in attempt to centralize symptoms (Fig. 6.4). Epidural steroids may be appropriate in those who fail to respond to treatment and may be helpful in reducing symptoms enough to allow for progression of a spine stabilization program. Treatment should progress with patient tolerance and return to play should

---

Box 6.1 Lumbar disc herniation/radiculopathy treatment algorithm

Initial phase (pain control):
Activity modification
Anti-inflammatory medication with muscle relaxants
Therapeutic modalities
Soft tissue mobilization
Epidural steroids
McKenzie program

Reactivation phase (correct postural, flexibility, and strength imbalance):
Continue McKenzie program
Active modalities – continuous low-level heatwrap therapy
Spinal stabilization – progressive
Nerve gliding techniques
Stretching hamstrings
Squat program
Address remaining issues pertaining to the entire kinetic chain
Advance to overall core strengthening
Sport-specific training

Maintenance phase (functional adaptations):
Continue with maintenance core stabilization
Upgraded sport-specific training with return to play
Comprehensive independent exercise program

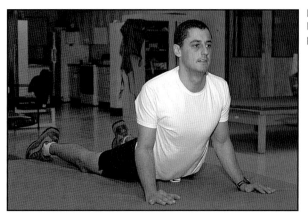

Figure 6.4
Press-up exercise to centralize pain in lumbar disc injury.

be dictated by both the clinical and functional measures. Surgery, although rarely necessary, may be appropriate for those with refractory symptoms with or without progressive neurologic loss.

Lumbar facet syndrome

The lumbar zygopophyseal joints are true synovial joints and are subject to inflammation. It is of key importance to understand the anatomy of these joints as it will clearly influence diagnostic and treatment decisions.[44] The lumbar facet joints maintain a sagittal orientation from L1–L4, with a more coronal orientation encountered at L5–S1. These joints are innervated by the posterior primary ramus, which supplies at least two zygopophyseal joints, with each joint receiving innervation from at least two spinal levels. The joints allow between 2 and 3 degrees of rotation at each segment within the lumbar spine and account for between 12 and 24% of compressive load, the remainder of which is absorbed by the intervertebral disc. The amount of compressive load increases as the intervertebral disc height decreases, such as is seen with degenerative disc disease. The facet syndrome may thus result from degeneration of the disc or the joint itself, positional overload such as may be seen with any repetitive overuse injury and secondary to trauma.[45,46]

The athlete often describes a sudden flexion/extension maneuver, often combined with rotation/side bending as the precipitating event. Lumbar facet syndrome commonly occurs in football, volleyball, gymnastics, figure skating, golf, and tennis, where end-range sagittal and transverse plane motion are combined. No significant research has been performed to identify the true incidence and prevalence of the facet syndrome, which is most likely secondary to the difficulty in obtaining reliable objective measures.

The athlete with facet syndrome may vary greatly in symptom presentation, and treatment may range from simple pharmacologic and non-pharmacologic measures to the use of osteopathic manipulation and steroid injection (Box 6.2). Athletes may respond quickly to manipulative treatment with or without the

Box 6.2 Lumbar facet syndrome treatment algorithm

Initial phase (pain control):
Activity modification
Anti-inflammatory medication with muscle relaxants
Therapeutic modalities
Soft tissue mobilization
Muscle energy techniques
High-velocity, low-amplitude manipulation
Consider intra-articular steroid injection into facet joint for refractory pain

Reactivation phase (correct postural, flexibility, and strength imbalance):
Active modalities
Spinal stabilization – progressive
Stretching hamstrings, hip flexors, quadriceps
Advance to overall core strengthening, including hip extensors, abductors
Address remaining issues pertaining to the entire kinetic chain
Sport-specific training

Maintenance phase (functional adaptations):
Continue with maintenance core stabilization
Upgraded sport-specific training with return to play
Comprehensive independent exercise program

use of medication, so this should be attempted prior to the use of interventional procedures. Return to play should be dictated by response to treatment and ability to perform all warm up drills without pain and with good biomechanics.

Lumbar spondylolysis/spondylolisthesis

Spondylolysis or fracture of the pars interarticularis can be related to an acute traumatic event or an overuse phenomenon causing stress fracture.[47] Micheli and Wood reported spondylolysis as the final diagnosis of 47% of adolescents between the ages of 12 and 18 years old presenting with complaints of low back pain.[38] Sports that require repetitive hyperextension will more commonly predispose to the development of a pars fracture. Rossi noted 63% of divers, 36% of weight lifters, 33% of wrestlers, and 32% of gymnasts had evidence for spondylolysis as compared to 5% of the general population.[48]

Spondylolisthesis is defined by a forward or backward subluxation of one vertebra on another. There are several types of spondylolisthesis: isthmic has an anatomic defect in the pars interarticularis; dysplastic types have structurally inadequate posterior elements; degenerative types are the result of significant degenerative changes of the zygopophyseal joints and deficient supporting ligaments; traumatic types are the result of fracture of the posterior elements other than the pars; and pathologic types are the result of metabolic, malignant, or infectious disease.[49] The Meyerding classification system separates slippages into 25% intervals, with a Grade I defined by a 0–25% slip, Grade II with a 26–50% slip, Grade III with a 51–75% slip, and Grade IV with a slip between 76 and 100%.[50] Spondylolisthesis is an uncommon occurrence in the competitive athlete, most likely secondary to superior dynamic muscular stabilization and skeletal maturity. Wiltse et al noted its occurrence in skeletally immature adolescent athletes between the ages of 9 and 14 years old and it was rarely seen in athletes above this age range.[49]

Athletes presenting with these fractures will complain of various symptoms, including localized lower back pain, worsening of pain with back extension, pain with standing, walking, or lying prone, with pain relieved with sitting, bending, or lying supine. On physical assessment, athletes may present with a hyperlordotic posture, tight hip flexors or hamstrings, weak abdominal muscles, pain, tenderness, and muscle spasm of the lower back. Spondylolysis is diagnosed with information noted in the history and physical examination, along with X-ray and/or specialized bone scan studies.[51] Treatment is somewhat controversial, with some advocating bracing for up to 23 hours per day.[38] Newer approaches utilize activity modification (avoidance of extension activities), in combination with stretching involved lower extremity musculature, and core muscle strengthening in neutral position while the fracture heals (Box 6.3). Newer research supports the concept that if this condition is discovered early in its course, a significant percentage of early fractures will heal.[52] As the fracture becomes older, bone healing becomes less likely. The ultimate goal of treatment is to return the athlete back to their sport pain-free and to prevent the likelihood of recurrence.

Box 6.3 Spondylolysis/spondylolisthesis treatment algorithm

Initial phase (pain control):
Activity modification – avoid extension activities
Analgesics if necessary
Therapeutic modalities for local muscle spasm
Utilize soft lumbosacral support for protection and proprioception

Reactivation phase (correct postural, flexibility, and strength imbalance):
Stretch hamstrings, hip flexors, quadriceps
Strengthen abdominal musculature
Spinal stabilization – progressive
Address remaining issues pertaining to the entire kinetic chain
Sport-specific training – modify technique

Maintenance phase (functional adaptations):
Continue with maintenance core stabilization
Upgraded sport-specific training with return to play
Comprehensive independent exercise program

Sacroiliac joint dysfunction

The sacroiliac (SI) joints are weight-bearing joints between the articular surfaces of the sacrum and ilium which are located on the lateral surface of the sacrum. They are part synovial joint and part syndesmosis, with the synovial portion being the anterior and inferior one-third of the joint.[53] There is hyaline cartilage on the sacral side and fibrocartilage on the ilial side. There are no muscles that directly control movement of the sacroiliac joints, but many indirectly affect movement. Sacroiliac joint movement is mainly passive in response to the action of surrounding muscles. The psoas and piriformis muscles pass anterior to the sacroiliac joints and imbalance of these muscles in particular may affect SI joint function. Imbalance in the length and strength of the piriformis strongly influences movement of the sacrum. Sacroiliac joint dysfunction occurs when there is an alteration of the structural or positional relationship between the sacrum upon a normally positioned ilium.[54] The sacroiliac joint plays a small but significant role in the cause of low back and buttock pain, although the true incidence is unknown. It has been reported to occur in elite cross country skiers, rowers, and gymnasts.[55–57] It is a true synovial joint with extensive innervation from the lumbosacral region, accounting for the difficulty differentiating sacroiliac joint dysfunction from that of surrounding structures. Various medical conditions such as rheumatologic disorders, infection, and neoplasms may also affect the joint and it is extremely important for the sports physician to rule out the possibility of sacral stress fracture. Johnson et al demonstrated sacral stress fractures in five collegiate athletes presenting with pain over the region of the sacroiliac joint.[58] It is therefore prudent to perform further diagnostic work-up in those subjects diagnosed with sacroiliac dysfunction who have a history of or risk factors for stress fracture or remain refractory to conservative care.

The diagnosis of sacroiliac joint dysfunction may be difficult and may be improved by using combinations of provocative maneuvers (e.g., Patrick's, Gaenslen's) and motion tests (e.g., standing flexion, Gillet's).[59,60] Provocative single- and double-blind joint injections may provide for improved specificity.[61,62] Treatment should include a similar paradigm as used with the facet syndrome, with the addition of sacroiliac bracing in those with hypermobility. Additionally, stretching and strengthening of the piriformis, gluteus maximus, and psoas should be included in the comprehensive rehabilitation program (Box 6.4). The program should progress from pain control phase through the reactivation and maintenance phases, as symptoms and function improve.

Box 6.4 Sacroiliac joint dysfunction treatment algorithm

Initial phase (pain control):
Activity modification
Anti-inflammatory medication with muscle relaxants
Therapeutic modalities
Sacral mobilization
Stretching of piriformis, gluteus maximus, and psoas
Consider sacroiliac bracing for hypermobile individuals
Muscle energy techniques
High-velocity, low-amplitude manipulation
Consider intra-articular steroid injection into sacroiliac joint for refractory pain

Reactivation phase (correct postural, flexibility, and strength imbalance):
Active modalities
Spinal stabilization – progressive
Stretching hamstrings, hip flexors, quadriceps
Advance to overall core strengthening, with attention towards hip extensors, piriformis
Address remaining issues pertaining to the entire kinetic chain
Sport-specific training

Maintenance phase (functional adaptations):
Continue with maintenance core stabilization, stretching program
Upgraded sport-specific training with return to play
Comprehensive independent exercise program

Sacral stress fracture

An atypical cause for low back and buttock pain in volleyball players is a stress fracture of the sacrum.[63] It is described mainly in an athletically active, premenopausal female population and is difficult to diagnose as plain X-rays are usually normal.[58,63] Triple-phase bone scan is the best way to diagnose these fractures.[63] The most significant risk factor for its occurrence has been described as an increase in impact activity due to a more vigorous exercise program.[58] It has been described in athletes participating in volleyball with the significant impact forces generated with landing from spikes, blocks, and serves as the probable etiology.[64] These stress fractures must be carefully evaluated, with historical information pertaining to a previous history of stress fracture, calcium intake, and evidence for the female athlete triad of anorexia, amenorrhea, and osteoporosis.[65] Biomechanical issues such as excessive pronation or supination of the foot, forefoot varus and valgus, leg length inequality, and reduced hip rotation have been

Box 6.5 Sacral stress fracture treatment algorithm

Initial phase (pain control):
Activity modification
Anti-inflammatory medication

Reactivation phase (correct postural, flexibility, and strength imbalance):
Stretching of piriformis, gluteus maximus, and psoas
Spinal stabilization – progressive
Advance to overall core strengthening
Address kinetic chain issues, including leg length discrepancy, hip rotation, foot mechanics
Sport-specific training

Maintenance phase (functional adaptations):
Continue with maintenance core stabilization, stretching program
Upgraded sport-specific training with return to play
Comprehensive independent exercise program

implicated in those at risk for recurrent stress fracture.[66] Athletes must be educated about the issue of stress fracture by allied health professionals and it is important for them to be told to report any localized continuous pain lasting for more than 2–3 days to their coach, trainer, or physician. Low bone mineral density has been implicated as a potential risk factor and screening with DEXA (dual-energy X-ray absorptiometry) scan may be appropriate to evaluate those who may be at greater risk for osteopenia and resultant stress fracture.[66,67] More research is necessary to further define this phenomenon. Most stress fractures respond to relative rest, correction of underlying biomechanical issues, and reduction in training intensity, especially the practicing of jumps with greater rotations (Box 6.5). A nutritional assessment is essential to clarify healthy eating attitudes and foods. Psychological support and counseling are equally as important to those female athletes identified as suffering from the female athlete triad or those with predisposing risk for this triumvirate of conditions.

CONCLUSION

Volleyball is a sport that requires strength, speed, endurance, and agility. The repetitive nature of the game, along with the requirements for high-velocity hitting and contact with the playing surface, may lead to significant spine-related problems. Athletes must be carefully evaluated, with treatment addressing not only the injured region but also the entire kinetic chain.

REFERENCES

1. Bahr R, Bahr IA: Incidence of acute volleyball injuries: a prospective cohort study of injury mechanisms and risk factors. Scand J Med Sci Sports 7:166–171, 1997.
2. Aagard H, Scavenius M, Jorgensen U: An epidemiological analysis of the injury pattern in indoor and in beach volleyball. Int J Sports Med 18(3):217–221, 1997.
3. Briner W, Benjamin H: Volleyball injuries: managing acute and overuse disorders. Sports Med 27(3):65–71, 1999.
4. Solgard L, Nielson AB, Moller-Madsen B, et al: Volleyball studies presenting in causality: a prospective study. Br J Sports Med 29:200–204, 1995.
5. Schutz, LK: Volleyball. Phys Med Rehabil Clin N Am 10(1):19–34, 1999.
6. Feltner ME, Fraschetti DJ, Crisp RJ: Upper extremity augmentation of lower extremity kinetics during countermovement vertical jumps. J Sports Sci 7(6):449–466, 1999.
7. Marshall RN, Elliot BC: Long-axis rotation: the missing link in proximal-to-distal segment sequencing. J Sports Sci 18(4):247–254, 2000.
8. Sakurai S, Ohstsuki T: Muscle activity and accuracy of performance of the smash stroke in badminton with reference to skill and practice. J Sports Sci 18(11):901–914, 2000.
9. Nicholas JA, Grossman RB, Hershman EB: The importance of a simplified classification of motion in sports in relation to performance. Orthop Clin N Am 8(3):499–532, 1977.
10. DeVita P, Hunter PB, Skelly WA: Effects of a functional knee brace on the biomechanics of running. Med Sci Sports Exerc 24(7):797–806, 1992.

11. Nadler SF, Wu KD, Galski T, et al: Low back pain in college athletes: a prospective study correlating lower extremity overuse or acquired ligamentous laxity with low back pain. Spine 23(7):828–833, 1998.

12. Osternig LR, Robertson RN: Effects of prophylactic knee bracing on lower extremity joint position and muscle activation during running. Am J Sports Med 21(5):733–737, 1993.

13. McNair PJ, Prapavessis H: Normative data of vertical ground reaction forces during landing from a jump. J Sci Med Sport 2(1):86–88, 1999.

14. Fairbank JCT, Pynset PB, Van Poortliet JA, et al: Influence of anthropometric factors and joint laxity in the incidence of adolescent back pain. Spine 9(5):461–464, 1984.

15. Renstrom AF: Mechanism, diagnosis, and treatment of running injuries. Instr Course Lect 42:225–234, 1993.

16. Clement DB, Taunton JE, Smart GW: Achilles tendinitis and peritendinitis: etiology and treatment. Am J Sports Med 12(3):179–184, 1984.

17. Knapik JJ, Bauman CL, Jones BH, et al: Preseason strength and flexibility imbalances associated with athletic injuries in female collegiate athletes. Am J Sports Med 19(1):76–81, 1991.

18. Teitz CC, Hermanson BK, Kronmal RA, et al: Evaluation of the use of braces to prevent injury to the knee in collegiate football players. J Bone Joint Surg 69A(1):2–9, 1987.

19. Nadler SF, Shumko J, Galski T, Feinber JH: Low back pain in college athletes: true incidence and proper screening. Proc N Am Spine Soc 110:62, 1995.

20. Nadler SF, Moley P, Malanga GA, et al: Functional deficits in athletes with a history of low back pain: a pilot study. Arch Phys Med Rehab 83:1753–1758, 2002.

21. Schaffle MD: Common injuries in volleyball. Treatment, prevention and rehabilitation. Sports Med 16(2):126–129, 1993.

22. Elliott BC: Back injuries and the fast bowler in cricket. J Sports Sci 18(11):983–991, 2000.

23. Green JP, Grenier SG, McGill SM: Low-back stiffness is altered with warm-up and bench rest: implications for athletes. Med Sci Sports Exerc 34(7):1076–1081, 2002.

24. Joseph J, Nightingale A: Electromyography of muscles of posture: thigh muscles in males. J Physiol 126:81–85, 1954.

25. Lyons K, Perry J, Gronley JK, et al: Timing and relative intensity of hip extensor and abductor muscle action during level and stair ambulation. Phys Ther 63:1597–1605, 1983.

26. Inman VT: Functional aspects of the abductor muscles of the hip. J Bone Joint Surg 29:607–619, 1947.

27. Jaramillo J, Worrell TW, Ingersoll CD: Hip isometric strength following knee surgery. J Orthop Sport Phys Ther 20(3):160–165, 1994.

28. Bullock-Saxton JE: Local sensation changes and altered hip muscle function following severe ankle sprain. Phys Ther 74(1):17–28, 1994.

29. Beckman SM, Buchanan TS: Ankle inversion injury and hypermobility: effect on hip and ankle muscle electromyography onset latency. Arch Phys Med Rehab 76:1138–1143, 1995.

30. Kankanaapa M, Taimela S, Laaksonen D, et al: Back and hip extensor fatigability in chronic low back pain patients with and without controls. Arch Phys Med Rehab 79:412–417, 1998.

31. Leinonen V, Kankanaapa M, Airakinen O, Hanninen O: Back and hip extension activities during trunk flexion/extension: effects of low back pain and rehabilitation. Arch Phys Med Rehabil 81(1):32–37, 2000.

32. Nadler SF, Malanga GA, DePrince ML, et al: The relationship between lower extremity injury, low back pain, and hip muscle strength in male and female collegiate athletes. Clin J Sport Med 10:89–97, 2000.

33. Nadler SF, Malanga GA, Feinberg JH, et al: The relationship between hip muscle imbalance and the occurrence of low back pain in collegiate athletes. A prospective study. Am J Phys Med Rehab 80(8):572–577, 2001.

34. McGill SM, Childs A, Liebenson C: Endurance times for low back stabilization exercises: clinical targets for testing and training from a normal database. Arch Phys Med Rehab 80(8):941–944, 1999.

35. Hodges PW, Richardson CA: Contraction of the abdominal muscles associated with movement of the lower limb. Phys Ther 77(2):132–142, 1997.

36. Hodges PW, Richardson CA: Delayed postural contraction of the transversus abdominis in low back pain associated with movement of the lower extremity. J Spinal Disorders 11(1):46–56, 1998.

37. Tertti MO, Salminen JJ, Paajanen HE, et al: Low-back pain and disk degeneration in children: a case-control MR imaging study. Radiology 180(2):503–507, 1999.

38. Micheli LJ, Wood R: Back pain in young athletes: significant differences from adults in causes and patterns. Arch Pediatr Adolesc Med 149:115–118, 1995.

39. Sward L, Hellstrom M, Jacobsson B, et al: Disc degeneration and associated abnormalities of the spine in gymnasts. A magnetic resonance imaging study. Spine 16(4):437–443, 1991.

40. Mundt DJ, Kelsey JL, Golden AL, et al: An epidemiologic study of sports and weight lifting as possible risk factors for herniated lumbar and cervical discs. The Northeast Collaborative Group on Low Back Pain. Am J Sports Med 21(6):854–860, 1993.

41. Nadler SF, Campagnolo DI, Tomaio A: High lumbar disc: diagnostic and treatment dilemma. Am J PM&R 77:538–544, 1998.

42. Malanga GA, Nadler SF: Nonoperative treatment of low back pain. Mayo Clin Proc 74:1135–1148, 1999.

43. Jensen MC, Brant-Zawadzki MN, Obuchowski N: Magnetic resonance imaging of the lumbar spine in people without low back pain. N Engl J Med 331:69–73, 1994.

44. Bogduk N, Engle R: The menisci of the lumbar zygopophyseal joints: a review of their anatomy and clinical significance. 9:454–460, 1984.

45. Mooney V, Robertson J: Facet joint syndrome. Clin Orthop 115:149–156, 1976.

46. Schwartzer AC, Derby R, Aprill CN, et al: Pain from lumbar zygopophyseal joints: a test of two models. J Spinal Disord 7:331–336, 1994.

47. Jackson DW, Wilse LL, Dingeman RD, Hayes M: Stress reactions involving the pars interarticularis in young athletes. Am J Sports Med 9:304–312, 1981.

48. Rossi F: Spondylolysis, spondylolisthesis, and sports. J Sports Med Phys Fitness 18(4):317–340, 1988.

49. Wiltse LL, Widell EH, Jackson DW: Fatigue fracture: the basic lesion in isthmic spondylolisthesis. J Bone Joint Surg 57A:17–22, 1975.

50. Wiltse LL Winter RB: Terminology and measurement of spondylolisthesis. J Bone Joint Surg 65A:768–772, 1983.

51. Read MTF: Single photon emission computed tomography (SPECT) scanning for adolescent back pain. A sine qua non? Br J Sports Med 28:56–57, 1994.

52. Morita T, Ikata T, Katoh S, et al: Lumbar spondylolysis in children and adolescents. J Bone Joint Surg (Br) 77-B:620–625, 1995.

53. Fortin JD: Sacroiliac joint dysfunction: a new perspective. J Back Musculoskel Rehab 3:31–43, 1993.

54. Lavignolle B, Vital JM, Senegas J, et al: An approach to the functional anatomy of the sacroiliac joints in vivo. Anat Clin 5:169–176, 1983.

55. Timm KE: Sacroiliac joint dysfunction in elite rowers. J Orthop Sports Phys Ther 29(5): 288–293, 1999.

56. Barakatt E, Smidt GL, Dawson JD, et al: Interinnominate motion and symmetry: comparison between gymnasts and nongymnasts. J Orthop Sports Phys Ther 23(5):309–319, 1996.

57. Lindsay DM, Meeuwisse WH, Vyse A, et al: Lumbosacral dysfunctions in elite cross-country skiers. J Orthop Sports Phys Ther 18(5):580–585, 1993.

58. Johnson AW, Weiss CB, Stento K, Wheeler DL: Stress fractures of the sacrum. An atypical cause of low back pain in the female athlete. Am J Sports Med 29(4):498–508, 2001.

59. Laslett M: The value of the physical examination in diagnosis of painful sacroiliac joint pathologies. Spine 23(8):962–964, 1998.

60. Cibulka MT, Koldehoff R: Clinical usefulness of a cluster of sacroiliac joint tests in patients with and without low back pain. J Orthop Sports Phys Ther 29(2):83–89; discussion 90–92, 1999.

61. Schwartzer AC, Aprill CN, Bogduk N: The sacroiliac joint in chronic low back pain. Spine 20:31–37, 1995.

62. Slipman CW, Sterenfeld EB, Chou LH, et al: The predictive value of provocative sacroiliac stress maneuvers in the diagnosis of sacroiliac joint syndrome. Arch Phys Med Rehab 79:288–292, 1988.

63. McFarland EG, Giangarra C: Sacral stress fractures in athletes. Clin Orthop 329:240–243, 1996.

64. Shah MK, Stewart GW: Sacral stress fractures: an unusual cause of low back pain in an athlete. Spine 27(4):104–108, 2002.

65. Zeni AI, Steet CC, Dempsey RL, Staton M: Stress injury to the bone among women athletes. Phys Med Rehab Clin N Am 11(4):929–947, 2000.

66. Korpelainen R, Orava S, Karpakka J, et al: Risk factors for recurrent stress fractures in athletes. Am J Sports Med 29(3):304–310, 2001.

67. Nattiv A: Stress fractures and bone health in track and field athletes. J Sci Med Sport 3(3):268–279, 2000.

CHAPTER

7

Biomechanics of Weight Lifting

Robert E Windsor
Frank JE Falco
Samuel Thampi
Frank King

INTRODUCTION

Athletic conditioning has evolved significantly over the past several decades. During the first half of the 20th century the role of weight lifting in training for other sports was very limited. Weight lifting was thought to create athletes that were "muscle bound," slow, and possibly predisposed to injury.[1,2] During that era, only weight lifters lifted weights and were generally not considered to be athletes. Beginning in the late 1960s, weight lifting enjoyed increasing popularity as an auxiliary means of athletic conditioning. Today, weight lifting has assumed a dominant role in training athletes in almost all sports.[3]

The medical field was also slow to accept weight training as a valid means of conditioning. In 1945, DeLorme described a conditioning program that emphasized the use of progressive resistance exercises.[4] The DeLorme technique required an individual to begin with a fraction of his 10-repetition maximum (10 RM) and increase the weight lifted throughout the training session until he could no longer lift the weight. In 1951, Zineoff described the "Oxford technique" of conditioning, which was a modification of the DeLorme technique.[5] The Oxford technique required an individual to begin a training session with the 10 RM after appropriate warm up.

The terms *weight lifting* and *weight training* are commonly, but incorrectly, used interchangeably. *Weight lifting* refers to the competitive sport of Olympic weight lifting and power lifting. *Weight training* refers to a technique of using resistance exercises to promote overall fitness. Body building is a competitive sport that emphasizes the development of a large symmetrical, well-proportioned physique.[3,6,7]

HISTORY OF WEIGHT LIFTING

The earliest mention of resistance exercises is a drawing on the funerary chapel in Beni-Hassan, Egypt.[8] This drawing depicts three people in various stages of lifting a heavy bag overhead for exercise. In 1896 BC there is record of strength competitions taking place in what is now known as the British Isles. In the sixth century BC, archeological data indicate that Milo of Crotone hoisted a heifer calf on his shoulders daily and walked the length of the Olympic stadium until the calf was 4 years old. Milo is often credited with the development of progressive resistance exercises and was a six-time Olympic champion.[8,9]

In the second century AD, a celebrated physician named Galen developed a system of resistance training using increments such as halters, or hand weights, to increase strength. His system also included heavy lifting, dumbbell exercises, and person-to-person isometric contraction exercises. With the fall of the

Roman empire and the beginning of the Dark Ages, weight training was lost for approximately 1000 years. Essentially, all physical training during this time was focused on warfare.[8]

In 1531 Sir Thomas Elyot made reference to Galen's system of exercises. In 1544 Joachim Camerius wrote the *Dialogue de Gymnasius*, which encouraged boys to engage in strength competitions, lift weights, and climb ropes. The latter part of the 16th century and the 17th century saw a gradual rebirth of the strength training philosophy, and by the 18th century, strong-man feats began springing up across London.[8]

Strength training did not become popular in Europe until the early 19th century. The Prussians had been defeated by Napoleon in 1811 and were not allowed to arm themselves. A Prussian nationalist named Friedrich Ludwig Jahn began training Prussian soldiers using resistance exercises to emphasize strength development so that they would be better able to defend themselves. As this trend spread, "strong-man" competitions sprang up across Germany as well. One such strong man, Fredrick Muller (known as "the Great Sandow") defeated the English strong-man team known as "Samson and the Cyclops" in 1889. This made him the most renowned strong man in England and caused England to become the center of strong men in Europe. In 1892 Florence Ziegfeld recruited the Great Sandow to the United States and in 1893 the Great Sandow performed at the Chicago World Fair. This ushered in the popularity of weight training in the United States.[8]

Modern-day amateur weight lifting had its birth in 1891, when the German Athletic Association was founded. It brought a large number of the local weight clubs under the guidance of a single governing body. Its first competition was in Cologne in 1893 and its first "World Championship" in Vienna in 1898. By 1900 it had over 300 clubs and 12 000 members.[8]

Beginning in 1896, three of the first four modern Olympics included a weight lifting competition. There was a rebirth of this sport in 1920, and it has continued until the present day. The first US National Powerlifting Championship was held in 1964, and in 1965 it was divided into a seniors and juniors competition. In 1969 the first National Collegiate Powerlifting Championship was held.[8]

Body building also became a growing sport around the turn of the century. Eugene Sandow sponsored physique contests for his students and awarded them gold, silver, and bronze statuettes. The first physique contest held in the United States was in 1904. It was held in New York City and offered large cash prizes to the winners. The first Mr America contest was held in 1939 and the first Mr Universe contest in 1947.[8]

DESCRIPTION OF DIFFERENT WEIGHT LIFTING STYLES

Body building is an artistic sport that emphasizes extreme muscularity, symmetry, and aesthetics. Body builders routinely engage in power lifting-type activities and emphasize a high repetition and moderate weight program. In addition, there is a greater emphasis on overall fitness and aerobic conditioning than in power lifting or Olympic lifting.[6,8]

Olympic weight lifting emphasizes speed, agility, and strength. It consists of the clean jerk and the snatch lifts. The clean jerk is a lift in which the weight bar is lifted from the floor to the shoulders and subsequently overhead. The snatch lift is a lift in which the weight bar is lifted from the floor directly overhead without stopping at the shoulders.[6,8]

Power lifting emphasizes extreme power development, with relatively little emphasis on speed or agility. Power lifting consists of the squat, bench press, and dead lift. The squat lift begins by holding the weight bar across the posterior–superior aspect of the shoulder girdles. The lifter then squats down to where the anterior thigh passes inferior to the horizontal plane of the patella in the squat position and then stands up. The bench press begins by a weight lifter lying supine on a bench and holding a weight bar in his hands, with his shoulders flexed 90 degrees and the elbows completely extended. The bar is then slowly lowered to the chest and held there until it has become motionless prior to raising it to its starting position. The dead lift involves lifting a weight bar from the floor to waist level and then lowering it to the floor under control.[6,8]

BIOMECHANICS OF POWER LIFTING

The biomechanics of power lifting most closely resemble lifting biomechanics utilized in the workplace and during activities of daily living. Thus, a more detailed description of power lifting follows.

Proper power lifting technique is crucial to timely advancement in strength and prevention of injuries. There is a paucity of biomechanical data published on power lifting. Although there are several accepted techniques for each lift, only the conventional methods will be described.

Squat

In the squat (Fig. 7.1), the lifter's heels should be slightly wider than shoulder width and the hips should be externally rotated to 30–45 degrees. The hips should not externally or internally rotate substantially during the lift, so that the knees flex in the same direction the feet are pointing. This helps maintain the lower extremities in physiologic position and thus decreases the torsional forces to the knees, hips, pelvis, and lumbar spine.[8]

The weight bar should be placed on the posterior-superior aspect of the shoulders and should not be allowed to roll significantly. The hands should be placed in a comfortable position, with the thumb on the same side of the bar as the fingers (monkey grip) (Fig. 7.2). This seems to prevent injuries of the upper extremity if the bar rolls or if the lifter has to "dump" the weight for any reason.

Lumbar lordosis should be maintained throughout the lift to aid stability, facilitate erector spinae contraction, and possibly reduce the load on inert soft tissues.[10–12] The angle created by the coronal plane of the lifter's trunk and the horizontal plane of the floor (trunk–floor angle) should be as large as possible during the lift and at no time should it be less than 45 degrees.[13–15] The degree of forward lean of the trunk during the squat is directly proportional to the trunk extensor torque and indirectly proportional to the thigh extensor torque. Highly developed lifters attempt to minimize trunk lean and thus minimize trunk extensor torque while maximizing thigh extensor torque. McLaughlin mentions a constant point during the lift at which the thigh–floor angle reaches 30.3 degrees, at which point the lifter is least able to generate

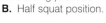
Figure 7.1
Squat lift.
A. Starting position.
B. Half squat position.

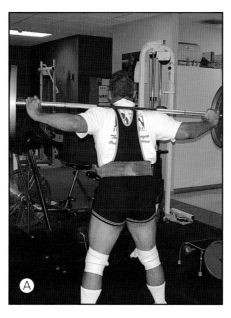
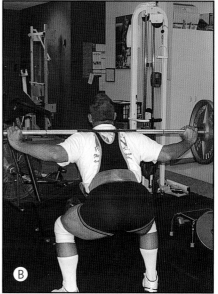

Illustration continued on following page

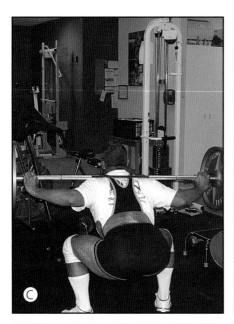

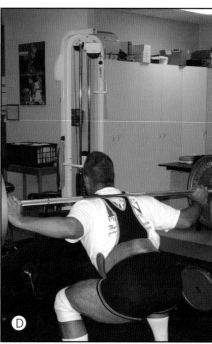

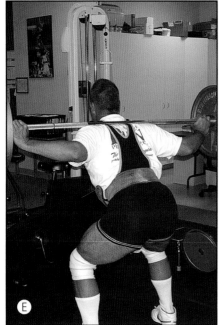

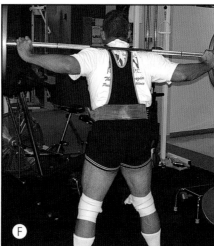

Figure 7.1
Continued
C. Full squat position.
D. and **E.** Rising from full squat position.
F. Returning to starting position.

Figure 7.2
Squat lift monkey grip. Notice that the thumb is positioned on the same side of the bar as the fingers.

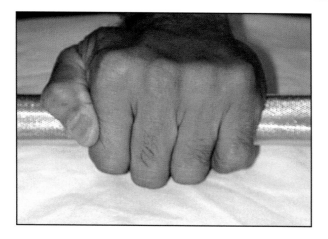

vertical force. This point is known as a "sticking point."[15] The maximum amount of weight a lifter is able to lift through this point of the event is generally equal to his one-repetition maximum (1 RM).

Center of gravity should be kept 5–7 cm, anterior to the heel–floor interface. If the center of gravity is maintained in the proper position, then the ankles will not dorsiflex beyond 30 degrees, the knees will not flex beyond 120 degrees, and proper trunk mechanics can be maintained throughout the lift.[16]

Bench press

In the bench press (Fig. 7.3) the lifter should keep his feet flat on the floor and his buttocks, shoulders, and head flat on the bench throughout the lift. Lumbar lordosis should be maintained and the scapulae should be kept in the fully retracted and "locked" position. This provides for maximum stability during the lift and may help prevent injuries to shoulder girdle and lumbar spine musculature.

Figure 7.3
Bench press.
A. Starting position.
B. Pause position.
C. Press to starting position.

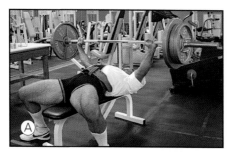
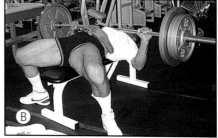
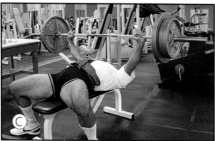

The lifter begins the lift by supporting a weight bar in his hands with his shoulders flexed 90 degrees and his elbows completely extended. Hand position on the bar should be as wide as comfortable for maximum power production.[17] The lifter should have his thumbs in the opposed position ("club grip") (Fig. 7.4) to prevent the bar from rolling out of his hands and falling on his chest. The bar is then slowly and smoothly lowered to the chest and "paused" until it is no longer moving, prior to lifting it back to its starting position. The path of the bar during descent should take a gentle arc, with the concavity toward the head, and during ascent the path should be similar, with the concavity toward the feet.[18] The bar should come to rest 2–5 cm superior to the sternoxiphoid junction. When the bar is on the chest, the shoulders should achieve a maximum abduction of 45 degrees. This degree of abduction initially increases as the bar is lifted from the chest and then decreases after the sticking point has been passed. The sticking point has been determined to be 12 cm or less from the surface of the chest.[17] Shoulder abduction at the termination of the lift is dependent on the lifter's hand position on the bar.

Dead lift

At the beginning of the dead lift (Fig. 7.5), the lifter stands over the bar while it rests on the floor. The feet should be positioned slightly narrower than shoulder width in a neutral position, and the legs should be touching the bar during the quiet standing position. The lifter stoops and grasps the bar immediately outside of his legs with his dominant forearm pronated and his non-dominant forearm supinated (reverse grip) (Fig. 7.6). Care should be taken during the stooping process to keep the bar as near the heel–floor

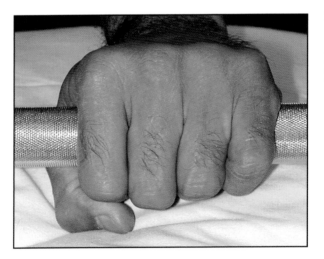

Figure 7.4
Bench press club grip. Note that the thumb is positioned on the opposite side of bar to the fingers.

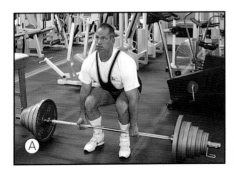
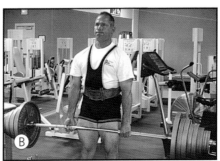

Figure 7.5
Dead lift.
A. Starting position.
B. Finishing position.

Figure 7.6
Dead lift reverse grip. Note that dominant forearm (in this case the left forearm) is pronated and the non-dominant forearm supinated.

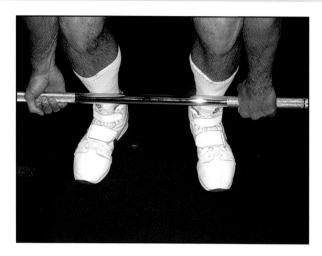

interface as possible (i.e., minimize ankle dorsiflexion); the torso is in an erect posture similar to the squat; and the head is up (i.e., cervical spine slightly extended beyond neutral).[19] Prior to lifting the weight off the floor, the lifter should "pull the slack out" (i.e., fully extend the elbows and fully depress the shoulder girdles). This will help prevent injuries that may occur to soft tissues as a result of a sudden jerking force.

Once lift-off has occurred, there is a natural tendency to extend the knees faster than the hips, thus creating excessive forward lean. This tendency should be resisted. The lifter should attempt to shift his center of gravity posteriorly in an attempt to offset the anterior moment created by the loaded bar.

In addition, the lifter should strive to maintain the upright trunk posture and "head-up" position while concentrating on extending his hips and dragging the bar up the anterior aspect of his legs.[19] Once the sticking point (infrapatellar region) has been passed, the ankles should begin to dorsiflex while the hips and knees continue to extend. The bar should continue to be dragged up the anterior aspect of the thighs until the lifter is in an erect posture. The bar should then be lowered in a controlled fashion using knee and hip flexion while keeping an upright trunk and head-up position.

TYPICAL TRAINING METHODS OF POWER LIFTING

Prophylactic conditioning

The novice power lifter typically has several "weak links" in his musculoskeletal chain that are at risk for injury. These links should be identified and strengthened prior to launching into a rigorous power-lifting program. Typically, the novice should focus on overall flexibility, strengthening the rotator cuff and abdominal musculature, power lifting technique, and muscle balance.[3,6,9,20,21]

Overall flexibility may minimize mechanical stress placed on vulnerable tissues.[1,21] A good flexibility program should include the shoulder girdle musculature, calves, hamstrings, quadriceps, iliotibial band, hip adductors, hip flexors, gluteal musculature, and abdominal obliques (Figs 7.7 and 7.8). This program should be performed immediately prior to and at the termination of each workout. It should emphasize slow, sustained stretching and avoid bouncing, which may injure the musculotendinous unit.

Typical power-lifting routines strive to increase shoulder girdle internal rotation and flexion strength, which may create a strength imbalance in the rotator cuff. To offset these changes, the rotator cuff should be trained twice weekly, with emphasis on external rotation and abduction (Fig. 7.9). This will help maintain strength and balance in the rotator cuff and thus dynamic stability in the glenohumeral joint during lifting.

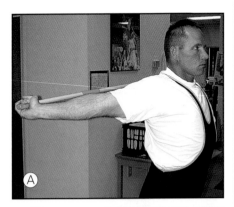

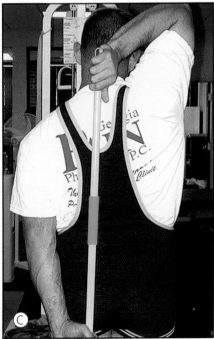

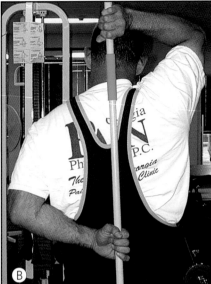

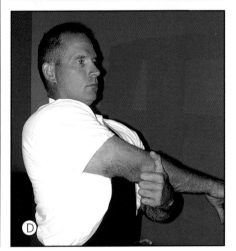

Figure 7.7
Shoulder girdle stretching exercise routine.
A–C. Stretching anterior shoulder girdle.
D. Stretching posterior shoulder girdle.

Specific prophylactic conditioning should also include the abdominal obliques (Fig. 7.10). The abdominal muscles may be trained daily without fear of overtraining. Strong abdominal oblique and transverse abdominal contraction during lifting has been demonstrated to help stabilize the lumbar spine as well as to create an extension moment at the lumbar spine.[22–24] This is via their attachment to the lumbodorsal fascia and the mechanical arrangement of this fascia.[2,12,24–31]

A beginning power-lifting program is a general weight-training program that emphasizes overall fitness and also power-lifting technique. Heavy power lifts are not emphasized in this phase, since a novice power lifter is at increased risk for injury until he has had the opportunity to develop proper technique and sufficient remodeling of his bones, entheses, and musculotendinous junctions to withstand the load of heavy weights.[32–39]

As the lifter matures and his lifting techniques improve, he can gradually begin to increase the weight lifted and decrease the number of repetitions per set. During this phase he should gradually begin wearing

Figure 7.8
Lower limb
stretching exercise
routine.
A. Calves.
B. Hamstrings.
C. Iliotibial band.
D. Hip adductors.
E. Hip flexors.

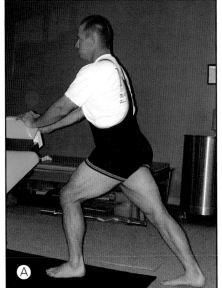
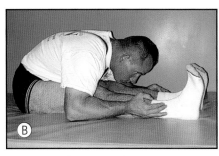
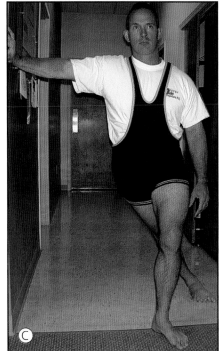
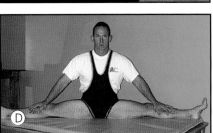
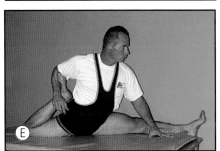

a weight belt (Fig. 7.11). These belts appear to support the lumbar spine by augmenting the abdominal mechanism and creating an extension moment at the lumbar spine.[40] Once the lifter has demonstrated technical proficiency and adequate overall conditioning, then he may begin a serious power-lifting program.

Cycle training

A serious adult power lifter has typically been training for 1–2 years. He trains in cycles that last 8–10 weeks and coordinates these cycles with competitions. Generally, the bench press and squat are trained

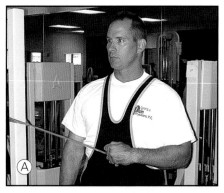

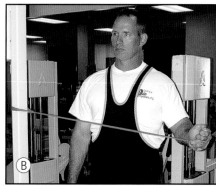

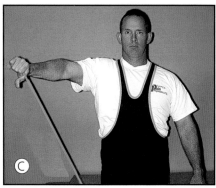

Figure 7.9
Rotator cuff strengthening exercise.
A. and **B.** External rotator strengthening.
C. Abductor strengthening.

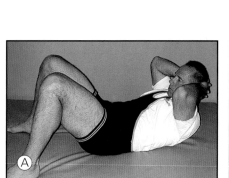

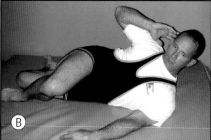

Figure 7.10
Abdominal strengthening exercise.
A. Rectus isolation.
B. Oblique isolation.

twice per week and the dead lift is trained once per week, although some lifters train squat only once per week and dead lift once every other week. The lifter will typically alternate "heavy" and "light" days, with the "heavy" days emphasizing heavier weights and fewer repetitions and the "light" days emphasizing lighter weights and more repetitions. The heavy days are designed to stress the muscle maximally to provide strength and a growth stimulus, whereas the light days are designed to allow the muscles to continue to heal and yet still receive a training stimulus. A lifter involved in cycle training seeks to achieve a 1 RM (within the cycle) once every 2 or 3 weeks. During weeks 2 and 3 prior to a major competition, the lifter generally eliminates or significantly curtails the light day to allow for maximum healing of overtrained or injured muscles.[34,41,42] During the week prior to competition, the lifter emphasizes rest and mental preparation for the upcoming competition.

Figure 7.11
Weight belt.

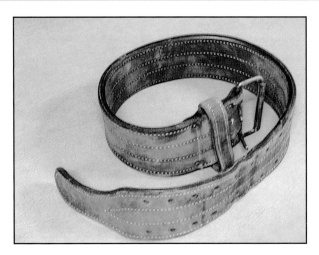

Auxiliary lifting techniques

The elite power lifter has been training vigorously for many years and has reached a very highly developed state. He is able to employ auxiliary lifting techniques that should not be attempted by others. These include lifts based on the "overload principle," such as heavy "walk outs" and "half squats," "heavy negative bench press," and "heavy partial dead lifts." These auxiliary lifts are generally performed with 110–130% of the 1 RM and should be performed once per week to once per month during weeks 3 through 8 prior to a major competition. These lifts should not be performed more frequently than once per week and should not be performed in the 2 weeks prior to a major competition, since muscles do not seem to be able to recuperate quickly enough. The intention of these lifts is to stimulate the bones, tendons, and contractile mechanism maximally to become stronger.

In between lifting cycles, the power lifter assumes a modified body-building routine. The emphasis is placed on overall fitness, including muscle balance, flexibility, and cardiovascular conditioning. Heavy joint-loading activities such as squats and dead lifts are still performed with significantly less weight and intensity. This is a healing phase.

SPINE INJURIES DURING WEIGHT LIFTING

Weight lifting has previously been described as one of the sports in which low back injuries most commonly occur. Low back injuries are more common in weight lifters than in power lifters.[43] In women undergoing strength training and running, back injuries are among the most common, and weight lifting accounts for the majority of lost training days.[44] Weight lifting-induced spine injuries are common and predictable in their scope; however, there is very little published about these injuries. As a result, much of the following information is drawn from the experience of one of the authors who is a physician treating spine injuries and a previously world-ranked power lifter. Power lifting will be used as a model since it comes closest to reflecting the methods used by the majority of strength athletes and industrial workers.

The incidence of spine injuries in weight lifting has not been well defined. In the adolescent population, all weight-lifting-induced musculoskeletal injuries combined range from 7.1% to 39.4%, depending on the definition of injury.[7,18,45] Low back injury related to weight lifting has been reported to be as high as 50% in adolescent weight lifters.[43] No similar data are available for the adult population. The authors estimate that the incidence of weight-lifting-induced spine injury lasting greater than 1 week in non-competitive males between the ages of 35 and 50 years old ranges from 10% to 20%. However, we estimate the incidence of these injuries in a similar population of competitive elite power lifters to be nearly 100%. The lumbar spine is most commonly involved.[43]

The types of spine injuries suffered while lifting weights are predictable. They include myofascial strain, zygapophyseal joint (Z-joint) sprain, chronic Z-joint dysfunction, disc injury with and without radiculopathy, spinous process fracture, vertebral body fracture, and possibly pars interarticularis fracture.[18,46–49] Myofascial strains and Z-joint injuries make up the major portion of these injuries and are usually self-limited. The remainder of these injuries may cause prolonged pain, dysfunction, and interference with training.

Spine injuries generally have one or more predisposing factors, including improper warm up, muscle strength or length imbalance, poor technique, overtraining, or skeletal imbalance such as leg length discrepancy or scoliosis. Other skeletal abnormalities that may predispose to injury include zygapophyseal tropism, equinous deformity, subtalar hyperpronation, tarsal coalition, and pelvic asymmetry.

Myofascial strain

True myofascial strain typically occurs in the superficial spinal erectors at the thoracolumbar or lumbosacral junction. The injury usually occurs during the dead lift or squat. The pain and dysfunction that occurs from this injury is usually self-limited and resolves spontaneously within 1–2 weeks with anti-inflammatory modalities and modified activities. There may or may not be an associated ecchymosis.

Zygapophyseal joint injury

A true Z-joint sprain or chronic Z-joint dysfunction with pain typically occurs in the mid-thoracic or thoracolumbar region. These injuries may also occur in the lumbar spine but are much more likely to be associated with a concomitant disc injury. A Z-joint sprain is usually the result of rotational movement during ascent in the squat or dead lift. Pain and dysfunction from this injury may last from several weeks to several months and occasionally may develop into a chronically painful condition. Z-joint dysfunction with pain may be the result of Z-joint sprain that has created a chronically dysfunctional joint or abnormal biomechanics resulting from scoliosis, leg length discrepancy, or zygapophyseal tropism. When these injuries occur acutely, they usually involve only one side and only 1 or 2 levels.

Rehabilitation of Z-joint injuries is dependent on their presentation. If an injury is acute and is associated with minimal pain and has not been preceded by other similar injuries, then it will generally resolve spontaneously within 2–4 weeks with anti-inflammatory modalities, modified rest, and progressive mobilization of the injured joint. The deep paraspinal and abdominal musculature should be adequately rehabilitated via a standard stabilization-type exercise outlined in other areas of this book.[50–52]

This exercise protocol should be followed by progressive conditioning of the superficial paraspinal muscles and lower extremities via sports-specific activities such as partial dead lifts, squats, and Roman-chair hyperextensions. Additionally, predisposing factors and technique errors should be sought and corrected.

If the injury is chronic, recurrent, or severe, it will probably take longer to improve and may not totally resolve. Rehabilitation efforts are similar to those mentioned above, although they generally need to be more intensive and may require the judicious use of zygapophyseal cortisone injections if an inflammatory component to the injury is suspected. Occasionally, in severe chronic cases, a diagnostic zygapophyseal-joint nerve block followed by Z-joint ablation may be required.[1]

Disc injuries

Disc injuries usually occur in the lower lumbar spine and less commonly at the thoracolumbar junction. They are generally also the result of rotational movements during ascent in the dead lift or squat. These injuries can usually be managed by conservative means and rarely require surgery.[52,53] Traditional weight-lifting equipment is not known to be associated with lumbar or cervical disc herniation; however, there is a possible association between the use of free weights and cervical disc herniation.[54]

Acute rehabilitation efforts focus on control of inflammation with cryotherapy and anti-inflammatory medication. Heating modalities should be avoided for the first several days.[55,56] Pain should not be managed with narcotics unless the pain is severe. If narcotics are indicated, they should be used for a limited time only and in a scheduled manner. The patient should remain mobilized as much as possible and bed rest should be employed for no longer than 2 days if at all.[57] Ideally, the patient should interrupt his workout schedule as little as possible, except to "work around the injury" and reduce training intensity. During this phase of recovery, the patient should emphasize open-chain aerobic conditioning, abdominal crunches, and non–disc-loading upper-extremity and torso activities such as light pec-deck, standing cable triceps extensions, and preacher bench curls. McKenzie program activities should be used acutely to centralize radicular pain and help normalize segmental motion.[58,59]

Epidural steroid injection (ESI) should be used if inflammatory radicular pain exists.[60] The authors do not use the "trial if three ESIs" concept. Performing ESIs under fluoroscopic guidance dramatically reduces the need for repeat injections. As a rule, if the first ESI does not work, then the third will not either.[61] Additionally, the "blind" (non-fluoroscopic) placement of an epidural needle during ESI has been demonstrated to be improper 25% of the time.[62]

Once radicular pain has resolved and segmental motion has improved, standard stabilization activities should be employed. In the experienced weight-trained athlete, this program can usually progress rapidly. Once the athlete is able to demonstrate adequate lumbar stability, gentle sports-specific disc-loading activities should be instituted. A weight belt should be worn at all times during this phase to augment the abdominal mechanism and lumbar extension moment.[40] Progression of activity should take place cautiously but as quickly as clinically acceptable. The athlete must be informed of typical warning signs and told of the importance of peripheralizing pain and neurologic signs. Home program activities should be performed on a daily basis and include McKenzie and stabilization activities.

Spinous process fractures

Spinous process fractures occur almost exclusively during the squat. These fractures generally involve C7 or TI.[63] They typically occur as the result of the weight bar suddenly rolling down the neck in an uncontrolled fashion during either ascent or descent. They may also occur at the top of the squat. This may occur if the lifter has rapidly ascended through the squat and the bar is allowed to bounce while resting on the back of the neck. This injury is usually heard and felt by the athlete. It is associated with the acute onset of localized pain and swelling and may be described by the athlete as a crunching or breaking sound and feeling. During either mechanism the injury may be prevented by not allowing the bar to roll or bounce and keeping the shoulder girdles adequately retracted and elevated to pad the spinous processes with contracted trapezius musculature. Usually there are no long-term consequences to this injury. It should be treated in the short term with anti-inflammatory medication and copious ice. Squats should be avoided for approximately 2 weeks, during which time the lower extremities should be conditioned with activities that do not place stress on the neck, such as leg presses, hack squats, leg extensions, and leg curls. Approximately 2 weeks after the injury, the lifter should begin light squats again and advance over time as pain allows. During the next 4–6 weeks emphasis should be placed on the prophylactic measures mentioned above.

Vertebral body injuries

Weight-lifting-induced vertebral body injuries are rare. There are four cases mentioned in the literature of weight-lifting-induced lumbar apophyseal ring fractures in adolescents.[47] In adults, weight-lifting-induced vertebral body compression fractures are probably even more rare and are usually associated with other injuries. We have seen only two: both cases involved elite lifters who were attempting maximum squat lifts and occurred when the lifters bounced at the bottom of the lift. Both lifters sustained a Grade

I LI vertebral body compression fracture as well as other injuries. Associated injuries in both cases included patellar tendon ruptures and anterior cruciate injuries. One case included a dislocated ankle and bilateral open tibial fractures. These cases point out that care of other injuries may be rate-limiting step in the overall recovery of the athlete who suffers from a weight-lifting-induced compression fracture. In addition, they demonstrate the importance of proper technique.

Care of a vertebral body compression fracture should include placing the athlete in a thoraco-lumbosacral orthosis (TLSO) extension brace for approximately 3 months and significantly curtailing his activities for at least 2–4 weeks. The brace should be worn continuously for the first 3–4 weeks, at which time the athlete may be permitted to remove it only while bathing. During this period, pain control may require the judicious use of narcotics. At 2–3 weeks, narcotic medication should no longer be required and the athlete should increase his activities as pain permits, while avoiding all axial and flexion loading forces.

Initially, all spine-loading activities should be avoided. If other injuries permit, open-chain aerobic conditioning is acceptable within the limits of pain. Approximately 6 weeks after the injury, the athlete is generally able to perform his activities of daily living in the brace without significant pain. At this point, it is acceptable to begin gentle conditioning activities of the upper and lower extremities that do not significantly load the spine and do not cause pain. In addition, at this point it is acceptable to begin gentle isometric abdominal conditioning activities within the brace. Conditioning activities should continue to be advanced within the limits of pain until the brace is removed at 3–4 months.

Once the brace has been removed, initial rehabilitation efforts should emphasize regaining segmental motion of the spine in general and the injured segments specifically. In addition, gentle stabilization activities should be initiated. Once the athlete has completed stabilization activities, it is acceptable to begin conditioning activities of the superficial paraspinal muscles. Approximately 6 months after the injury, the patient may begin very light squats and dead lift activities, advancing as tolerated.

Other injuries

As of the writing of this chapter, we have seen neither reports in the literature nor clinical cases of weight-lifting-induced fractures of the pars interarticularis. However, weight lifting does appear to be highly associated with its development, since its reported incidence in weight lifters is 36.2% compared to 5–10% for the normal population.[18]

We have treated six elite power lifters with a symptomatic spondylolisthesis. Of this group, four lifters had defects at L5 with a Grade I slip and the other two lifters had defects at L4 with a slip. Two lifters had a Grade I slip and the other two lifters had a Grade II slip. No defects were acute at the time of presentation and no athletes gave a history of a traumatic event. All athletes had a degenerative disc at the level involved but no herniations were demonstrated by either a computed tomography (CT) scan or magnetic resonance imaging (MRI). All the power lifters had been complaining of low back pain at the segment involved for greater than 2 years and all had activity related unilateral or bilateral radicular pain. When they were not in a heavy portion of their training cycle, they all had tolerable low back pain only. However, when they began to train heavily, their back pain would increase and radicular pain would develop.

All six of these athletes were extremely competitive; therefore, relative rest was not an acceptable option to them. Flexion and stabilization activities were of no benefit in any of these cases. Four of the six athletes were able to achieve partial, temporary relief with McKenzie extension activities. The other two athletes were able to get partial, temporary relief with manual mobilization of the involved segment. These athletes were followed for 9–21 months and all continued to compete despite the above-mentioned symptom complex.

LUMBAR STABILIZATION IN POWER LIFTING

Initially, the injured power lifter should be treated appropriately for the type, age, and severity of an injury as outlined above and in other areas of this book. When the active phase of injury rehabilitation begins it should include cardiovascular conditioning, appropriate stretching, extremity strengthening that does not present a substantial axial or rotational load to the lumbar spine, and the initial phases of lumbar stabilization outlined in other parts of this book. It is especially important to review proper lifting mechanics and breath control. By following these precautions, intraspinal pressures may be minimized and further injury may be avoided.

Conditioning should be advanced as rapidly as tolerated by the athlete. Signs that advancement may be taking place too rapidly include peripheralization of pain, return of dural tension sign, neurologic change in one or both lower extremities, or possibly worsening of dyskinetic segmental motion of the lumbar spine.

Once the lumbar stabilization program has reached the intermediate stages and the athlete is tolerating it without difficulty, sports-specific stabilization should begin. Initially, we recommend alternate extremity bench press-type activities with the athlete standing, pushing on either Theraband tied to the wall at shoulder level, or using a cable system with the pulley at shoulder level. The athlete should keep one foot forward and should keep the lumbar spine in a neutral posture. The athlete should be advanced in weight (or tension), repetitions, and time.

Once the athlete has been advanced at least twice in the standing bench press-type activities and is tolerating it without difficulty for at least three sessions, then Roman chair activities should be initiated. In this exercise, the athlete places his anterior pelvis prone on one pad and his posterior ankles under the other pads of the Roman chair and alternately eccentrically flexes and concentrically extends his lumbar spine against gravity. He should begin with at least two sets of 10 and advance in repetitions and sets as tolerated. After he has progressed to at least three to four sets of 20 repetitions without difficulty, weight should be applied to his posterior shoulder girdles or cervical spine.

Once the athlete is performing three to four sets of 20 repetitions with 20–30 lb without difficulty, it is time to progress to alternating one-arm lifts bent over supported rows. In this exercise the athlete bends at the waist with one foot forward. He places one hand on a flat utility bench and grasps a dumbbell that he can manage easily that is resting on the floor. While keeping the lumbar spine in a neutral posture, the dumbbell is lifted to the chest with a coupled scapular retraction and shoulder extension activity and then lowered back to the floor. Once again, this should be advanced until the athlete can perform 20 repetitions for three to four sets on each side at least three times per week.

Once this activity is well tolerated and the weight has been advanced at least twice, it is time to begin partial dead lifts out of a rack. Initially, the bar should begin approximately 4–6 inches above the knees. Four to six sets of no more than 8–10 repetitions should be performed. Initially, this activity should occur with the bar only. Weight should be added and the bar should be progressively lowered toward the floor as tolerated. This activity must be advanced slowly and should be performed no more frequently than twice per week.

Once the dead-lift program has begun and is progressing without difficulty, then partial squats may begin. This program should also begin with the bar only. Initially, only quarter squats should be performed and only weight should be increased. Four to six sets of no more than 8–10 repetitions and no fewer than 4–6 repetitions should be performed. This program should occur no more frequently than twice per week. It is generally acceptable to progress to half squats once the squat program has progressed for six to eight training sessions without setback, the weight has been advanced at least five times, and both the therapist and athlete are comfortable with progressing to the next phase.

Once both the partial dead lifts and partial squats are being performed for at least 4–6 repetitions with at least 50% of the athlete's previous 1 RM with acceptable technique, minimal low back pain, and no lower extremity pain, it is usually acceptable to progress to the full technique. Of course, with the progression from one phase to the next the weight should be reduced accordingly to evaluate how well the athlete will be able to handle it. Once it is determined that the athlete will do fine with the weight, then it is acceptable to progress with caution.

The most common reasons for an athlete's failing to progress through a program is attempting to advance too rapidly, failing to follow through with the core stabilization activities, and having unrealistic expectations about how rapid recovery will be. Once the athlete has recovered, the main identifiable reasons for relapse are not maintaining a flexibility program, proper warm-up activities, proper lifting technique, and at least a basal stabilization program.

SUMMARY

Weight training has permeated almost every aspect of athletics and has become an integral part of most sports-specific training. In addition, the weight-lifting sports of power lifting, body building, and Olympic lifting have become popular and well-defined sports.

Very little research exists on the kinetics and biomechanics of weight lifting. As a direct result, coaches and athletes are developing programs largely from empirical data. More research is needed on proper lifting technique, biomechanics, and injury epidemiology in order to best prevent injury and maximize performance gained through weight training.

REFERENCES

1. Silvers H: Lumbar percutaneous facet rhizotomy. Spine 15:36, 1990.
2. Tesh K, Dunn J, Evans J: The abdominal muscles and vertebral stability. Spine 12:501, 1987.
3. DiNubile N: Strength training. Clin Sports Med 10:33, 1991.
4. DeLorme T: Restoration of muscle power by heavy resistance exercises. J Bone Joint Surg 27A:645, 1945.
5. Zineoff A: Heavy-resistance exercises; the "Oxford technique." Br J Phys Med 14:129, 1951.
6. Fleck S, Kraemer W: Resistance training: basic principles (part 1 of 4). Phys Sportsmed 16:160, 1988.
7. Risser W: Musculoskeletal injuries caused by weight training. Clin Pediatr 29:305, 1990.
8. Todd T: Brief history of resistance exercises. In: Pearl B, Moran G, eds. Getting stronger. Bolinas, CA: Shelter Publications; 1986.
9. Stover C: Physical conditioning of the immature athlete. Orthop Clin North Am 13:525, 1982.
10. Farfan H: The biomechanical advantage of lordosis and hip extension for upright activity: man as compared with other anthropoids. Spine 3:336, 1978.
11. Hart D, Stobbe T, Jaraiedi M: Effect of lumbar posture on lifting. Spine 12:138, 1987.
12. Styf J: Pressure, in the erector spinae muscle during exercise. Spine 12:675, 1987.
13. Capozzo A, et al: Lumbar spine loading during half squat exercises. Med Sci Sports Exerc 17:613, 1985.
14. McLaughlin T: A kinematic model of performance of the parallel squat as performed by champion powerlifters. Med Sci Sports Exerc 9:128, 1977.
15. McLaughlin T, Lardner T, Dillman C: Kinetics of the parallel squat. Res Q 49:175, 1978.
16. Landers J, Bates B, Devita P: Biomechanics of the squat exercise using a modified center of mass bar. Med Sci Sports Exerc 18:469, 1986.
17. Madsen N, McLaughlin T: Kinematic factors influencing performance and injury risk in the bench press exercise. Med Sci Sports Exerc 16:376, 1984.
18. Johnson K: Low-back pain in sports. Phys Sportsmed 21:53, 1993.
19. Brown E, Abani K: Kinematics and kinetics of the dead lift in adolescent power lifters. Med Sci Sports Exerc 17:554, 1985.
20. Grimby G: Progressive resistance exercises for injury rehabilitation. Sports Med 2:309, 1985.
21. Hershman E: The profile of prevention of musculoskeletal injury. Clin Sports Med 3:65, 1984.
22. Gracovetsky S, Farfan H, Lamy C: The mechanism of the lumbar spine. Spine 6:249, 1981.
23. Macintosh J, Bogduk N, Gracovetsky S: The biomechanics of the thoracolumbar fascia. Clin Biomed 2:78, 1987.
24. McGill S, Norman R: Potential of lumbodorsal fascia forces to generate back extension moments during squat lift. J Biomed Eng 10:312, 1988.
25. Davis P: The use of intra-abdominal pressure in evaluating stresses on the lumbar spine. Spine 6:90, 1981.

26. Gracovetsky S, Farfan H, Helleur C: The abdominal mechanism. Spine 10:317, 1985.

27. Grew N: Intraabdominal pressure response to loads applied to the torso on normal subjects. Spine 5:149, 1980.

28. Grillner S, Nilsson J, Thorstensson A: Intra-abdominal pressure changes during natural movements in man. Acta Physiol Scand 103:275, 1978.

29. Harman E, et al: Intra-abdominal and intra-thoracic pressures during weight lifting and jumping. Med Sci Sports Exerc 20:195, 1987.

30. Hemborg B, et al: Intraabdominal pressure and trunk muscle activity during lifting – effect of abdominal muscle training in healthy subjects. Scand Rehab Med 15:183, 1983.

31. Mairiaux P, et al: Relation between intra-abdominal pressure and lumbar moments when lifting weights in the erect posture. Ergonomics 27:883, 1984.

32. Aggrawal N, et al: A study of changes in the spine of weight lifters and other athletes. Br J Sports Med 13(2):58, 1979.

33. Brown A, McCartney N, Sale D: Positive adaptation to weight-lifting training in the elderly. Am Physiol Soc 69(5):1725, 1990.

34. Fleck S, Kraemer W: Resistance training: physiological responses and adaptations (part 2 of 4). Phys Sportsmed 16:108, 1988.

35. Gleeson P, et al: Effect of weight lifting on bone mineral density in premenopausal women. J Bone Miner Res 5:153, 1990.

36. Gracovetsky S, Farfan H, Lamy C: A mathematical model of the lumbar spine using an optimized system to control muscles and ligaments. Orthop Clin North Am 8:135, 1977.

37. Granhed H, Jonson R, Hansson T: Mineral content and strength of the lumbar vertebrae: a cadaver study. Acta Orthop Scand 60:105, 1989.

38. Granhed H, Jonson R, Hansson T: The loads on the lumbar spine during extreme weight lifting. Spine 12:146, 1987.

39. Hutton W, Adams M: Can the lumbar spine be crushed in heavy lifting? Spine 7:586, 1982.

40. Lander J, Simonton L, Giacobbe K: The effectiveness of weight-belts during the squat exercise. Med Sci Sports Exerc 22:117, 1990.

41. Fleck S, Kraemer W: Resistance training: physiological responses and adaptations (part 3 of 4). Phys Sportsmed 16:63, 1988.

42. Kraemer W, Fleck S: Resistance training: exercise prescription. Phys Sportsmed 16:69, 1988.

43. Raske A, Norlin R: Injury incidence and prevalence among elite weight and power lifters. Am J Sports Med 30:248–256, 2002.

44. Reynolds KL, Harman EA, Worsham RE, et al: Injuries in women associated with a periodized strength training and running program. J Strength Cond Res 15:136–143, 2001.

45. Brady T, Cahill B, Bodnar L: Weight training-related injuries in the high school athlete. Am J Sports Med 10:1, 1982.

46. Alexander M: Biomechanical aspects of lumbar spine injuries in athletes: a review. Can J Appl Sci 10:1, 1985.

47. Browne T, Yost R, McCarron R: Lumbar ring apophyseal fracture in an adolescent weight lifter. Am J Sports Med 18:533, 1990.

48. Granhed H, Morelli B: Low back pain among retired wrestlers and heavyweight lifters. Am J Sports Med 16:530, 1988.

49. Yoganandan N, et al: Microtrauma in the lumbar spine: a cause of low back pain. Neurosurgery 23:162, 1988.

50. Robinson R: The new back school prescription: stabilization training, part 1. Spine State Art Rev 5:341, 1991.

51. Saal J: Rehabilitation of football players with lumbar spine injuries (part 2 of 2). Phys Sportsmed 16:117, 1988.

52. Saal J: The new back school prescription: stabilization training, part 2. Spine State Art Rev 5:357, 1991.

53. Saal J, Saal J: Nonoperative treatment of herniated lumbar intervertebral disc with radiculopathy. Spine 14:431, 1989.

54. Mund DJ, Kelsey JL, Golden AL, et al: An epidemiological study of sports and weight lifting as possible risk factors for herniated lumbar and cervical disc. Am J Sports Med (21)6:854–860, 1993.

55. Duncombe A, Hopp J: Modalities of physical therapy, Vol 5. Phys Med Rehab State Art Rev 5:493, 1991.

56. Shelton G: Principles of musculoskeletal rehabilitation. In: Mellion M, ed., Sports injuries and athletic problems. Philadelphia: Hanley & Belfus; 1988.

57. Deyo R, Diehl A, Rosenthal M: How many days of bedrest for acute low back pain? A randomized clinical trial. N Engl J Med 315:1064, 1986.

58. Donelson R, Silva G, Murphy K: Centralization phenomenon. Spine 15:211, 1989.

59. Mackler L: Rehabilitation of the athlete with low back dysfunction. Clin Sports Med 8:4, 1989.

60. Benzon H: Epidural steroid injections for low back pain and lumbosacral radiculopathy. Pain 24:277, 1986.

61. El-Khoury G, et al: Epidural steroid injection: a procedure ideally performed with fluoroscopic control. Radiology 168:554, 1988.

62. White A, Derby R, Wynne G: Epidural injections for the diagnosis and treatment of low-back pain. Spine 5:78, 1980.

63. Herrick R: Clay-shoveler's fracture in power-lifting. Am J Sports Med 9:29, 1981.

CHAPTER

8

The Spine and Bicycling: New Perspectives

Laurie L Glasser

INTRODUCTION

The invention of the wheel encouraged the development of many different types of new vehicles for transportation. The first "bicycle" was invented in China in 2300 BC and the bicycle was used subsequently in Egypt and India. Interestingly, this vehicle was initially banned because it was deemed to intrude on "domestic sanctity."[1] In the early 1800s a bicycle was invented which was composed of two wheel sets connected by a piece of wood and propelled by a cyclist pushing the ground. The Penny Farthing bicycle, invented in the late 1800s, resembled today's tricycle, in that it was propelled by pedals on the front wheel. In the early 1900s the chain-driven bike was developed. Despite the technological advances of the past 100 years, both the mechanism of propelling the bike forward as well as common cycling injuries have not significantly changed.[2]

Bicycling is one of the most popular recreational sports.[3] However, it can be associated with fractures, strains and sprains, contusions and non-traumatic overuse injuries.[4–10] Many injuries are preventable given proper positioning on the bike and an accurate understanding of the biomechanics of cycling.[11]

Bicycle-related spine pain has probably been underreported. The incidence of spine pain in long-distance cyclists varies from 17% to 70%.[3,5,12–16] In one survey of 518 recreational cyclists, 49% of the respondents reported neck pain and 30% reported back pain. Previously it was thought that the spine was fixed during cycling, which would have protected the low back from injury. New research has brought that belief into question. In addition, the prevalence of non-cycling related back pain approaches 80% in the US population.[17–19] Chronic spine pain can be unrelated to bike riding; discogenic low back pain is quite common.[20] Therefore, careful clinical assessment is necessary to determine the relationship of a rider's back pain to cycling.

Muscular strains and ligamentous sprains cause the majority of bicycle-related back pain. Most recreational cyclists will experience stiffness or aching after long rides but most pain will resolve with rest, ice and a nonsteroidal anti-inflammatory drug (NSAID). In some cyclists, spine pain can become chronic and severe enough to interfere not only with the sport of bicycling but also with other activities of daily living.[4] One contributing factor to spine pain and cycling is based on one simple fact: the bicycle is a symmetric object and individuals are not. Injury often occurs when muscular or ligamentous asymmetries are compounded by hours of forceful, repetitive pedaling.[2]

The complete differential for spine pain is obviously much more complicated and can include any common structural defect (such as spondylosis, disc-related problems, facet syndrome, sacroiliac joint dysfunction, spinal stenosis, spondylolysis, spondylolisthesis), myofascial pain, osteoporosis, neoplasm, malingering, trauma, rheumatological, or other medical etiologies.[21]

SPINE-RELATED PAIN AND THE BIOMECHANICS OF CYCLING

Obviously, a cyclist moves the bicycle forward by pushing the pedals. One complete circular phase is called the pedal cycle, which comprises the *power phase* (top dead center to bottom dead center or 0 degrees to 100 degrees) and the *recovery phase* (bottom dead center to top dead center). Efficient well-trained road cyclist's aim for between 60 and 120 pedal revolutions per minute, placing each extremity under the power phase cycle between 3600 and 7200 times per hour. Mountain bikers tend to pedal in the bottom portion of this range because of the difficulties navigating the terrain at higher revolutions.[2,7,8]

Power phase

The maximal pedal force is during the power phase of cycling (0 degrees to 180 degrees) and peaks between 90 degrees and 110 degrees.[11,22]

The power phase (or push phase) is initiated by the hip flexors contracting to prepare for the push. The quadriceps (and other knee extensors), adductor magnus, and gluteal muscles supply the force in the early power phase. The hamstrings (and other hip extensors) and calf muscles add force during the late power phase. As the gluteals extend the hip to push the leg down on the pedal during the power phase, the paraspinal muscles are recruited to stabilize the gluteal and hamstring muscles.[8] Plantar flexors of the foot contract further during the power phase to assist with the push of the pedals.

Decreased flexibility in the gluteal and hamstring muscles causes increased tension on the iliotibial band as well as the paraspinal muscles. Tight gluteals or hamstrings can also create hyperextension of the back as the paraspinal muscles attempt to stabilize the lower back and pelvis.[2] Proper positioning on the bike allows appropriate leg extension, maximizing the forces of the gluteus maximus and biceps femoris.[8,22]

Recovery phase

The iliopsoas and hamstrings initiate the recovery phase (bottom dead center to top dead center). With the use of toe clips or clipless pedals the dorsiflexors exert a strong force, pulling the pedal upward. The gluteus medius provides stability at the hip joint. In the late recovery phase, the knee extensors are recruited to prepare for the power phase.

For optimal force, the plantar flexors, knee extensors, and hip extensors must be flexible and strong. If the iliopsoas group is tight, the pelvis is prevented from rotating posteriorly, which can lead to abnormal lumbar mechanics.[11]

RIDING POSITION

The position of the spine during bicycling is quite different from the normal standing position. Preserving ergonomic lumbar lordosis during cycling may be one of the most important determinants in preventing spine pain. With a loss of lumbar lordosis there is extra stress on the lumbar spine and the neck is forced into a hyperextended position to compensate. Too much lordosis of the lumbar spine also causes spine pain.

Cyclists can ride from positions ranging from an almost upright position to a very forward flexed position. In a more upright position, most recreational riders have an easier time maintaining a proper amount of lumbar lordosis and keeping the neck in a more neutral position. The downside of riding in an upright position is that wind resistance is increased, markedly decreasing cycling speed.[4,15,23]

Many competitive cyclists tend to tuck the lumbar and thoracic spine into a kyphotic position, leading to a progressive loss of lumbar lordosis and an increased thoracic kyphosis. The cervical spine is then forced into a compensatory hyperextension, exacerbating spine pain. Elite cyclists are able to maintain lordosis of the lower (L5–S1) lumbar spine even in the most tucked position. This lordosis may be maintained by increasing the load of the arms, thereby decreasing the load on the spine.[4,24]

In many sports there is an inherent protection of spine stability by increased intra-abdominal pressure. In cycling, this protection of stability is often absent because the abdominal muscles must remain relaxed for maximum cycling power. It isn't possible to compress the abdomen during cycling and maintain a normal respiratory pattern. Muscular imbalances of the flexor to extensor muscles of the lower extremities contribute more to lumbar pain in cyclists than in other athletes, as cyclists cannot compensate by increasing abdominal pressure.[4,24]

Nachemson has done extensive work on intradiscal pressures in many positions and activities. His studies involved placing pressure transducers in the discs of living patients and asking them to perform several postures and exercises. From his work we know that pressures are lowest in the supine position, higher while standing, even higher while sitting, and highest with extreme forward flexion. Nachemson did not specifically study intradiscal pressures while cycling.[18,25] However, based on these classic studies, it has been previously assumed that all activities involving forward flexion of the lumbar spine increase the size of the intervertebral canal and foramina, and increase dural sac and nerve root tension. This classic teaching states that with lumbar spine flexion, the posterior ligamentous complex of the vertebrae is tensed, leading to a higher incidence of annular bulging and, with the addition of rotatory and torsion forces, can produce annular tears and disc herniations.[26] In addition, since the sinovertebral nerve provides innervation to the posterior longitudinal ligament, vertebral body, and outer aspect of the annulus fibrosis, as these areas are tensed, back pain can result from reflex muscle contracture as a result of the short axon reflex mediated by the sinovertebral nerve.[24]

Classic teaching would lead one to assume that the biomechanics of bicycle riding would be expected to result in disc injury. One small study of elite cyclists attempted to address the biomechanics of intervertebral disc pressures, specifically in lumbar flexion during cycling.[24] Assumptions about intradiscal pressures were made based on roentgenograms specifically focused on the angles of the vertebra during various cycling positions. Radiography has been previously shown to be valuable in quantification of spinal kinematics. The radiographs were performed in three positions: sitting with hands on the upper part of the handgrips, sitting with hands on the lower part of the handgrips, or with the hands and forearms supported on the triathlon aero handlebars. Three intensities were also studied: rest (sitting on the bicycle without pedaling), moderate pedaling intensity, and peak pedaling intensity.

Competitive cyclists generally ride in a seated and forward flexed position; however, these athletes likely partially support the body during cycling by distributing weight to the arms, which decreases intradiscal pressure. In addition, especially in elite athletes, even though the lower spine appears to be in a kyphotic position during cycling, the L5–S1 segment stays in the physiologic lordotic position through all positions of cycling at all intensities.[24]

In Usabiaga's study, electromyographic readings on the elite cyclist's abdominal musculature, para-vertebral musculature, and thoracic musculature were also performed.[24] Lumbar muscle tone increased proportional to pedaling intensity but increased less when the hands were on the upright part of the handlebars. The abdominal muscles remained relaxed regardless of pedaling intensity. When racing time trials to decrease air resistance, a cyclist leans far forward in a non-ergonomic angle on an aerobar to achieve greater speed.[3] In these highly trained cyclists, riding on the aerobar did not significantly change lumbar muscle tone. Thoracic muscle tone was position-dependent and increased more with the aerobar and with cervical extension.[24]

Theoretically, poor position, lack of abdominal support, road vibration, and forward flexion are potential risk factors for increased disc injury; however, there is no study to show that bicycle riders have an increased risk of disc problems compared to the general population. Part of the explanation may be because the weight-bearing component of forward flexion is eliminated during cycling, and load on the spine is decreased by distributing the load to the arms of the cyclist.[20] In addition, adaptation to different bike positions seems to affect hip flexion far more than the amount of lumbar spine flexion. The elite cyclists were able to maintain a physiologic lordosis at L5–S1 despite extremes of forward flexion.

Finally, it is important to note that Usabiaga's study population only included a small sample of highly trained experienced cyclists; therefore, the generalization of these results to recreational cyclists is limited. Additional follow-up studies using a larger sample size would be important.

BIKE FIT

The daily activities of most individuals comprise accumulations of too much postural forward flexion: sitting, improper ergonomics, leaning forward to do deskwork. Cycling requires flexibilities not present in the average individual: an anteriorly tilted pelvis, flexible hamstrings, and gluteals. Although guidelines to a proper bicycle fit follow, a bicycle fitter or sports medicine professional needs to fit the bike to the individual's morphology and range of motion limitations rather than sticking to one particular "cookie-cutter" formula.[10,15]

The body contacts the bicycle in three areas: hands, seat, and feet. The relative positions of these contacts determine comfort and efficiency on the bike. There are many variables that determine these positions; crank length, distance from crank center or bottom bracket to seat, seat angle, seat tube angle and seat offset, distance from seat to handlebar, relative height of seat and handlebar, handlebar width, and handlebar drop on road style handlebars.

To truly understand the factors that contribute to spine pain and the reasoning behind changing riding ergonomics, it is first important to define the concepts that influence bike fit.[4,10,15]

The most common bike fit errors include improper saddle height, improper handlebar reach (long and low), and misalignments of pedal and shoe. Easily adjustable parameters include type and height of saddle, saddle angle, height of handlebars, the distance between the saddle and the handlebars (fore and aft position), length of crank, and foot position. The bike frame cannot be adjusted if the frame is not the correct size for the rider; there is really no way to adjust the bike so that the rider can ride with the proper ergonomic posture and maintain proper lumbar lordosis.[4,8]

Although there are guidelines for appropriate fit, adjustments should be individualized to a cyclist's morphology. For example, the optimal crank arm length, seat height, and longitudinal foot position on the pedal usually increase as the height and size of the cyclist increases, whereas the seat tube angle usually decreases as the rider's size increases. In addition, a cyclist's range of motion deficits will change how he or she should be positioned on the bike. Finally, the type of riding will influence position on the bike.[27] In addition, educating a cyclist in improving gear-shifting techniques and using appropriate cadence improves cycling efficiency and decreases injuries.[8,15]

Fore and aft position (distance from the saddle seat to the handlebars)

The distance from the seat to the handlebars is called the fore–aft distance. This depends on the length of the top tube but can be modified by the position of the saddle and handlebar height.[7–10,28] The fore–aft position may be the most important part of fitting a bike because it determines how the rider's body is balanced on the bicycle. This balance will determine how comfortable the cyclist is on the bike and how efficiently the cyclist will be able to ride.

To begin approximately assessing fore and aft position, the rider can start with the saddle in the forward-most position that allows him to lift his hands off of the handlebar and maintain the torso position without strain. Another way to roughly begin estimating fore and aft position is to place the pedals at 3 o'clock and 9 o'clock. When the ball of the foot is on the pedal, a plumb line should drop from the anterior mid patella to the center of the pedal axle.[10] The plumb line method to determine fore and aft position should not be taken as doctrine: it is only an estimate, because the fore and aft position is determined more by how the cyclist intends to ride than by any other parameter.

When the seat is shifted slightly backward, there is more force on the cranks, and therefore an increased ability to climb. Mountain bikers (who tend to climb more than road or tour bikers) usually set the fore–aft position 1–2 cm behind the pedal axles. Other riders who prefer a slightly backwards seat position are those individuals over 6 feet tall, long-distance riders who do a lot of climbing and riders who ride around 90 rpm.

In contrast, riders under 6 feet tall who spin at 95 rpm or faster and like to sprint usually prefer a fore–aft position directly over the pedal axles. This allows a more forward handlebar position. The further forward the handlebars, the more power the cyclist has for sprinting, standing, and accelerating with high-speed control.

Although climbing leverage is decreased with a more forward seat, another benefit of this position would be to open the hip angle for those riders who have less-flexible hips.

Proper fit of the bike involves a compromise of power and comfort. If the saddle is well back for balance, the handlebars will need to be back as well. But to get power to the pedals while out of the saddle, the handlebars should be forward of the cranks. There is a balance between being fit for a comfortable seated position and reach to the handlebar, and a forward handlebar position for those times when more standing is required. The difference between an uncomfortable and a comfortable long ride can often be corrected with only an inch or two correction in the fore–aft position.

Handlebar position

The range of handlebar positions available for a given handlebar stem depends on the height, angle, and reach (extension) of the handlebar stem. As in all fit parameters, the optimum handlebar position depends on the type of riding. Proper handlebar stem height can place the stem from 0 to 4 inches below the seat. Short distance road races require a cyclist to use a lower handlebar position for a more aerodynamic position. For mountain biking, a handlebar stem height of 1–2 inches below the seat places more weight on the forward wheel, so that it is easier to steer on climbs. Touring bicyclists sometimes have their handlebar stems placed at a height equal to their seat.

A quick estimate of the proper handlebar stem height can be approximated by having the cyclist sit on the bike with the arms bent and the hands in the "hands low" position on the drop bars. A plumb line should be dropped from the tip of the cyclist's nose to approximately the center of the handlebar stem. A quick test of fit is with the rider's hands on the drops with the elbows slightly bent; the handlebar should block the view of the front axle. The stem is too short if the axle is noted to be in front of the bar in this position. Conversely, the stem is too long if the rider's view of the front axle is behind the handlebar.

The most important fit parameter of handlebar stem height and reach is comfort. Most riders are comfortable in the position that allows their forearms to be horizontal with their elbows at 90 degrees and the hands on the drop handlebars at the forward-most position. When handlebars are the right height, the rider cans look ahead without neck hyperextension. If the handlebars are too high (higher than the seat), body weight is shifted too far over the rear of the bike.

A lower handlebar height usually produces a more aerodynamic position and allows the cyclist to be able to "pull up" under hard acceleration. However, too low a handlebar stem height can cause compensatory neck hyperextension. Also, handlebars that are placed too low can force a cyclist to excessively reach for the bars. This will increase lumbar flexion, pelvic rotation, and hamstring tension of the cyclist. The back (paraspinal muscles) will be placed under a greater load and can become hyperextended to compensate.[2]

A higher handlebar height (with a more forward seat) results in a more upright, less aerodynamic position for the cyclist. It has been generally thought that a cyclist with back pain should ride upright because this position increases hip flexion, decreases the tension of the gluteus maximus muscle, and therefore tension on the lumbar spine. One common bike-fitting error is overcompensation by raising the handle bar position too high for an individual cyclist. Back pain can actually be increased from excessive handlebar height, as the lumbar spine becomes hyperlordotic (extended) to engage the gluteals and hamstrings. The gluteals and hamstrings are most efficiently recruited if the torso is flexed approximately 45 degrees to the thighs.[6,10,15,29]

Seat height

There is controversy over the optimum seat height for power and efficiency. Mountain bikes used for off-road riding usually require a seat height that is slightly lower than a road bike, increasing stability and maneuverability. A basic clinical estimate of fit is to have the cyclist mount his bicycle on a trainer and pedal while centered in the saddle. For most people this results in a saddle height that leaves some bend in the knee at the bottom of the pedal stroke, when the pedal stroke has the balls of the feet over the axle of the pedals. The saddle height can be estimated to be the height where the heels maintain contact with the pedals without hip rocking at the bottom of the pedal cycle. Some riders naturally pedal toes down, whereas others have the foot in a more level position. It is also important to look at ankle range of motion and an individual cyclist's pedaling style. For example, if a cyclist maintains his foot in slight dorsiflexion for most of the pedal stroke, but has to "reach" or plantar flex his foot at the bottom of the pedal stroke, the seat is slightly too high.

Another formula to determine optimum seat height was developed by Greg LeMond's coach using wind tunnel tests. LeMond believes that 0.8333 multiplied by inseam length (floor to crotch height) of the cyclist is optimum: 2–3 mm should be subtracted from that equation if the cyclist uses clipless pedals.[10]

Other researchers have demonstrated that a relatively higher seat height of 115% of crotch height can decrease lower extremity loads in the case of rehabilitation of lower extremity injuries.[28] Still other researchers have measured saddle height and oxygen consumption and conclude that the optimum seat height for utilizing oxygen most efficiently is 106–109% of crotch height.[8,24] An alternative method of addressing the proper seat height focuses on the angle of the knee while the cyclist is seated and the pedal is in the bottom dead center position. Knee flexion in this position should be between 15 and 27 degrees; most cyclists do well between 22 and 27 degrees of knee flexion.[10,21]

The cyclist can experiment within a few millimeters to find a comfortable position within the range of "optimum"; however, rapid changes in saddle height are highly associated with injury. It is not recommended to correct saddle height by more than about 6 mm every few rides.[10]

Saddle angle and type of saddle

Most research supports the level seat angle as the preferred position. If the nose of the saddle has too much of a decline, it is likely that the cyclist will place too much stress on the upper extremities to prevent "sliding off" the front of the saddle. Women usually prefer a slightly tilted-up seat and men usually prefer a slightly tilted-down seat. The seat should not be tilted in any direction greater than 3 degrees.[10]

Some authors believe that seat angle also has a tremendous impact on the biomechanical forces to the pelvis and spine; however, it is generally felt that other parameters of fit are more important than saddle angle. For example, if the hamstrings are tight the pelvis won't appropriately rotate and increased forces will be exerted into the delicate perineal structures, regardless of saddle angle. Salai's controversial work concluded that an anterior 10–15 degree inclination angle would decrease tension on the anterior longitudinal ligament and therefore decrease back pain.[3] This has not been widely accepted in the application of research to individual cyclists.

The type of saddle may also be important in decreasing back pain. A recent small study evaluated a "novel" saddle, which supported the weight of the body on the ischial tuberosities while relieving pressure on the perineal structures. In this "anatomically correct" saddle, the posterior aspect of the saddle was broad and the pudendal area was gutted. This design decreased bicycle-related back pain, saddle sores, chafing, and painful pubic bones.[30] Finally, women's saddles should be wider than men's, since a woman's pelvis is wider. Many women's saddles have a cutout or low-density section in the center to take pressure off the pubic bone. Proper fit on the bike is far more important than the type of saddle on the bike.

Some saddle adjustments are very important in decreasing back pain, however. In those cyclists with a prominent leg length discrepancy or a scoliotic deformity causing pelvis asymmetry, altering the thickness of one side of the seat can balance paraspinal muscle function.

Frame size

Although the seat tube length always specifies frame size, choosing a bike strictly by seat tube length ignores other important measurements. The top tube length and seat tube angle are also important for good fit (Fig. 8.1).

Figure 8.1

Seat tube length, top tube length, and seat tube angle are important for good fit. a, seat tube length (measured "center to top"); b, seat tube angle; c, head tube length; d, head tube angle; e, steering axis; f, bottom bracket height; g, top tube length; h, chainstay length.

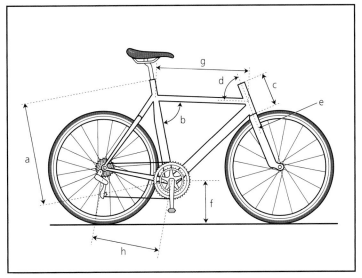

Frame size is a parameter of bike fit that is not adjustable once a bike is purchased. To roughly estimate frame size for a road bike (or the center to top tube length) a guide of 0.67 × the inseam length is commonly used. Another method is to stand flatfooted straddling the bike frame. Racing frames should have a minimum of 1 inch (2.2 cm) of clearance between the cyclist and the frame. Mountain bike frames should have a minimum of 3 inches (7.6 cm) of clearance between the rider and the top tube of the frame. In fact, most mountain bikers prefer a frame size that is approximately 10–12 cm smaller than a road bike frame.

It is important to consider both riding style and an individual's morphology when choosing frame size. For example, a rider that wants to cruise a bike path, getting a good view of surrounding scenery, will have a different frame size, bike type, and fit approach than a racer who needs to be positioned for optimum aerodynamics and speed.

For example, if a rider has short arms or a short torso, he or she would want a relatively short top tube. This would mean that the frame size may be a bit smaller than would be calculated by the above formula or measurements.

If a rider has shorter legs and a longer torso, standard formulas would calculate too small a frame size. Too small a frame will result in too small a top tube for a rider, with most of his mass and length from the waist up. An inadequate top tube length would require this rider to lean too close to the handlebars, altering the center of gravity. An individual with most of her mass from the waist up needs a longer frame with a longer top tube length to facilitate proper balance on the bike.

Finally, if an individual's femur is longer than average for height, this individual may benefit from a slack seat tube angle (about 72 degrees). Proper frame geometry will improve riding comfort, efficiency, and proper weight distribution between the front and rear wheels (ideally 45% front/55% rear).

COMMON NON-TRAUMATIC SPINE-RELATED BICYCLING INJURIES

Musculoskeletal

Musculoskeletal asymmetries, weaknesses, and inflexibilities limit the ability to ride a symmetrical bicycle with force over time. Common muscle weaknesses include the quadriceps, hamstrings, gluteus medius, and the lumbar extensors. Tight inflexible quadriceps tend to pull the pelvis forward, which can cause back pain. Hamstrings help stabilize the knee joint under forceful extension of the leg during pedaling and then assist to clear the leg across the back of the pedal stroke. Tight hamstrings tend to cause a backward pelvic tilt, leading to back pain. The gluteus medius helps to guide femoral direction and stability in pedaling and prevents the knee from drifting too far in a valgus direction. The pelvic musculature and lumbar extensors form a stable and essentially immobile support from which the force of the lower extremities and hip musculature is transmitted to the pedals. A poorly positioned pelvis can contribute to back pain. Weakness of trunk musculature results in abnormal joint-loading and extremity/spine motion during cycling.[2,22]

Improper fit

Positioning and proper fit on the bike is critical to preventing muscular injuries. By changing parameters, the bicycle can be adjusted to emphasize maximum efficiency or to minimize injury. Maximum efficiency and minimal injury are not always mutually exclusive. In the long term, a comfortable, healthy cyclist will be most efficient.

A good bike fit should consider individual musculoskeletal challenges and body type. Once the bicycle is properly fitted, the cyclist should know the specific measures so the fit can be corrected following any crashes or damage to the bike during shipping.[10]

Neck pain

Neck pain is also common in bicyclists. Neck pain can be caused by road vibration transmitted through the handlebars to the upper spine, neck hyperextension, cervical muscular fatigue, improper fit, or poor riding technique. Neck hyperextension is commonly caused by wearing an improperly fitting helmet, which limits the upper field of vision, or by improper bike fit.[15] Unconditioned athletes are more likely to fatigue their cervical spine extensors. Common bike fit errors associated with neck pain include excessively long or low handlebars or a saddle with too much of a downward tilt. Raising the handlebars or using handlebars with a shallower drop can decrease neck hyperextension and sometimes eliminate neck pain. Other treatment recommendations include daily isometric exercises with the neck in flexion, extension and lateral deviation to strengthen the neck musculature, as well as scapular stabilizer strengthening. Many people also benefit most from chin retractions and scapular pinching. The cyclist would be instructed to perform these exercises periodically during breaks in rides. Off the bike, strengthening the extensor muscles of the neck can be performed with prone posterior neck lifts with light resistance.[4,5,31] In addition, changing riding technique can sometimes decrease pain. Riding with locked elbows transmits more road vibration to the neck. Unlocking the elbows and varying hand position can decrease neck pain.[15]

Other structural etiologies of neck pain in cyclists

If these simple interventions are ineffective, it is important to look for other etiologies for the pain, such as cervical degenerative disc disease, cervical radiculopathy, cervical spondylosis, or other medical etiologies referring to the thorax.[15] A common structural etiology of chronic neck pain in cyclists is cervical facet syndrome exacerbated by neck hyperextension.[4]

Upper back pain

Trigger point spasm in the upper back (usually in the left levator scapula and upper left trapezius) is commonly seen in the cyclist, probably caused by the cyclist repetitively looking over his left shoulder to avoid approaching cars.[15]

Increased load on the arms and shoulders used to support the rider can increase neck and upper back pain. Dropped handlebars in the "hands low" position can exacerbate the pain. Specific treatment recommendations might include shortening the handlebar reach, moving the seat forward, or using less handlebar drop. In addition, having the cyclist unlock his elbows, changing the mirror placement on the helmet, or switching to a more upright handlebar can also improve neck pain.[15]

Mid and low back pain

Muscle fatigue of the trunk extensor muscles and lack of endurance in an unconditioned or deconditioned athlete are important areas to address as etiologies of muscular mid or low back pain.[32] The lumbar and thoracic musculature, which are not directly involved in pedaling, are groups of stabilizing muscles that allow more force to be transferred from the hip and leg muscles to the crank.[7] The muscles of the lower back are recruited to some extent during uphill riding, large gear riding, and sprints, or in cyclists who ride in an excessively upright position.[9] Isokinetic trunk extensor weakness and decreased aerobic capacity are other important factors in the development of low and mid back pain.[33]

Lower back pain in cyclists can be caused by inflexible hamstrings, inflexible gluteals, riding with too low a cadence, quad bias pedaling, poor back extensor strength, and poor bike fit with too long or too low handlebars.[4,10,32,33]

Sacroiliac joint dysfunction

Sacroiliac (SI) motion dysfunction is another type of cycling-induced back pain. Clinically, SI dysfunction is usually associated with a dull ache in the buttock region and around the area of the PSIS (posterior superior iliac spine). Altered lower extremity biomechanics, which can be repetitively aggravated in cycling, can place abnormal forces on the SI joint in its direction of motion, the sagittal plane.[24]

When a cyclist is in the "tucked position," the angle of both the sacrum and the inclination of the lumbar spine angle become increasingly horizontal as compared to standing. The combination of the change of the angle of the SI joint, the relatively fixed position of the pelvis on the bike saddle, and the rapidly changing hip angles that occur during pedaling lead to increased forces on the SI joint.[24]

Aging, degeneration, and gradual loss of SI cartilage can also contribute to decreased SI motion. Muscular control is important in stabilizing the SI joint, especially strength of the quadratus lumborum, erector spinae, glutei and piriformis. Other treatment recommendations can include a sacroiliac injection, brace, or mobilization.[21]

PERTINENT EXAMINATION OF THE CYCLIST

History

Obtaining the history from a cyclist should include specific cycling questions, including the portion of the pedal cycle that correlates with the cyclist's pain, the type of terrain, the gears used, and how the cyclist was fitted.[2] Important clues as to the etiology of back pain can be obtained by asking if there have been any recent adjustments to the fit of the bike or any changes in riding terrain. The sports medicine physician should also review the bike-training log to look for any dramatic changes in the athlete's training schedule.[16]

Common causes of new-onset back pain in a cyclist often include a recent seat adjustment. The seat may have been raised to adjust the bike for a different orthopedic problem but the handlebars weren't raised enough to compensate for the new seat height. Maintaining proper lumbar lordosis and avoiding hyperflexion of the lumbar spine can markedly decrease the incidence of bicycle-induced back pain.[4]

In addition, it is important to ascertain whether the cyclist recently changed his training to include more standing climbs or sprinting. In this case, back pain can occur because of muscular strain of the stabilizing muscles of the lumbar spine. It could be helpful to instruct the cyclist to decrease their weekly mileage by 10% until the back pain disappears. During this time, the cyclist should also be told to ride in lower gears with higher cadence and to avoid climbing. This will decrease the forces on the gluteals and hamstrings, decreasing the amount of force to the lumbar stabilizers and hopefully decreasing pain.[2]

The physician should determine the location of the pain, the nature of the pain (acute or insidious), the frequency of the pain (constant or intermittent), and the mechanism of injury (traumatic or non-traumatic). The character of the pain (sharp, dull, associated with numbness, or tingling) and the relevant past history of previous injuries are also important to note. Finally, an associated medical history should be obtained to address the possibility of spinal infection, i.e., rule out night sweats, fever, drug use, and history of carcinoma or HIV.[2,6,31]

Physical examination

Off bicycle examination

It is important to observe the patient walking to evaluate the biomechanics of gait, looking for clues that could affect riding and to observe the gross curvature of the spine. Some individuals have a kyphotic thoracic posture, which can lead to hypermobility of the thoracic spine and hypomobility of the lumbar spine while cycling. Pronation or supination of gait during ambulation can be translated to cycling-related injuries – some cyclists require orthotics.[2,4]

Flexibility of hip flexors, tensor fascia lata, hamstrings, and gluteals should be assessed. Tight gluteals and hamstrings can cause hyperextension of the back. Even hip flexor tightness affects cycling. Although the hip flexors are in a contracted position during cycling, a tight hip flexor can affect the fluidity of flexion of the hip. Therefore, flexible hamstrings, hip flexors, and gluteal muscles are paramount to avoiding back injuries.

In addition, it is important to test neck muscular strength because strong neck extensor muscles are important to prevent a hyperextended neck. Core abdominal strength should be addressed, as a strong mid-section can help to protect the back from injury.[4,22]

On bicycle examination

Observe the cyclist on the bike, assessing bike fit and pedal stroke. The average relatively inflexible recreational cyclist will probably have tight hamstrings, hip flexors, and gluteals, which would obviously require a different bike fit than for a flexible, elite cyclist.

One important observation for the on-bicycle examination is the amount of knee extension during the pedal cycle. Too much knee extension for the length of the cyclist's hamstring muscles can cause the hamstrings to pull on the pelvis, hyperextending the back. A cyclist with tight hamstrings and gluteals should be adjusted to ride in a more upright position. The overall bike fit should be observed and adjusted to the individual, taking into account the type of riding done and the limits of the range of motion of the cyclist.[29]

SPORTS-SPECIFIC REHABILITATION FOLLOWING AN INJURY

Diagnosis

The first part of treating an injury is defining the etiology of the injury. If the injury is from overtraining, relative rest and a change in training must be part of the program. Too many miles, too many hours, or too much intensity without appropriate recovery is a common cause of injury. A general rule is that increasing miles or distance should be accompanied initially by decreasing the intensity. Conversely, if an athlete is working at a high intensity, miles and time need to decrease.[29,34]

Strengthening

It is important to strengthen the three groups of muscles that stabilize the spine:
- The spine extensors and gluteal muscles are used to extend the spine and legs.
- The spine flexors (primarily the abdominal and iliopsoas muscles) are used to flex the spine and provide anterior stabilization of the spine. The iliopsoas also flexes the hip. The abdominal obliques and spine rotators stabilize the spine when upright, rotate the spine, and help maintain proper posture and spinal curvature.
- The scapular stabilizers support the upper spine and allow weight to be partially distributed to the upper body while cycling.

In the absence of a specific resistance program, spine stabilizers weaken with age. Daily activity, and even cycling, does not provide adequate strengthening of all the above muscles. Therefore, spinal and scapular stabilization exercises are helpful to perform during both the biking season as well as during off-season.[7-10]

Commonly, tight hamstrings, gluteals, or chronically shortened hip flexors are present in cyclists with low back pain. Although the iliopsoas muscle is chronically contracted during cycling, chronic spasm in the psoas restricts a fluid range of motion. Therefore, soft tissue mobilization of the psoas improves functional mobility.[22]

As biking does not contribute to abdominal strength, many cyclists with low back pain have weak abdominals and core strength. While riding a bicycle, weak abdominals allow the back to become hyper-lordotic, which can lead to strained muscles and sprained ligaments.[8]

Stretching

Biking involves repetitive motion in which the muscles are partially contracted and are often not fully stretched. This can lead to muscular tightness. Pedaling alone is not enough to keep most muscles loose. To counteract this tightening, the cyclist should be taught various stretching techniques. Stretches can include periodically grabbing the brake hoods, getting off the saddle, and using the arms, back, and body weight to drive the pedals. The shift in position will stretch the back muscles and prevent stiffness and fatigue.[9]

Stretching, both on the bike during long rides and off the bike, decreases fatigue and improves performance. Stretching should focus on the lower paraspinals, gluteals, tensor fascia latas, iliopsoas, quadriceps, and hamstring and calf muscles (Figs 8.2 and 8.3).

On long rides, it is recommended to stretch at least every hour. It is important to practice safety in on-the-bike stretching: avoiding stretching in traffic or on bumpy roads.

Rehabilitation program

A beginning rehabilitation program for a low back injury should usually include trunk stabilization and spinal and lower extremity flexibility exercises, including stretching to the lower paraspinals, gluteals, tensor fascia latas, hip flexors, quadriceps, hamstring, and calf muscles. Finally, other functional restrictions, structural tightness, or weaknesses should be addressed and corrected.

Once the initial phase of treatment has been completed, an emphasis on activities that imitate cycling is initiated. These exercises include one-legged work, first on the floor and then on the cycle using high resistance. Coordination is improved with high-resistance exercises such as single leg pedaling and riding with the bike trainer elevated to mimic hills and by performing seated and standing sprints.

The last phase of rehabilitation should include both interval training and fast cycling. The theory behind this is that by practicing fast cycling a cyclist will naturally become more economical and relaxed while riding both at fast speeds as well as at slower speeds.[35]

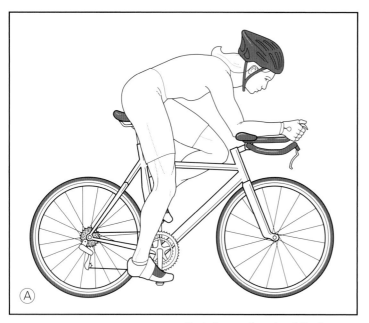

Figure 8.2
On bicycle stretches. Stretching before and after biking is important. Even while riding a bike, some simple stretches can be performed. These exercises should be performed only when riding alone at a relatively low speed, as a high level of concentration is necessary to prevent falling off the bike. (Reproduced with permission from Burke.[9])

A. Middle and upper back stretch: while on the saddle with the hands on the bar, round the back while lowering the head slightly. Hold for 5 seconds, then straighten. Relax; repeat stretches interspersed with pedaling to maintain speed.

Illustration continued on following page

Education

Educating the cyclist in proper pedaling techniques can both treat and prevent common biking injuries. The cyclist should be taught to make circular motion while pedaling: i.e., the pedals should have equal cadence in the downstroke as well as the upstroke. Common pedaling errors include quad bias pedaling or "pedaling squares" – the cyclist applies extensive force on the downstroke and then less force on the upstroke. The ideal cadence for endurance bicycling is 80–100 rpm. Injuries can occur at prolonged low or higher cadences.[10]

Economy of pedal stroke

Teaching a cyclist to pedal smoothly and correctly can also help prevent injury by making the pedal stroke ergonomically effective. Pedaling smoothly ("spinning circles") is more ergonomically efficient than pushing big gears ("riding squares"). Oxygen utilization is improved by 10% just by improving pedal force application from top dead center to the bottom of the pedal stroke.[27,36,37]

Force delivery is often improved by getting the athlete to think about "pushing through" at the top and "pulling back" at the bottom of the pedal stroke. This pedal stroke "economy" will result in a lower demand on the musculature of the leg in the power phase at constant pedal power or greater speed for the same power phase effort. Since the physiological strain felt by the body is directly related to VO_{2max}, the economical cyclist will have an advantage and will be able to ride faster while experiencing less fatigue.

Biomechanical improvements can also improve economy and contribute to the rehabilitation of the athlete. Any factor that uses energy not contributing to propelling the bicycle forward should be avoided. Examples of inefficient energy use include fighting the bicycle, gripping the handlebars too tightly, using too much upper body energy while climbing, or riding in non-aerodynamic positions.

Figure 8.2

Continued

B. Lift up from the breastbone and look upward to extend the spine. Hold for 5 seconds.

C. Lower and middle back stretch: keep a hand on the bar next to the stem; reach around and place the back of the arm across the lower back. Twist the upper body toward the arm behind the back. Hold for 5 seconds. Relax; repeat stretches interspersed with pedaling to maintain speed.

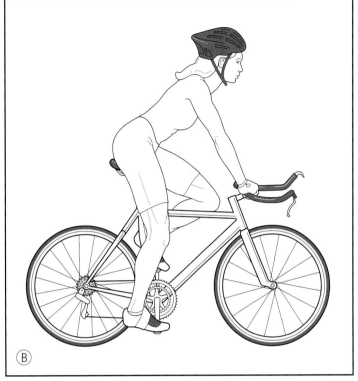

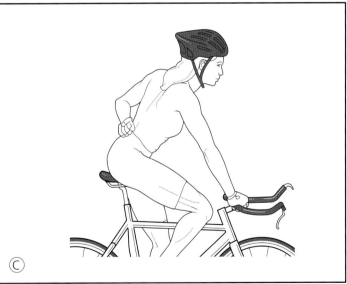

Illustration continued on following page

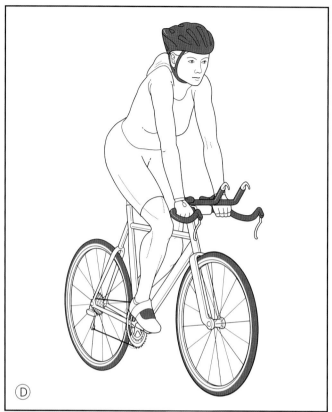

Figure 8.2
Continued
D. Shoulder and neck stretch: lift both shoulders to ears until tension is felt. Hold for 5 seconds and then lower to the original position.
E. Neck stretch: turn the chin to the shoulder for a few seconds, repeat to the other side. Move the shoulder slightly back to accommodate the chin while moving the opposite shoulder slightly forward. Hold for 5 seconds, and then do the other side. This will loosen the middle back and make it easier to rotate behind while cycling.

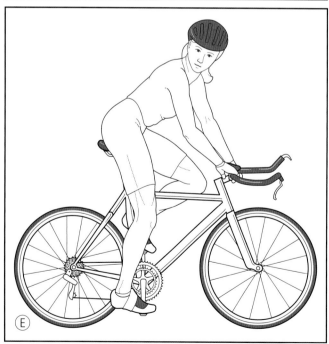

Illustration continued on following page

Figure 8.2
Continued

F. Gluteus maximus, calf, and hamstring stretch: with the forward pedal in the 9 o'clock position, stand, raise the hips, straighten the legs, and drop the heels. Hold for 5 seconds. Then rotate the crank arm 180 degrees and repeat.

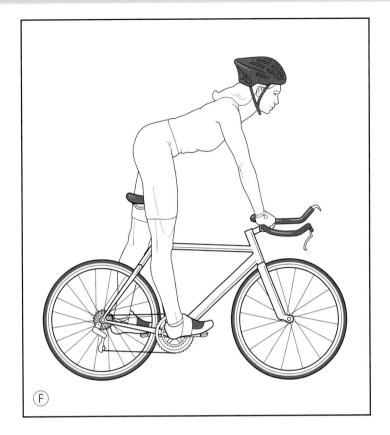

Medical interventions

Other medical treatments to rehabilitate the athlete include NSAIDs, physical therapy, trigger point injections, Lidoderm patches, Therma Care, lifestyle modifications, proper rest, stress reduction, proper sleep, manual mobilization, inferential current, and TENS machine.[38]

SPORTS-SPECIFIC TRAINING AND PREVENTION TECHNIQUES

Training

To train for peak performance the elite cyclist should address his individual strengths and weaknesses, focus on consistency with training, and avoid overtraining. Overall performance is enhanced by a cyclist's ability to be aware of his individual strengths and weaknesses. For example, if the cyclist is a poor climber, he should focus on building anaerobic power. Many athletes neglect their weaknesses and concentrate on their strengths, preventing them from improving their abilities.[29]

Overtraining

In addition, it is very important to be consistent in training. Performance is improved by doing *less* more often than by doing *more* less often. Finally, there is an optimum training threshold. As the athlete passes

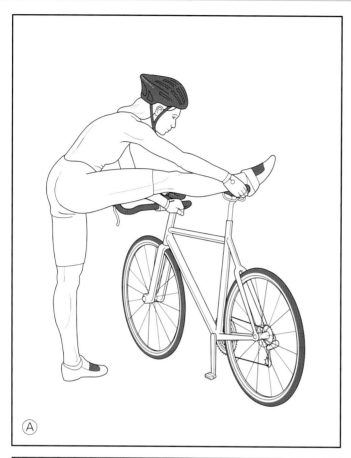

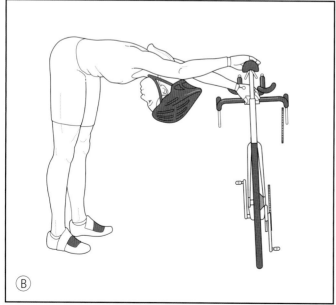

Figure 8.3
Stretching off the bike is also important.
(Reproduced with permission from Burke.[9])
A. Hamstrings stretch: place one ankle on top of the seat or rear tire and keep the other hand on the back edge of the saddle and the other on the stem. The leg should be almost straight but not locked and the foot should be pointed directly ahead. Bend until a stretch in the hamstrings is felt. Hold for 15–30 seconds. Repeat on the other leg.
B. Arms, back, shoulders, neck, and hamstring stretch: Stand 3–4 feet from the bicycle with the feet shoulder-width apart. With the knees bent and the hips over the feet, lower the upper body and move the chin to the chest until tension is felt. Hold for 20–30 seconds.

Illustration continued on following page

Figure 8.3
Continued

C. Quad stretch: stand on the left side of the bike and place the right hand on the saddle for balance. Reach behind with the left hand and grasp the top of the right foot. Slowly pull the foot toward the middle of the buttocks until a stretch is felt in the quadriceps and knee. Hold for 20–30 seconds. Grasp the handlebar stem with the left hand and repeat.

D. Hips and groin stretch: hold the bar top with one hand. Bend and lift one leg, bringing the knee toward the chest and place the foot on the saddle, top tube, or rear tire. Keep the other leg straight and the foot forward. Hold for 15–20 seconds. Repeat.

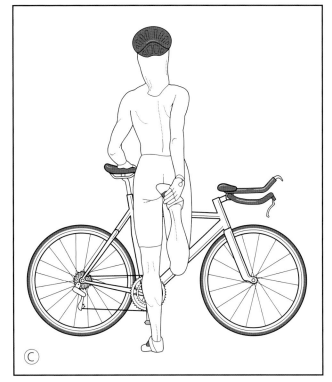

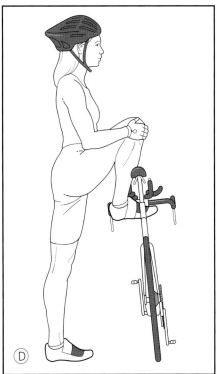

Illustration continued on following page

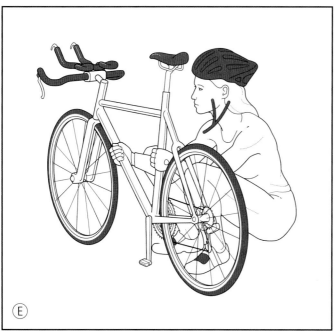

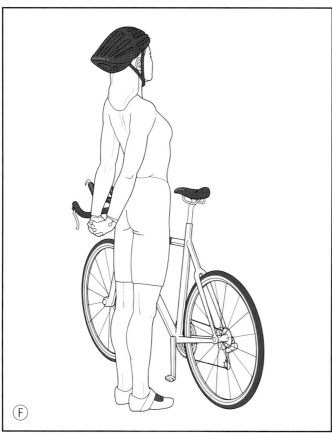

Figure 8.3
Continued

E. Knee and lower back stretch: stand 2 feet from the bike with the feet shoulder-width apart and the toes pointed slightly outward. Grasp the middle of the seat tube and down tube. Slowly squat, keeping the heels planted and the middle of the knees over the feet. Hold for 20–30 seconds. The cyclist should avoid this stretch if he has any meniscal injury or if this stretch produces any pain.

F. Shoulder, spine, and upper back stretch: lean the bike against the hips or rest the bike against a stable object. Interlace the fingers behind the arms backward until a stretch is felt through the front of the shoulders. Hold for 15–20 seconds.

the limits of his adaptation capability, the gains actually decline. Overtraining symptoms include muscle soreness, weight loss, increase in morning heart rate, a feeling of heaviness in the legs, constipation or diarrhea, inability to complete training, and a feeling of fatigue. The athlete may also experience emotional clues of overtraining such as irritability, loss of appetite, anxiety, or sleep disturbances.

The elite athlete should use a daily training diary to record morning pulse rate, body weight, and sleep patterns. If an increase in morning pulse is greater than 10%, or a sleep deficit is greater than 10% or a decrease in body weight is greater than 3%, then there is evidence for overtraining and the athlete should use training time that day to nap or rest.[8,29]

Heart rate monitors

One way to prevent overtraining during workouts would be to incorporate heart rate monitors into the work out. Wireless heart rate monitoring helps the athlete train at the optimum level of effort: hard enough to improve fitness and performance without overtraining. One way to use a heart rate monitor is to determine the heart rate at which the lactate build-up sensation occurs and train below that heart rate. If an athlete feels a perceived exertion at a heart rate that is lower than his usual lactate threshold, then he knows to take it easier that day. On easy days, the athlete should ride at a heart rate that is 25% below anaerobic threshold. The athlete should incorporate at least one or two easy days into his routine. On hard workout days, the elite or competitive cyclist should usually concentrate on distance work. It has been described that maximum training benefits are realized if the first few hours of training are at, or slightly below, their lactate threshold and the last 2 hours of training include at least two 10-minute intervals which are at their lactate threshold. All cyclists, from beginning amateurs to professionals, can benefit from using heart rate monitors to learn more about the way their body reacts to training demands.[37]

Overuse injury prevention

Overuse injuries occur when excessive force is maintained to a soft tissue over time. Overuse injuries may also occur as a result of an improperly rested acute injury. Common cycling overuse injuries occur cycling at too high of an intensity for a prolonged period of time or by using too large of a gear too early. The cyclist should be educated to listen to warning signs of pain that persists.

Key points in preventing bicycle-related back pain:
1. maintain appropriate, ergonomic pelvic rotation during riding
2. maintain hamstring, gluteal, and hip flexor flexibility
3. maintain ergonomic alignment of spine
4. maintain core-strength.[34]

Off-season training

Strengthening/periodization
If a cyclist doesn't ride during the off season, he or she needs to do some aerobic cross training, which will result in similar tissue adaptations. The "off season" should be thought of more as unstructured training. Cross training should stress activities that will load the soft tissues. Swimming is an excellent cross-training activity to strengthen the upper back while improving aerobic conditioning. The freestyle, breaststroke, and backstroke are better than the butterfly, which strains the lower back. Running, in-line skating, or snow shoe-ing are also other excellent cross-training activities.[35]

A periodization plan improves fitness by focusing on developing one aspect of fitness at a time, then progressing to another skill. The premise of this training regimen is that training variables are varied to allow for rest and regeneration to improve overall performance. One example of periodization is to focus on muscle hypertrophy exercises for 6 weeks, then change to basic strengthening exercises for 4 weeks, power exercises for 4 weeks, then muscular endurance exercises for 4 weeks.[35]

Weight training in conjunction with on-the-bike resistance work increases peak power, which increases an athlete's sustainable power output. The movements in the gym start in broad ranges of motion and progress to ranges similar to what a cyclist would use. For instance, when using a leg press machine in the gym, the knee angles used in pedaling should be mimicked. The connective tissues are stressed to improve the athlete's ability to sustain heavy muscular loads. Weight training will benefit the cyclist by increasing strength and power, to exert more force into the pedals, improving endurance and therefore preventing injury.[35]

On-the-bike resistance training on an indoor trainer has advantages for cyclists because the actual cycling motion is used to increase strength. Some techniques to increase power on the trainer include sprinting on a gear against very high resistance or attempting to maintain cadence against increasing resistance. Speed, or the rapid application of force, is what leads to an increased ability to produce peak power.[20]

Strengthening the back and abdominal muscles and improving overall fitness can decrease the incidence and duration of low back pain episodes. A high level of cardiovascular fitness provides protection against back injury.[17,19]

Weather, gear, and cycling

In the fall and spring months, the cyclist should be instructed to wear a long-enough jersey to cover the lower back in cool weather so that the muscles will be warm and less susceptible to injury. In winter months, clothing is critical to preventing hypothermia. The cyclist should be instructed to insulate the head and neck by wearing a knit cap/face mask that extends down the neck under the helmet and a helmet cover to keep the wind off the head and neck. Forty percent of body heat is lost from an inadequately protected head and neck. The inner layer of clothing should be a fabric that wicks moisture away from the skin and ventilates excess water perspiration. The other garments should provide insulation weather protection from wind and wetness. Hands should be covered with mittens instead of gloves. Mittens are much warmer than gloves because they trap all of the hand's warmth in a single compartment. If needed, the athlete could wear a pair of full-fingered thin liner gloves underneath his mittens to promote extra warmth.

While riding in cold weather, the athlete should cycle into the wind on the way out, and with the wind on the way back. The theory is that a tailwind will be helpful at the end of the ride. Riding into a headwind while tired can cause fatigue, decrease in speed and resultant chilling, or even hypothermia in extreme cases. In fact, hypothermia is a common and serious cold weather injury, which results in a drop of the body's core temperature. Fatigue, damp clothing, and wind chill are factors contributing to hypothermia. Although temperature is a factor, it doesn't have to be very cold for an individual to experience hypothermia. If a cyclist wears clothing that doesn't breathe, along with cotton undergarments that get wet from sweat, and then slows down for some reason (i.e., riding into the wind or climbing), heat loss and resultant hypothermia can rapidly occur. Early warning signs of hypothermia include shivering, muscle weakness, and loss of coordination.[35]

Taping

This chapter has repeatedly emphasized how important maintaining lumbar lordosis is to preventing cycling-related back pain. A simple taping procedure can be employed to provide an excellent feedback mechanism to train the cyclist to maintain proper lumbar lordosis while cycling. Prior to riding, the cyclist can have a partner apply a 1- or 2-inch wide adhesive tape from the sacrum to the thoracolumbar junction while the cyclist is standing in ergonomic lumbar lordosis. Then, if the cyclist loses lumbar lordosis while riding, the tape will pull on the skin to provide valuable feedback to the cyclist.[4]

CONCLUSION

This chapter has reviewed literature outlining biomechanical and training factors that can contribute to bicycling-related injuries. Maintaining an ergonomic position on the bike will require an anteriorly tilted pelvis and flexible hamstrings and gluteals. The cyclist should attempt to maintain lumbar lordosis, avoid thoracic kyphosis, and keep the neck in neutral while riding. The bike should be properly fitted. In addition, improving riding mechanics and pedal stroke and addressing any strength or flexibility deficits will assist in decreasing cycling-related spine pain. Specific therapeutic exercises have been addressed which can assist the lumbar spine in remaining neutral and avoiding cervical hyperextension. Hopefully, these suggestions can not only improve a cyclist's riding enjoyment but also decrease bicycling-related spine and musculoskeletal pain.

REFERENCES

1. Ericson M: The biomechanics of cycling. A study of joint and muscle load during exercise on the bicycle ergometer. Scand J Rehab Med Suppl 16:1–43, 1986.
2. Sanner WH, O'Halloran WD: The biomechanics, etiology and treatment of cycling injuries. J Am Podiatr Med Assoc 90(7):354–376, 2000.
3. Salai M, Brosh T, Blankstein A, et al: Effect of changing the saddle angle on the incidence of low back pain in recreational bicyclists. Br J Sports Med 33:398–400, 1999.
4. Schofferman J: Chronic and recurring low back pain and neck pain in bicycle riders. SpineLine Nov./Dec.:15–19, 2002.
5. Wilber CA, Holland CJ, Madison RE, et al: An epidemiological analysis of overuse injuries among recreational cyclists. Int J Sports Med 16:201–206, 1995.
6. Mayer PJ: Helping your patients avoid bicycling injuries. J Musculoskel Med 5:31–40, 1985.
7. Burke ER: Back: the overlooked cycling muscles. Bicycling 1:84–85.
8. Burke ER: Cycling. In: Watkins RG, ed., The spine and sports. St. Louis: Mosby; 1996:502–596.
9. Burke ER: Fast and loose. Bicycling 32(6):80–84, 1991.
10. Burke ER: Proper fit of the bicycle. Clin Sports Med 13(1):1–14, 1994.
11. Gregor RJ, Broker JP, Ryan MM: The biomechanics of cycling. In: Holloszy JO, ed. Exercise and sport sciences reviews. Baltimore: Williams and Wilkins, 1991:127–169.
12. Weiss BD: Nontraumatic injuries in amateur long distance bicyclists. Am J Sports Med 13(3):187–192, 1985.
13. Weiss BD. Clinical syndromes associated with bicycle seats. Clin Sports Med 13(1):175–186, 1994.
14. Williams MM, Hawley JA, Black R, et al: Injuries among competitive triathletes. NZ J Sports Med 3:2–6, 1988.
15. Mellion MB: Common cycling injuries: management and prevention. Sports Med 11(1): 52–70, 1991.
16. Cipriani, D, Swartz JD, Hodgson CM: Triathlon and the multi-sport athlete. J Orthopaed Sports Phys Ther 27(1):42–50, 1998.
17. Lahad A, Malter AD, Bergh AO, et al: The effectiveness of four interventions for the prevention of low back pain. J Am Med Assoc 272(16):1286–1291, 1994.
18. Nachemson AL: The lumbar spine. An orthopaedic challenge. Spine 1(1):59–68, 1976.
19. Cady LD Bishoff DP, O'Connel ER: Strength and fitness and subsequent back injuries in firefighters. J Occup Med 21:269–272, 1979.
20. Saal JA, Saal JS: Intradiscal electrothermal therapy for the treatment of chronic discogenic low back pain. In: Lauerman WC, Miller MD, eds. Clinics in sports medicine: the spine and sports, 21(1). 2002:167–187.

21. LeBlanc KE: Sacroiliac sprain: an overlooked cause of back pain. Am Fam Phys 11:1459–1463, 1992.

22. Timmer CA. Cycling biomechanics: a literature review. J Orthopaed Sport Phys Ther 14(3):103–114, 1991.

23. Jeukendrup AE: High-performance cycling. Champaign, IL: Human Kinetics Publishers; 2002.

24. Usabiaga J, Crespo R, Iza I, et al: Adaptation of the lumbar spine to different positions in bicycle racing. Spine 22(17):1965–1969, 1997.

25. Carolsson CA, Nachemson A: Neurophysiology of back pain: current knowledge. In: Nachemson A, Jonsson E, eds. Neck and back pain: the scientific evidence of causes, diagnosis and treatment. Philadelphia: Lippincott, Williams and Wilkins; 2000:149–159.

26. Watkins RG: Lumbar disc injury in the athlete. In: Lauerman WC, Miller MD, eds. Clinics in sports medicine: the spine and sports, 21(1). 2002:147–165.

27. Shennum PL, DeVires HA: The effect of saddle height on oxygen consumption during bicycle ergometer work. Med Sci Sports Exerc 8:119, 1976.

28. Browning RC, Gregor RJ, Broker JP, et al: Effects of seat height changes on joint force and moment patterns in experienced cyclists. [Abstract of article. J Biomech 21(10):871,1988].

29. Carmichael C: Training tips for cyclists and triathletes. Boulder, CO: Velo Press; 2001.

30. Keytel LR, Noakes TD: Effects of a novel bicycle saddle on symptoms and comfort in cyclists. SAMJ 92(4):295–298, 2002.

31. Huurman WW: The spine in sports. In: Mellion MB, ed. Office management of sports injuries and athletic problems. Philadelphia: Hanley and Belfus; 1988:199–212.

32. Moffroid M, Reid S, Henry SM, et al: Some endurance measures in persons with chronic low back pain. J Sports Phys Ther 20(2):81–87, 1994.

33. Keller A, Hellesnes J, Brox JI: Reliability of the isokinetic trunk extensor test, Biering–Sorensen test and the Astrand bicycle test: assessment of intraclass correlation coefficient and critical difference in patients with chronic low back pain and healthy individuals. Spine 26(7):771–777, 2001.

34. Holmes J, Pruitt A, Whalen A: Lower extremity overuse in bicycling. Clin Sports Med 13:187–205, 1994.

35. Burke EF: Off-season training for cyclists. Boulder, CO: Velo Press; 1997.

36. Shennum PL, DeVires HA: The effect of saddle height on oxygen consumption during bicycle ergometer work. Med Sci Sports 8:119–121, 1976.

37. Edwards S, Reed S: The heart rate monitor book for cyclists. Boulder, CO: Velo Press; 2002:125–228.

38. Nadler SF, Steiner DJ, Erasala G, et al: Continuous, low-level heat wrap therapy provides more efficacy than ibuprofen and acetaminophen for acute low back pain. Spine 27(10):1012–1017, 2002.

FURTHER READING

Fuhrman G: Resistance training for cyclists. NSCA's Performance Training Journal 1(5):2000. (www.nsca-lift.org/perform)

Gonzalez HG, Hull ML: Multivariable optimization of cycling biomechanics. [Abstract of article. J Biomech 22:1151–1161, 1989].

CHAPTER

9

Football Injuries

Robert Clendenin
J Keith Nichols

INTRODUCTION

Football is the ultimate contact sport. The spine is frequently injured as a result of acute or repetitive trauma or training injuries. Only the knee, ankle, and shoulder are injured more frequently. The forces generated by collisions on the football field and potential for injury increase as the size, strength, and speed of the player grows each year.

There are an estimated 1.4 million football players at the high school, college, and professional levels, with thousands more participating in leagues each year.[1] Contact sports have a higher rate of injury than non-contact sports. Football has the highest rate of injury and highest percentage of day lost injuries among organized athletics. One recent study found that 76.7% of high school football players missed playing time due to injuries each season.[2]

Risk of injury increases with age, body weight, and the level of play. Eighth grade football players have four times the risk of injury than do fourth graders.[3] Sixty-five percent of football injuries are the result of direct contact. Players being hit or tackled have the greatest time lost from participation, followed by those players hitting or tackling.[4]

This chapter will discuss injuries to the spine seen specifically in contact football. These injuries will be divided anatomically into the cervical, thoracic and lumbar divisions, with emphasis on presentation, diagnosis, treatment, and prevention.

POSITION-SPECIFIC INJURIES

Football can be divided into offensive positions and defensive positions. Offense consists of linemen and the skill positions, which include the quarterback, running backs, and receivers. The offensive linemen have a greater incidence of lumbar injury secondary to the specific forces that occur during blocking. Run blocking involves a compressive force applied to a flexed spine, increasing axial compression of the intervertebral discs, which predisposes them to a higher incidence of disc injuries, including internal disc disruption and herniated nucleus pulposus. Pass blocking increases stress on the posterior element secondary to repetitive hyperextension, with or without rotation, leading to a higher incidence of posterior element injuries.

Receivers have a higher incidence of traumatic neck injuries secondary to direct blows to the helmet when tackled or striking the ground. Receivers are relatively unprotected as they reach or dive for the football. Receivers also have a higher incidence of contusions and/or spinous process fractures of the thoracolumbar spine from direct blows to the back from a helmet and/or shoulder pad. The receiver's spine is often exposed and left unprotected in turning away from the defense to catch a forward pass.

Running backs function as blockers, runners, and receivers, and therefore are prone to both cervical and lumbar spine injuries. Injuries to the lumbar spine and cervical spine are similar to that previously mentioned for linemen and receivers. Running backs have repetitive collisions at higher rates of speeds, which lead to a greater force applied to the cervical spine, predisposing them to a higher incidence of stingers and/or traumatic cervical injuries.

Quarterbacks are most often injured during the process of passing. Most injuries occur when a quarterback is hit from the blind side, causing an acceleration/deceleration cervical spine injury similar to that seen in individuals involved in rear end motor vehicle collisions. They also have a high incidence of contusions and/or spinous process fractures from the direct blow to the spine from a helmet.

Defensive positions consist of linemen, defensive backs, and linebackers. Defensive linemen have a high incidence of posterior element injuries due to repetitive hyperextension. Defensive backs have the highest incidence of neck injuries, usually a result of tackling head first. Linebackers have a higher incidence of stingers from repetitive high-impact, high-velocity collisions occurring during tackling.

CERVICAL SPINE

Anatomy and biomechanics

The cervical spine serves as a bridge and supporting structure from the head to the torso. There is a fine balance between the strength and stability needed to protect the spinal cord and the flexibility needed for head movement. It is this freedom of motion that places the cervical spine at risk for catastrophic injury when subjected to the extreme, unpredictable mechanical stresses of contact football.

The cervical spine consists of seven vertebrae and eight cervical nerve roots. Intervertebral discs between each vertebrae act to absorb shock. The first cervical vertebrae, or the atlas, consists of a ring with two lateral masses that articulate with the two occipital condyles of the skull. The motion of nodding occurs at this joint.

The second cervical vertebrae, or axis, resembles the lower cervical vertebrae, except that the odontoid process sits on top and articulates with the anterior arch of the atlas. The axis bears the actual load of the head and atlas and transfers that load to the cervical spine.[5] The C1–C2 joint (Fig. 9.1) provides 50% or more of total axial rotation.[6]

The third through seventh cervical vertebrae are considered normal cervical vertebrae. They provide a load-bearing function through a three-column system consisting of the vertebral body anteriorly and the paired facet joints posteriorly. In contrast to the lumbar spine, the facet joints and cervical intervertebral discs equally distribute the vertebral load.[7] The lower cervical spine provides most of the flexion and extension and up to 50% of the rotation.

The intervertebral discs function to absorb shock and to increase mobility. The cervical discs also give the cervical spine its lordotic curve by their wide anterior and narrow posterior shape. This lordotic curve causes the load bearing to fall on the posterior edge of the vertebral body above C4–C5 and anterior edge below.

Biomechanics of cervical injury

Cervical injuries in football may be caused by improper tackling, clothes lining or face masking, a knee to head blow, head butting, or acute hyperextension or hyperflexion forces.[8] These are most common in defensive players, particularly linebackers and defensive backs. There have even been cases reported of cervical fractures after collision with spring-loaded tackling or blocking dummies.[9]

Figure 9.1
The cervical vertebrae: C1–C2, the atlanto-axial joint and the normal C3–C7 vertebrae.

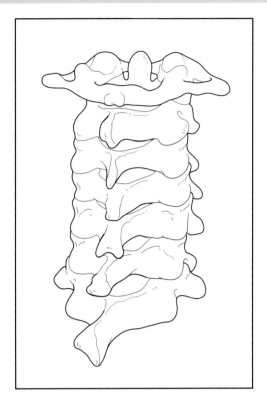

The cervical spine is normally protected by the lordotic curve and the ability of the neck musculature and intervertebral discs to moderate these compressive forces. When the neck is straightened it loses its ability to dissipate force and the compression is directly transmitted to the spinal structures. Torg has been a leader in identifying axial compression as the major cause of catastrophic cervical injury.[10] This occurs when a force is applied directly to the top of the helmet as the initial point of contact with the neck straightened. This causes the cervical spine to bear the force between the head, which is stopped, and the trunk, which is still moving forward. This can lead to cervical spine failure secondary to fracture, dislocation, and spinal cord injury. Axial loading has been validated in numerous studies including cadaver models.[11–13] (See also Fig. 2.1, page 35.)

The improvement in the safety of football helmets led to an increase of neck injuries due to the use of the head and neck as a weapon. This led to changes in 1976 at both the college and high school levels that banned the intentional use of the crown of the helmet to strike an opponent or the use of the helmet as the initial point of contact. This change produced a dramatic decrease in the frequency of catastrophic neck injuries. The rate of quadriplegia for 100 000 high school players fell from 1.92 in 1976 to 0.33 in 1995. The rate for 100 000 college players likewise fell from 10.67 to 1.33 over the same time period.[14]

Cantu and Mueller reviewed spinal cord injuries directly caused by football between 1977 and 1998. They found 200 cervical cord injuries, with 142 (71%) playing defense and 53 (26.5%) injured while tackling in a head-down position causing axial loading. Defensive backs had the highest rate of injury among positions.[15]

Onfield evaluation

The worst fear of every team physician is of the player that fails to get up after a play and lays motionless on the field. The risk of serious cervical spine injury is very small, but the results can be catastrophic. Every team physician, trainer, or EMS (Emergency Medical Service) responder must be trained in and aware of the proper evaluation and supportive treatment and technique of immobilization in such a patient. The failure to recognize a serious spinal injury or improper handling or movement of the cervical spine can lead to deterioration in neurologic status.

The unconscious player's vital signs must be checked and cardiopulmonary resuscitation (CPR) begun if absent. If vital signs are present, then the unconscious patient must be treated with the assumption that he has an unstable cervical spine. Likewise, any conscious patient with significant bilateral extremity weakness or paresthesias, especially in the lower extremities, with neck pain and loss of active motion, must be immobilized and transported by spine board for X-ray evaluation. The player should be placed on a spine board by a minimum of five people, with the captain maintaining control of the head and neck at all times (Fig. 9.2).

The consensus is that both the helmet and shoulder pads should remain in place until the player reaches the hospital. The recommendation is based on studies that reveal significant movement in cadaver spines with unstable cervical lesions during removal of protective football equipment.[16,17]

The removal of the helmet only has been found to cause an increase in cervical lordosis and extension and removal of shoulder pads only to cause increase in cervical flexion. A cervical collar should be applied with the helmet in place. The helmet should then be immobilized to the spine board with the use of tape or a strap. The properly fitted helmet using BTLS (basic traumatic life support) immobilization should allow less than 3% of head movement when immobilized in this fashion.[18]

Initial X-rays should be performed with the helmet and pads in place. If these are inadequate,[19] then the equipment may be removed using the National Athletic Trainer Association technique. This technique involves four people and has been shown to produce no abnormal motion in normal spines.[20] Cervical computed tomography (CT) scans and flexion extension X-rays may be used if initial films are negative.

The patient with transient resolved neurologic symptoms and full painless cervical range of motion may return to play.

Stingers/burners

The most common cervical spine injury in football is the stinger or burner. The career incidence ranges from 49 to 56%, with an equally high rate of recurrence.[21,22]

The player will normally present with his arm adducted after a blow or fall to the shoulder or neck. There will be an immediate onset of burning or tingling down the arm, usually to the thumb or index finger. There may be weakness in the C5–C6 distribution.

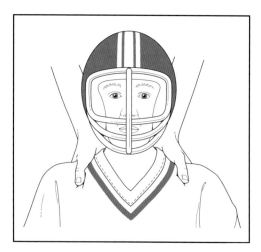

Figure 9.2
To prevent head and neck movement, firmly grip the clavicle/sternal area and rest the head on the forearms.

Shoulder injuries such as dislocation or cervical radiculopathy may present in a similar fashion.

The cervical spine should be painless with normal motion. The symptoms usually are transient and the player may return to action when symptom-free if he has normal strength and sensation with pain-free neck range of motion.[23] When neurologic symptoms persist, the player should be withheld from contact and further evaluation undertaken including a complete cervical spine series (anteroposterior, lateral, flexion and extension, oblique, and odontoid views), cervical magnetic resonance imaging (MRI), and electrodiagnostic studies if necessary.

There are three main biomechanical models of injury. The first injury model is a stretch to the upper trunk of the brachial plexus, with the head in a laterally deviated position, caused from a blow depressing the shoulder at the same time that the head is laterally deviated in a contralateral direction. The second injury model is compression of the nerve root in the neural foramen, caused by neck hyperextension with or without lateral flexion. The third injury model is a blow or contusion directly to the brachial plexus at Erb's point (Fig. 9.3).

Players with cervical stenosis measured by an abnormal Torg ratio have been found to have a high incidence of extension type-stingers.[23,24,24a] Kelly et al[25] also found increased risk in players with foraminal stenosis, measured using the foraminal/vertebral body ratio:

0.65 players with stingers and 0.72 normal controls

Post-injury rehab should focus on neck strengthening and stretching in a chest-out posture. This causes slight flexion of the cervical spine, which opens the lateral foramen and also helps to unload part of the weight of the head from the cervical spine. The thoracic outlet is also opened by altering the alignment of the scalene muscles and clavicle to the neck.[26]

Prevention is accomplished by use of properly fitted shoulder pads with some minor adaptations. Shoulder pads should fit tightly to the chest and have a modified A-frame shape.[27] Some restriction of neck movement can be achieved with the use of lifters or a cowboy-type collar under the shoulder pads and a neck roll outside of the pads.

Figure 9.3
Potential areas of
injury of stingers/
burners:
A. Neural foramen.
B. Upper trunk of
    the brachial
    plexus.

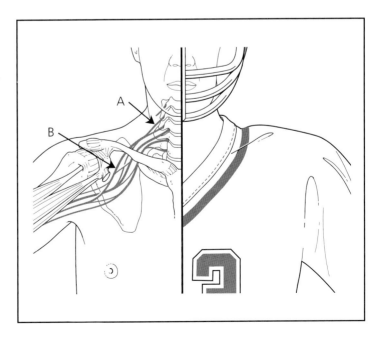

Fractures

Cervical spine fractures are a rare but potentially devastating injury not to be missed by the team physician. The athlete may present with weakness, dysesthesias, or paresthesias in the extremities, with neck pain and loss of motion. The C5–C6 level is the most commonly injured and the C1–C2 level is the most often not diagnosed. Axial compression is the most common mode of injury, although hyperflexion or hyperextension may also produce fractures.

The severity may range from stable fractures that require no more treatment than a soft collar to unstable fracture dislocation with spinal cord injury. Cervical X-rays including anterior–posterior, lateral, and odontoid views should be obtained. A CT scan is more sensitive if plain films are negative and is particularly helpful to rule out upper cervical fractures. Flexion/extension lateral films are used to rule out an unstable ligamentous injury. There are three findings on flexion/extension films that suggest instability:

1. an increase in the atlantodens interval of greater than 3.5 mm
2. anterior vertebral subluxation greater than 20% of the vertebral body or 3.5 mm
3. an angle of 11 degrees or greater between the inferior plates of adjacent vertebral bodies (Fig. 9.4).

Cervical disc disease

Cervical disc injuries in a football player may present acutely and may be confused with a stinger or cervical fracture. The most common presentation though is one of gradually increasing pain in the neck and shoulder blade with activity which may or may not develop a radicular component. The discs are placed under stress not only by the direct contact received in football but also may be the result of cumulative trauma which occurs in the weight room and on the training field.

MRI is the most useful diagnostic tool and should be utilized in a player with radicular symptoms. Players with significant disc abnormalities associated with neurologic symptoms should be withheld from contact, although they may continue with low-impact aerobic activities. Most disc pain is mediated through inflammation, and corticosteroids and inflammatory agents should be utilized initially. Epidural injections allow for placement of a greater concentration of steroid at the site of inflammation. These injections must be performed under fluoroscopy, both for greater efficacy and for greater safety. Stojanovic

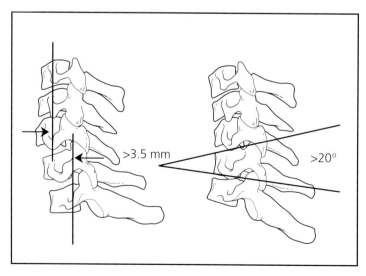

Figure 9.4
Lateral flexion/extension X-rays are necessary to evaluate ligament injury that causes potential instability.

>3.5 mm

>20°

et al found in a recent study that the loss of resistance technique was not adequate when compared to fluoroscopically controlled injection.[28] Intermittent cervical traction with Mackenzie's exercises should also begin immediately and progress to strengthening of the cervical paraspinal muscles and stabilizers as tolerated. Return to play is allowed when the player is neurologically intact and has normal pain-free cervical motion. Players who do not respond to conservative treatment and have clear anatomic abnormalities on MRI should be referred for surgical evaluation.

Transient quadriparesis

Transient quadriparesis or cervical cord neuropraxia (CCN) is a rare transient neurologic injury of the cervical spinal cord that occurs in the absence of a structural abnormality. The rate of occurrence is about 7.3 per 100 000 football players.[29] The key to the presentation of CCN is that there is neurologic dysfunction in more than one extremity. Torg et al, in a study of 110 cases of CCN, found that the most common presentation was involvement of all four extremities (80%), with the least common being the lower extremity alone or the ipsilateral arm and leg (less than 5%).[30] Sensory changes including numbness, burning pain, tingling, or loss of sensation are present and may or may not be associated with weakness or paralysis. These symptoms normally resolve within 15 minutes (74%)[30] but may persist for up to 48 hours. There is no significant neck pain associated with CCN. The differential would include cervical spine injury, radiculopathy, or cervical stinger.[29] There is a case of atraumatic quadriparesis in a college football player in the literature with transverse myelitis.[31]

Torg et al identified a correlation between cervical stenosis and transient quadriparesis in skeletally mature football players.[32] Stenosis is defined as a Torg ratio of less than 0.8 on plain X-rays or a mid-sagittal canal diameter of less than 12 mm on MRI.

The Torg ratio (spinal canal/vertebral body) is the distance from the mid-point of the posterior aspect of the vertebral body to the nearest point on the corresponding spinolaminar line divided by the anterior-posterior width of the vertebral body on lateral X-ray.[10] This ratio eliminates the errors seen with absolute measurements caused from image magnification, variations in technique, and anatomy. This ratio is highly sensitive for CCN (93%) but has a low predictive value (0.2%) and thus is not useful for screening purposes.[32] (See Fig 2.4 page 37.)

Pediatric transient neuropraxia appears to have no correlation with cervical stenosis and is thought to be the result of increased cervical spine mobility secondary to immature cervical spine supporting musculature.[33]

The mechanisms of transient neuropraxia are secondary to a brief acute decrease in anterior-posterior diameter of the spinal cord caused by hyperflexion or hyperextension. Penning[34] described a "pincher mechanism" causing cord compression. With the spine in hyperflexion, the distance between the anterior superior aspect of the spinolaminar line of the superior vertebral body and posterior superior aspect of the body of the adjacent vertebra is diminished. With extension, the distance between the posterior inferior aspect of the superior vertebral body and the anterior superior aspect of the spinolaminar line of the subjacent vertebra is decreased. This subjects the cord to compression with transient disturbance in neurologic function.

The prognosis of CCN is excellent, with full recovery the normal outcome. Work-up includes plain X-rays and MRI to rule out cervical fracture or cord injury. The player may return to full contact if imaging studies are negative and full neurologic recovery has been obtained. There is no absolute contraindication to return to full contact after an episode of CCN and the player is thought to be at no higher risk for a permanent catastrophic neurologic injury.[32]

It is important to counsel the patient that there is an overall high rate of recurrence (62%) of CCN after returning to contact football.[30] This rate of recurrence is high enough that many players choose not to return to contact football. The rate of recurrence can be estimated by the sagittal diameter of the spinal canal. Players with MRI evidence of cord injury, ligament instability, or neurologic symptoms lasting greater than 36 hours, and multiple episodes should not return to contact football.[10]

Spine-tackler spine

Spine-tackler spine is a diagnosis carried by a specific subset of football players who are at high risk for catastrophic cervical injury. Torg et al first identified these players in a 1993 study of the National Football Head and Neck Injury Registry.[35] These players had four identifying factors:

1. congenital stenosis (Torg ratio of less than 0.8)
2. loss of lordotic curve or straightening of the cervical spine
3. pre-existing post-traumatic radiographic abnormalities
4. history of utilizing spear-tackling head-first techniques.

These players should avoid any sport with the possibility of axial loading to the cervical spine.

Soft tissue injury

Cervical spine soft tissue injuries in football can be compared to whiplash injuries seen after a motor vehicle accident. They include an acceleration-type injury, as the trunk is struck and moved forward, causing the C-spine to go into extension. Likewise, as a player is tackled, the momentum of the trunk is stopped and the head and neck momentum continues onward, causing a flexion of the cervical spine.

The structures affected include the interspinal ligaments, synovial lined facet joints, and paraspinal and parascapular musculature. Treatment includes early use of modalities to prevent secondary edema and rapid mobilization to prevent loss of motion. When the pain persists, judicious use of trigger point and facet injections may quicken the player's return to action. Strengthening should begin as soon as it is tolerated, with an isometric program. This can be advanced to isotonic strengthening, as tolerated, using a high-repetition/low-weight protocol. Return to play is allowed when the cervical motion approaches normal range.

Return to play

There is a wide variation of opinions of which cervical spine injuries can be safely allowed to return to contact football and which cannot. The results of a recent questionnaire published in *Spine* indicate there is consensus only that return to contact sports carries a higher risk than non-contact sports.[36] The following guidelines in Box 9.1, published by Torg and Ramsey-Emrhein in 1997, provide a framework for this decision.[37] This decision should also be augmented by the experience of the physician and by the choice of a well-educated athlete.

THORACIC SPINE

Serious injuries to the thoracic spine are rare in football. The thoracic spine is immobile compared with the cervical and lumbar spines and is adherently more stable due to its attachment to the rib cage bilaterally. Most thoracic injuries are ligamentous sprains or contusions from direct contact.

Thoracic spine compression fractures have been reported in the literature and are thought to be a result of axial loading to the shoulders with the spine forwardly or laterally flexed.[38] These fractures present with non-specific complaints of back pain or stiffness and are often made worse with deep breathing. Physical

---

Box 9.1 Guidelines for return to play

No contraindication to participation:

1. Spina bifida occulta.
2. Type II Klippel–Feil congenital one level fusion.
3. Developmental spinal canal stenosis (Torg ratio less than 0.8).
4. Resolved burner.
5. Mild ligament sprain without laxity.
6. Healed stable vertebral body compression fracture.
7. Healed stable end plate fracture.
8. Healed "clay shoulders" fracture.
9. Healed intravertebral disc bulge.
10. Stable one-level surgical fusion.

Relative contraindication of participation:

1. Recurrent acute and chronic burners.
2. Developmental canal stenosis with episodes of cervical cord neuropraxia – intervertebral disc disease – MRI evidence of cord compression.

3. Ligament sprain with mild laxity (less than 3.5 mm AP displacement and less than 11 degrees rotation).
4. Healed non-displaced Jefferson fracture.
5. Healed stable mildly displaced vertebral body fracture without a sagittal component or neural ring involvement.
6. Healed stable neural ring fracture.
7. Healed intervertebral disc herniation.
8. Stable two-level surgical fusion.

Note: return to play in the above two categories assumes the athlete is asymptomatic with normal cervical motion and neurologic function.

Absolute contraindication to participation:

1. Odontoid agenesis, hypoplasia, or os odontoideum.
2. Atlanto-occipital fusion.
3. Type I Klippel–Feil mass fusion.
4. Developmental canal stenosis with ligament instability – cervical cord neuropraxia with signs or symptoms lasting more than 36 hours – multiple episodes of cervical cord neuropraxia.
5. Spear-tacklers spine.
6. Atlanto-axial instability.
7. Atlanto-axial rotary fixation.
8. Acute cervical fracture.
9. Ligament laxity (greater than 3.5 mm AP displacement or 11 degrees rotation).
10. Vertebral body fracture with a sagittal component.
11. Vertebral body fracture with associated posterior arch fracture and/or ligament laxity.
12. Vertebral body fracture with displacement into the spinal canal.
13. Healed fracture with associated neurologic findings or symptoms, pain, or limitation of cervical range of motion.
14. Intervertebral disc herniation with neurologic signs or symptoms, pain, or limitation of cervical range of motion.
15. Cervical fusion at three or more levels.[30]

examination will usually reveal point tenderness at the level of injury. Neurologic deficits are rare. X-ray work-up will reveal anterior vertebral body wedging on the lateral view.

Treatment is with bracing for approximately 12 weeks with an extension-type TLSO brace. Return to play is allowed with radiographic healing and when the player is pain-free.

LUMBOSACRAL SPINE ANATOMY

The lumbosacral spine is composed of five lumbar vertebrae, the sacrum, and a coccyx. When the lowest lumbar vertebra has some or all of the radiologic features of the first sacral segment, it is termed sacralization.[39] Lumbarization occurs when the first sacral segment has the radiographic appearance of a lumbar vertebra. The lumbar vertebral bodies increase in size from L1 to L5 and make up 25% of the height of the entire spine. The shape of the spinal canal evolves from an oval on its side at L1 to a triangular shape at L5.[40]

Contained within the vertebral column spinal canal is the spinal cord. In adults the cord may extend to the discs between L1 and L2, although it can end somewhat higher at the body of L1 or lower at the body of L3. The nerve roots then continue distally as the cauda equina. The spinal nerves exit below their corresponding numbered vertebrae, e.g., the L5 nerve root exits below the L5 vertebra through the L5–S1 intervertebral foramina.

There are six major ligaments in the lumbar spine: the anterior longitudinal ligament, posterior longitudinal ligament, ligamentum flavum, supraspinous ligament, interspinous ligament, and the capsular ligament (Fig. 9.5).[17]

The intervertebral discs consist of two distinct components: a paracentrally located nucleus pulposus surrounded by an outer annulus fibrosis. The nucleus is composed of a mucoid material with a high water content. The water content decreases with age from 88% in preadolescence to 70% in the elderly. The annulus fibrosis is composed of collagen fibers arranged in sheets known as lamella. The lamella are arranged in concentric rings that surround the nucleus pulposus. The lumbar disc is normally more thick anteriorly than posteriorly. Each disc is bound superiorly and inferiorly by a vertebral end plate.

The musculature of the back acts on the lumbar spine, to produce forward movement, flexion, extension, lateral bending, and rotation. There are three major groups of intrinsic back muscles in the lumbar spine, consisting of the erector spinae muscle group, transverse spinalis, and the segmental muscles. The erector spinae consists of three columns of muscles from the medial to lateral: from the spinalis, the longissimus, and iliocostalis. Unilateral contraction of the erector spinae causes lateral flexion of the vertebral column to the same side with some rotation to that side. Bilateral contraction produces extension of the spinal column. The transverse spinalis consists of the semispinalis, multifidus, and rotator muscles. They incline medially and superiorly and fill in the concavity between the tips of the transverse processes and the spinous processes. Unilateral contraction produces rotation to the opposite side, with bilateral contraction, causing extension of the spinal column. The segmental muscles consist of the interspinalis and intertransversarii (Fig. 9.6).

The abdominal musculature have a significant role in lumbar spine movement.

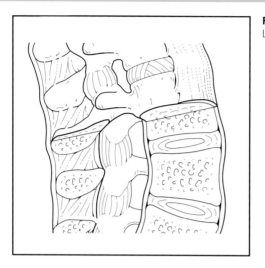

Figure 9.5
Lumbar vertebral ligament.

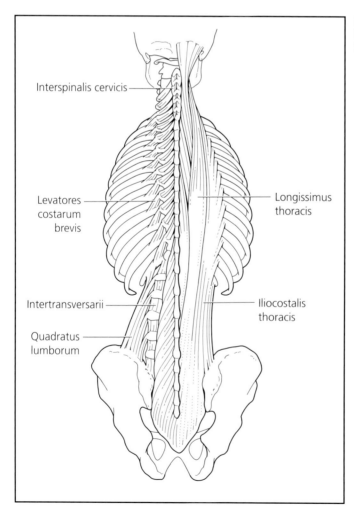

Figure 9.6
Muscular attachments of
the spine.

Interspinalis cervicis

Levatores
costarum
brevis

Longissimus
thoracis

Intertransversarii

Iliocostalis
thoracis

Quadratus
lumborum

The abdominal muscles consist of the rectus abdominalis, transverses abdominus, internal oblique, and external oblique. The abdominal muscles are the significant flexors and the lateral flexors of the trunk and also assist in rotation.

BIOMECHANICS

The basic motion segment of the spine consists of two adjacent vertebral bodies, their intervertebral discs, and their two apophyseal joints. This is referred to as the three-joint complex. Each motion segment can be divided into an anterior and posterior element. The anterior element consists of the vertebral bodies, the discs, and the anterior and posterior longitudinal ligaments. The anterior element provides stability and is the weight-bearing and shock-absorbing component of the spine. The posterior element consists of the neural arches, which protect the neural structures and control spinal movements. Each vertebral body is connected to the vertebral body above and below by a pair of zygapophyseal joints. The zygapophyseal joints are almost in sagittal plane to the lumbar spine, which facilitates flexion and extension but limits rotation. Normal range of motion of the lumbar spine is 60 degrees of flexion, 25 degrees of extension, and 25 degrees of right and left lateral bending; 75% percent of lumbar flexion and extension occurs at L5–S1, 20% at L4–L5, and the remaining 5% at other levels. Morphologic changes occur in the lumbar spine with flexion, extension, lateral bending, and axial rotation. The size of the vertebral canal and intervertebral foramen increases with flexion and decreases with extension.[41,42] Lateral bending decreases foraminal width, height, and area at the bending side but increases these dimensions at the opposite side of bending.[42] Axial rotation also decreases the foraminal width and area at the rotation side but increases the foraminal height and foraminal area at the opposite side.[42]

FOOTBALL INJURIES

Football can place significant compressive, shear, torsion, and rotational forces on the lumbar motion segments, leading to injury. Interior linemen are most often affected, most probably because of repetitive extension loads during blocking. Gatt et al found compression, shear, and lateral bending forces to be 7, 2.6, and 1.4 × body weight, respectively, at the L4–L5 motion segment while hitting a blocking sled.[43] These loads exceeded those determined during fatigue studies that cause pathologic changes in both the lumbar disc and pars interarticularis. Edwards et al applied compressive–flexion and compression–extension loads to cadaveric lumbar motion segments and found that the highest stresses are measured along the posterior and posterior lateral annulus, not the nucleus which corresponds to common sites of disc degeneration and herniation.[44]

Spondylolysis/spondylolisthesis

Football players, especially interior linemen, are involved in activities that involve repeated forceful hyper-extension of the spine, which delivers significant forces to the pars interarticularis. Repetitive forces at the pars may result in spondylolysis and, ultimately, spondylolisthesis. There is a 6% overall incidence of spondylolysis in the general population. Several investigations of football players have noted an incidence ranging from 15% to 50%. Spondylolysis refers to a bony defect in the pars interarticularis. Forward slipping of a vertebra on its adjacent vertebra can occur, with bilateral spondylolysis, and this results in spondylolisthesis. Five different types of spondylolysis and spondylolisthesis have been described:
  1. dysplastic
  2. isthmic
  3. degenerative
  4. traumatic
  5. pathologic.

Isthmic is the most common form of spondylolisthesis and is the type most commonly seen in the athletic population. The most common site for a pars defect is L5, followed by L4 and L3, respectively. Spondylolisthesis, therefore, most commonly occurs at L5–S1, followed by L4–L5 and L3–L4.

Patients usually present with complaints of a dull backache which may radiate to the buttocks and/or thighs. With high-degree slips, neural impingement can occur, resulting in radicular symptoms such as neurologic deficits in the lower extremities. The majority of radiculopathies are L5 in origin from a L5–S1 spondylolisthesis. Symptoms are usually aggravated by activities such as extension and rotation, which increase stress on the pars.

The physical examination can reveal spasm to the lumbar paraspinals as well as the hamstrings. The patient may have a limited straight leg raise. The majority of patients have no evidence of neurologic dysfunction but a full neurologic evaluation is indicated in all patients presenting with low back pain. Palpation of the back may reveal tenderness of the paraspinals as well as the sacroiliac joints. Lumbar extension is usually limited secondary to pain.

The initial radiographic work-up should include plain films consisting of AP, lateral, and oblique views. Spondylolysis is graded from I to IV by dividing the adjacent vertebral body into quadrants. Grade I is less than 25% slippage, Grade II less than 50%, Grade III less than 75%, and Grade IV less than 100% (Fig. 9.7). If the superior vertebra completely dislocates anteriorly, it is referred to as a spondyloptosis. If an athlete's pain is not resolved in 3–4 weeks, a bone scan should be ordered. Bone scans may show increased activity on one or both sides in patients with normal plain films. Single-photon emission

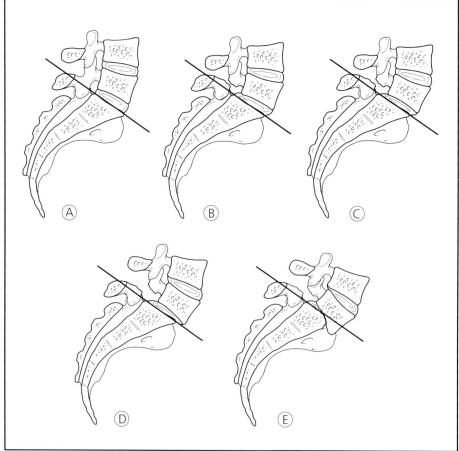

Figure 9.7
Lumbar spondylolisthesis. Note varying degrees of slippage.
A. Grade I.
B. Grade II.
C. Grade III.
D. Grade IV.
E. Grade V.

computed tomography (SPECT) imaging is most reliable in the early diagnosis of stress reaction of the pars and may show a pars defect that is not apparent on radiographs or bone scans.

Initial treatment consist of avoiding aggravating activities and rest. There is no true consensus on management, with treatment ranging from decreasing activity to rigid immobilization. As the patient improves, a rehabilitation program that focuses on lumbar stabilization, abdominal strengthening, and hamstring stretching can be initiated. If a patient continues to have pain and is unresponsive to decreased activity, a Boston brace, lumbosacral corset, or thoracolumbosacral orthosis (TLSO) should be considered. The main treatment objective is to stop the pain with whatever amount of inactivity it takes. Once the athlete's symptoms are resolved, competition is permitted after appropriate reconditioning. No permanent restrictions are placed on athletes with asymptomatic spondylolysis and spondylolisthesis.

Disc herniation

Disc herniations are not uncommon in football players. The injury usually occurs with flexion and rotation of the lumbar spine during contact activities. Patients typically present with severe back and leg pain, with the leg pain being more pronounced than the back pain. The most common radiculopathies in decreasing order of frequency are S1, L5, L4, and L3, resulting from L5–S1, L4–L5, L3–L4, and L2–L3 herniations, respectively. Some common radicular syndromes are listed in Table 9.1.

The evaluation should include a full neurologic examination, consisting of strength, sensation, and reflexes of the lower extremities. Sciatic tension tests – including sitting straight leg raise, supine straight leg raise, contralateral straight leg raise, and femoral nerve stretch – should be performed. Assessment of bowel or bladder function is essential as any significant involvement requires immediate diagnosis and surgical consultation.

Plain films are initially obtained to rule out any associated bony pathology. The imaging study of choice in the diagnosis of lumbar radiculopathies is MRI. In patients presenting with clinical evidence of a lumbar radiculopathy, the MRI can be used to confirm the diagnosis. Some herniated discs may be missed by MRI. CT myelography can then be utilized for further evaluation. Electromyography is also very useful as it can localize the level of involvement.

Treatment ranges from conservative to surgical, depending on the degree of neurologic involvement. Hard neurologic findings on clinical examination in the presence of bowel/bladder dysfunction require immediate surgical intervention. In our practice, surgery is usually reserved for those patients with severe unremitting pain, upper motor neuron signs, and/or progressive neurologic deficits. The majority of radiculopathies will resolve with conservative treatment over a 3-month period of time. In the athlete,

Table 9-1 Common clinical features of lumbar radiculopathies

Disk level	Nerve root	Motor deficit	Sensory deficit	Reflex compromise
L3–L4	L4	Quadriceps, tibialis anterior, thigh adductors	Anterolateral thigh Anterior knee Medial leg and foot	Knee
L4–L5	L5	External hallucis longus, tibialis anterior, extensor digitorum longus and brevis, gluteus maximus	Lateral thigh Anterolateral leg Mid-dorsal foot	Medial hamstrings
L5–S1	S1	Gastrocnemius-soleus Gluteus maximus Toe flexors	Posterior leg Lateral foot	Ankle

time may be a factor in the decision to proceed with surgery, as surgery usually results in quicker relief of pain and return to full activities in a shorter time frame. Initial conservative care involves relative rest, analgesics, nonsteroidal anti-inflammatory drugs (NSAIDs), and at times the utilization of an antispasmodic medication. Epidural steroid injections can also be utilized for pain control. Physical modalities can be effective in the initial treatment to help reduce pain and reflex muscle spasm. As the athlete's symptoms improve, a back rehabilitation program can be initiated. Therapy should initially determine which exercises help to centralize pain and reduce radicular pain. Exercises that significantly increase low back pain or radicular pain should be avoided. Therapy should progress as symptoms dictate to involve abdominal, lumbar extensor strengthening. Aerobic activities such as running are allowed if they do not increase symptoms, as only a small percentage of the stress from landing on the ground is transmitted to the lumbar spine. Therapy should also include education to improve poor techniques or body mechanics. As the symptoms resolve, the athlete is progressively returned to full activity.

Zygapophyseal pain

Football players, especially interior linemen, are subjected to repeated and forceful lumbar hyperextension, which can result in injury to the zygapophyseal joints. The athlete usually presents with low back pain that can refer to the buttocks and thighs. There is no clear clinical identifying pain pattern that can reliably diagnose the zygapophyseal joints as the source of pain. Symptoms may be exacerbated by certain movements such as hyperextension, combined extension, and rotation, as well as rising from forward flexion. Initial work-up should include a full physical examination and appropriate imaging studies to exclude other sources of pain.

The current gold standard for diagnosing zygapophyseal mediated pain is anesthetizing the medial branches (medial branch blocks) innervating the suspected painful joints. Each zygapophyseal joint is duly innervated. Therefore, two medial branch blocks must be performed for each joint. There is a high false-positive response to single medial branch blocks; thus, dual blocks are recommended, which significantly decreases the false-positive rate. If the dual blocks each result in substantial pain relief, then radiofrequency lesioning is an appropriate recommendation. The initial treatment for acute zygapophyseal pain is relative rest, medication, and avoidance of exacerbating activities and physical modalities. Extension exercise may exacerbate the athlete's pain. Therefore, flexion and neutral postures and exercises should be emphasized. Aerobic activities that maintain the lumbar spine in flexion such as bicycling, stair climber machines, and walking on an inclined treadmill may be better tolerated by the athlete. Stretching of the lower extremities with particular attention to the hamstrings, hip flexors, and hip internal/external rotators should be included in the exercise program. Strengthening of the abdominal and gluteal musculature should be incorporated into the rehabilitation program as well. The athlete can be progressively returned to normal activities as symptoms dictate. The absence of pain during and following position-specific activities usually indicates that the player can successfully return to play.

Sprain/strain/contusions

Contusions of the lumbar spine in football are usually secondary to a direct blow such as when a helmet strikes the lumbar region during tackling. Pain, muscular spasm, and decreased range of motion can occur. Initial treatment includes relative rest and icing for the first 24–48 hours. If the contusion is severe, one must be aware of possible underlying injury to the kidney and/or spleen. If pain is still significant after 24–48 hours, then the application of heat and utilization of appropriate medication may be helpful. After the acute spasm resolves, a program of progressive stretching and strengthening can be initiated. The area can be protected from further contusion with the use of protective padding. The athlete is able to return to full contact as allowed by pain and discomfort.

Musculoligamentous sprains and strains of the lumbar spine may appear insidiously or have an acute onset. Treatment is similar to sprains and strains in the other areas of the body. Initial treatment consists of relative rest, ice, and medication if necessary for pain control. Rehabilitation focuses on stretching and strengthening of both the abdominals and lumbar paraspinals. Intensity and progression of activities should be guided by symptoms. In most cases, the injury is self-limited and healing occurs without long-term sequelae.

REFERENCES

1. Mueller FO, Blythe CS: Can we continue to improve injury statistics in football? Phys Sports Med 12:79–84, 1984.

2. Beachy G, Akau CK, Martinson W, et al: High school sports injuries, a longitudinal study at Punahou school: 1998 to 1996. Am J Sports Med 25:675–681, 1997.

3. Stuart JM, Morrey MA, Smith AM, et al: Injuries in youth football: a perspective observational cohort analysis among players age 9–13 years. Mayo Clin Proc 77:317–322, 2002.

4. Meeuwisse WH, Hagel BE, Mohtadi NG, et al: The distribution of injuries in mens Canada West university football: a five-year analysis. Am J Sports Med 28:516–523, 2000.

5. Mercer SR, Bogduk NB: Joints of the cervical vertebral column. J Orthop Sport Phys Ther 31:171–182, 2001.

6. Panjabi MM, Crisco JC, Vasquada A, et al: Mechanical properties of the human cervical spine as shown by three-dimensional load-displacement curves. Spine 26:2692–2700, 2001.

7. Pal GP, Sherk HH: The vertical stability of the cervical spine. Spine 13:447, 1988.

8. Schneider RC: Head and neck injuries in football. Mechanisms, treatment and prevention. Baltimore: Williams and Wilkins, 1973.

9. Torg JS, Quedenfield TC, et al: Collision with spring-loaded football tackling and blocking dummies. JAMA 236:1243–1244, 1976.

10. Torg JS, Guille JT, Jaffe SJ: Injuries to the cervical spine in American football players. J Bone Joint Surg Am 84–A:112–122, 2002.

11. Gosch HH, Gooding E, Schneider RC: An experimental study of cervical spine and cord injuries. J Trauma 12:570–576, 1972.

12. Bauze RJ, Ardran GM: Experimental production of forward dislocation in the human cervical spine. Bone Joint Surg Br 60:239–245, 1978.

13. Nightingale RW, McLelhaney JH, et al: Experimental impact injury to the cervical spine: relating motion of the head and the mechanism of injury. J Bone Joint Surg Am 78: 412–421, 1996.

14. Clarke KS: Epidemiology of athletic neck injury. Clin Sports Med 17(1):83–96, 1998.

15. Cantu RC, Mueller FO: Catastrophic football injuries: 1997/1998. Neurosurgery 47:673–675, 2000.

16. Palumbo MA, Hulstyn MJ, Fadale PD, et al: The effect of protective football equipment on alignment of the injured cervical spine. Am J Sports Med 24:446–453, 1996.

17. Donelson WF, Laverman WC, Heil B, et al: Helmet and shoulder pad removal from a player with a suspected cervical spine injury. Spine 23:1729–1733, 1998.

18. Waninger KN, Richards JG, Pan WT: An evaluation of head movement in backboard immobilized helmeted football, lacrosse, and ice hockey players. Clin Sports Med 11:82–86, 2001.

19. Davidson RM, Burton JH, Snowise M, et al: Football protective gear and cervical spine imaging. Ann Emerg Med 38:26–30, 2001.

20. Peris MD, Donaldson WF, Torers J, et al: Helmet and shoulder pad removal in suspected cervical spine injury. Spine 27:995–999, 2002.

21. Clancy WG Jr, Brand RL, Bergfeld JA: Upper trunk brachial plexus injuries in contact sports. Am J Sports Med 5:209–216, 1977.

22. Sallis RE, Jones K, Knoppler: Burners: offensive strategy for an unreported injury. Phys Sports Med 20:47–55, 1992.

23. Nissen SJ, Laskowski ER, Rizzo TD: Burner syndrome recognition and rehabilitation. Phys Sports Med 24:57–64, 1996.

24. Castro FP, Ricciardi J, Brunet ME, et al: Stingers, the Torg ratio in the cervical spine. Am J Sports Med 25:603–608, 1997.

24a. Meyer SA, Schulte KR, Callaghan JJ, et al: Cervical spinal stenosis and stingers in collegiate football players. Am J Sports Med 22:158–166, 1994.

25. Kelly JD, Aliquo D, Sitler MR, et al: Association of burners with cervical canal and foraminal stenosis. Am J Sports Med 28:214–217, 2000.

26. Watkins RG: Neck injuries in football players. Clin Sports Med 5:215–246, 1986.

27. Shannon B, Klimkiewicz JJ: Cervical burners in the athlete. Clin Sports Med 21:29–35, 2002.

28. Stojanovic MP, Vu TN, Caneris O, et al: The role of fluoroscopy in cervical epidural injections. An analysis of contrast dispersal patterns. Spine 27:509–514, 2002.

29. Torg JS, Pavlov H: Cervical spinal stenosis with cord neuropraxia in transient quadriplegia. Clin Sports Med 6:115–133, 1987.

30. Torg JS, Corcoran TA, Thibault LE: Cervical cord neuropraxia: classification, pathomechanics, morbidity, and management guidelines. J Neurosurg 87:843–850, 1997.

31. Ross DS, Swain R: Acute atraumatic quadriparesis in a college football player. Med Sci Sports Exerc 1663–1665, 1998.

32. Torg JS, Naranja RJ, Pavlov H: The relationship of developmental narrowing of the cervical spinal canal to reversible and irreversible injury of the cervical spinal cord in football players. J Bone Joint Surg Am 78:1308–1314, 1996.

33. Boockvar JA, Durham SR, Sun PP: Cervical spinal stenosis in sports-related cervical cord neuropraxia in children. Spine 26:2709–2713, 2001.

34. Penning L: Some aspects of plain radiography of the cervical spine in chronic myelopathy. Neurology 12:513–519, 1962.

34a. Schnirring L: C-spine management guidelines proposed. Phys Sports Med 26:15–16, 1998.

35. Torg JS, Sennett B, Pavlov H, et al: Sphere tacular spine: an entity precluding participation in tackle football and collision activities that expose the cervical spine to axial energy inputs. Am J Sports Med 21:640–649, 1993.

36. Morganti C, Sweeney CA, Albanese SA: Return to play after a cervical spine injury. Spine 26:1131–1136, 2001.

37. Torg JS, Ramsey-Emrhein, JA: Cervical spine and brachial plexus injuries. Return to play recommendations. Phys Sports Med 25:61–88, 1997.

38. Elattrache N, Fadale PD, Fu F, et al: Thoracic spine fracture in a football player. A case report. Am J Sports Med 21:157–160, 1993.

39. Esler AD: Bertolli's syndrome revisited. Transitional vertebra of the lumbar spine. Spine 14:1373, 1989.

40. Dupuis PR: The anatomy of the lumbosacral spine. In: Kirkaldy-Willis WH and Bernard TN, eds. Managing low back pain, 4th edn. Philadelphia: Churchill Livingstone; 1999:10–27.

41. Schnebel BE, Simmons JW, Chowning J, et al: A digitizing technique for the study of movement of interdiskal dye in response to flexion and extension of the lumbar spine. Spine 12:309–312, 1988.

42. Fujiwana A, An HS, Lim TH, et al: Multilogic changes in the lumbar intervertebral foramen due to flexion/extension, lateral bending, and axial rotation. Spine 26:876–882, 2001.

43. Gatt CJ, Hozea TM, Palumbo RC, et al: Impact loading of the lumbar spine during football blocking. Am J Sports Med 25:317–321, 1997.

44. Edwards WT, Ondway NR, Zheng Y, et al: Peak stresses observed in the posterior lateral anulus. Spine 26:1753–1759, 2001.

CHAPTER

10

Basketball and the Spine

Bryan Williamson
Robert Tillman

Narrowing down the possible spine injuries a basketball player is likely to sustain requires that the topic be narrowed by position as well as location within the spine. In interviewing multiple college- and professional-level athletes and trainers, it appears that most spine injuries involve extreme movements of the lumbar spine, including hyperextension, overloading of the lumbar spine during contact with another player, or hyperflexion. There is very limited published information that could be found regarding the number of spine-related injuries from basketball, or current types of treatment specific to spine-related basketball injuries. The most comprehensive study was sponsored by the National Athletic Trainers Association (NATA), which involved the data collection of the most prevalent injuries in the most popular sports, of which basketball was one sport in the study.[1] What is evident in the literature is that spine injuries are quite rare compared with most other categories of injury in the sport of basketball. Foot/ankle injuries account for 35–40% of injuries in both male and female high school basketball players. Hip/thigh/leg injuries account for 14–16% of male/female basketball injuries; knee injuries make up 10–13%, forearm/wrist/hand injuries account for about 10%, and face/scalp injuries account for 8–12%. Spine injuries appear to be very limited in basketball players, although no sport is without some occurrence of all types of injuries. What information was found supported the fact that most spine injuries are lumbar in nature, and involve hyperextension, overloading due to contact with another player, and to a lesser extent, hyperflexion.[2]

Lumbar hyperextension injuries can occur due to repeated hyperextension movements. This is seen most often in centers, forwards, and post players, who are often aggressively leaping and hyperextending while fighting to rebound the basketball. Most extremes of spine motion and player contact occur directly under or around the basketball goal, either during an attempted shot/score or rebound. Overloading the spine due to one player jumping and inadvertently landing on another player while either in the extended or flexed position can increase the complexity of the injury. The following example is a sequence of events that could lead to such an injury.

The play involves a head and or body fake, as the post or center attempts to deceive his defender into reacting by leaping too soon in an attempt to block or intercept the post/center's effort to score a basket down low in the "paint." The event involves timing by the offensive player. As the defender is drawn to jump too soon, the offensive player attempts to jump as soon as the defender is in the air, utilizing the split second that the defender has stalled in his leap, to jump himself while rotating toward the basket and score. If timing is off, or if the defender jumps forward toward the offensive player rather than vertically, impact occurs while the offensive player is exploding up and rotating from a crouched position. The defender lands, or loads the offensive player's back, while the offensive player is moving from a flexed to an extended and rotated torso position. The unexpected load, combined with the extension/rotation motion, can lead to a mechanical low back injury serious enough to prevent further play without medical and rehabilitative intervention.

DYNAMICS OF SPINE MOTION

Although cervical and thoracic injury and dysfunction are known to occur in basketball players, the most common spine injuries involve the lumbar spine. As a result, only the dynamics of lumbar joint mechanics are described below.

The lumbar zygapophyseal joints, while maintaining a flexed position, rotate and laterally flex in the same direction.[3,4] While maintaining or moving into a neutral or extended joint position in the lumbar spine, lateral flexion and rotation occur in the opposite directions.[5-7] As applied to the dynamics of the basketball player, when the post or center turns away from the basket and reaches to receive a pass, a flexed lumbar spine position is created. This allows flexion and gapping of the posterior lumbar segments. The player may "fake" a turn either right or left in this position in order to draw his defender standing between himself and the basket into the air, then prepares to explode up and rotate toward the basket to score. An understanding of lumbar arthrokinematics, including coupled motion of the facet during a transition from a lumbar flexed position into an extended and rotated position is necessary when discussing pathology related to mechanical dysfunction. This aggressive reversal of motion, topped with the weight of the defending player loading the offensive players back during the extension and rotation movement, leads to a combination of possible lumbar facet joint and surrounding connective, muscular, and interjoint tissue injuries. The combination of injuries has been previously labeled "The Manual Therapy Lesion,"[8] and the following tissue damage may occur:

1. A tear in one or more facet capsules due to the explosive and high-speed reversal of joint mechanics of the facets within the capsule(s) while moving from a flexed, to an extended and rotated position.

2. Damage to Type I mechanoreceptors[9-11] in the capsule. Type I receptors (also known as Golgi–Mazzoni corpuscles) are responsible for kinesthetic awareness of joint motion.[10,11] They are located in the most superficial layers of the facet capsule. Injury to the capsule itself leads to damage to the receptor system, and loss of the ability to recruit tonic muscle fibers such as the multifidi and rotatory muscles that directly cross and support the lumbar facet joints.[10,12]

3. Entrapment of the fibroadipose meniscoid[13] within the facet joint during the reversal of the flexed, gapped facet as it aggressively moves back into a closed pack, extended position within the capsule. The normally free-floating meniscoid which typically acts as a friction-reducing pad between the inferior and superior articular surfaces of the facet joint is now moved out of place within the capsule, and acts as a painful space-occupying lesion that is repeatedly impacted by the edge of the inferior articular process each time the athlete attempts to move into a fully upright or rotated position.

4. Acute sharp pain, a result of stimulation of the Type IV mechanoreceptors in the capsule and fibroadipose meniscoid structures. Type IV mechanoreceptors (also known as free nerve endings)[14] are stimulated to fire with the onset of tissue damage, and stimulate the CNS to propagate a pain response in the area surrounding the tissue damage. With pain and tissue damage comes tonic muscle guarding, inflammation, loss of mobility, and subsequent loss of the ability to play basketball. Prolonged tonic guarding due to repeated reirritation of the injury site in an attempt to play or practice leads to atrophy of tonic muscles surrounding the involved lumbar segments. Weakened tonic musculature surrounding the involved facet joints means correct, precise motion around a physiologic axis can no longer be controlled.

5. The inability to control a physiologic axis of motion or axis of rotation[15] around a segment leads to repeated interjoint and capsular damage, increased meniscoid locking, and progressive degeneration of the articular surfaces.

6. The inability to maintain a normal physiologic axis now leads to frequent severe episodes of low back pain, restricted trunk motion due to pain, muscle guarding, and joint entrapment, and loss of practice and playing time.

7. Alteration of facet joint motion into extreme rotation with extension under a load could even place abnormal shear stresses through the intervertebral disc, and play a role in either a circumferential tear of the annulus,[16,17] or the early onset of degenerative disc disease due to the asymptomatic occurrence of vertebral end-plate fractures.[18,19]

DIFFERENTIAL DIAGNOSIS OF RELATED LUMBAR SPINE PATHOLOGY

It is important prior to any rehabilitation process or clearance to participate further in basketball play or practice to rule out the lumbar pathology given in Box 10.1.

All of the factors given in Box 10.1 require radiographic and or magnetic resonance imaging (MRI) followed by physician interpretation of diagnostic tests. Pathology related to a heavy load being placed on the lumbar spine while transitioning into dynamic rotation and extension from a forward flexed, or at least mid-range lumbar spine position, can involve one or two types of tissue, or multiple types of tissue involvement.[16] Determining the extent of tissue damage involves a complete spine evaluation, followed by an organized rehabilitation program based on three factors:

1. mechanical and histologic assessment of the spine dysfunction
2. correlation of the physical assessment with available diagnostic studies
3. implementation of appropriate manual therapy, therapeutic exercise, and adjunct modalities as indicated.

Box 10.1 Lumbar pathology

1. Unstable spondylolisthesis
2. Pedicle fracture
3. Vertebral body compression fracture
4. Acute disc herniation

REHABILITATION

Rehabilitation of the injury described above begins with a complete physical evaluation of the athlete. Box 10.2 outlines the systematic steps through the evaluation process.

Special attention should be given to making the determination during the evaluation if the primary dysfunction is arthrokinematic, including joint movement and connective tissue integrity, or contractile, involving primarily a muscular component. The use of Cyriax's differential diagnosis concepts can be of much benefit at this point in the evaluation and determination of the clinical course of action for the athlete.

It is important to note that failing to assess any of the various aspects of a spine evaluation may lead to a non-specific tissue assessment, prolonged injury time, prolonged rehabilitation time, and increased down time for the athlete.

Box 10.2 The evaluation process

- Initial observation
- History & interview
- Visual inspection
- Active movement
- Passive movement
- Resisted muscle testing/Cyriax's differential diagnosis
- Palpation
- Reflex testing
- Sensory & neurologic testing
- Segmental joint play testing
- Assessment and diagnosis
- Contraindications to treatment
- Plan of care

CORRELATION OF FINDINGS

The basketball player who sustains a lumbar spine hyperextension and/or overload injury while dynamically moving into lumbar extension and rotation will often demonstrate the following characteristics upon physical examination:

1. Acute pain and muscle guarding.
2. Inability to return to an upright standing position.
3. Significant limitation to rotation in one direction; minimal or moderate limitation into rotation in the opposite direction.
4. Significant limitation into sidebending and rotation in opposite directions (e.g., athlete unable to stand fully erect; 75–90% limited into lumbar right rotation; 75–90% limited into lumbar left sidebending).
5. Palpation reveals aggressive muscle guarding of the lumbar multifidi. Palpation of the posterior superficial interspinous ligaments is painful.

6. Reflexes are either normal or hyper-reflexive.

7. Resisted examination often reveals significant pain and minimal weakness in one part of lumbar rotation, and minimal pain in two parts of lumbar rotation. Sidebending reveals the same type of finding. Significant pain and minimal weakness in sidebending to one side. Minimal pain and weakness to sidebending in the mid-range or end-range toward the opposite side.

8. Placing the athlete in a slightly lumbarflexed position and resisting the motion of extension and rotation reproduces symptoms, and is moderately weak.

9. Assessment of segmental mobility is difficult initially due to muscle spasm/guarding, but, as symptoms reduce, joint play often reveals the facet joint restriction on one side of the lumbar spine into rotation and extension. Loading/compression of the segment, especially with an extension component, reproduces significant pain and increased muscle guarding.

10. Nerve tension tests are most often either negative, or turn negative within 48 hours from the time of injury.

INVOLVED PATHOLOGY

A brief review of structural anatomy will show the tissues most often affected with overload to the lumbar spine during a dynamic extension and rotation movement. Posteriorly, the tissues most often in lesion include the facet capsule, fibromeniscoid interarticular pad or plica of the facet, the supraspinous ligament, interspinous ligament, and possibly the ligamentum flavum (Fig. 10.1). If the load of the defensive player falling onto the offensive player as he turns to attempt to score is too great, the lumbar rotary and extensor muscle groups, including the multifidus, longissimus, and erector spinae, are all at risk. Which of the above structures is in actual lesion is assessed upon complete physical evaluation (Box 10.2).

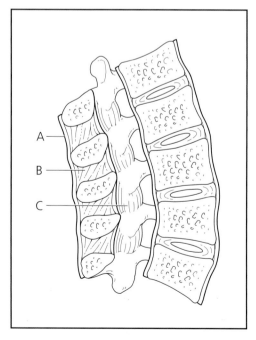

Figure 10.1
A. Supraspinous ligament.
B. Interspinous ligament.
C. Ligamentum flavum.

TREATMENT

Phase I

Goals

The goals of phase I treatment are:

- control of pain and muscle guarding
- stimulation of muscular and connective tissue healing through appropriate mechanical stress
- unloading of impinged/entrapped intra-articular and capsular structures.

Treatment

Phase I treatment is initiated if the player is in acute distress, unable to achieve an upright position, and has been cleared through diagnostic testing.

1. Use of superficial heat, cold, and e-stim to produce a high-intensity afferent stimulus to the dorsal horn for temporary symptom control.[20]

2. Manual therapy:
   - Position patient in sidelying, with the involved side of the lumbar spine off the treatment table. A pillow may be placed under the patient's side to increase lateral flexion away from the lumbar facet joints and tissue that need to be unloaded (Fig. 10.2).
   - Block the segment just above the area of lesion, and apply a mid to end-range mobilization into rotation of the segment above (Fig. 10.3). Due to multisegment innervation by the medial branch of the posterior primary rami, which innervates the facet joints up to three segments above and below a particular segment, an inhibitory effect can occur by mobilization of the facet above the segment in lesion, reducing pain and guarding at the area of injury. (See Ref. 21, Fig. 5 – the nociceptive receptor system.)

3. Therapeutic exercise:
   - This therapeutic exercise regimen follows the Medical Exercise Training (MET) rationale.[22,23] Initial goals for exercise include flushing of injury metabolites collected in the surrounding tissue, reduction of muscle guarding, prevention of muscle wasting, and stimulation of muscular and connective tissue healing processes through correctly dosed therapeutic exercise.

After evaluation of the patient to determine the extent of acute tissue injury, and performing manual therapy techniques to reduce or inhibit acute symptoms, the clinician has a short opportunity to initiate an exercise regimen that will work to achieve the above stated goals of initial MET. Activities such as 3–5 minutes of mid-range, below pain supine torso rocking (Fig. 10.4A and B), initiation of a bridging movement (Fig. 10.5), and mid-range pulley-resisted sidelying lumbar rotation with a resistance that the

Figure 10.2
Positioning of the athlete to unload facet joint surfaces and reduce stress on surrounding soft tissues.

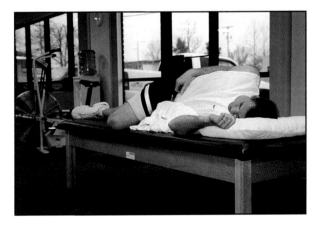

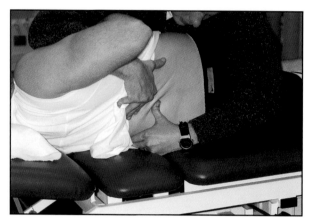

Figure 10.3
Mobilization of the spine segment above the segment in lesion.

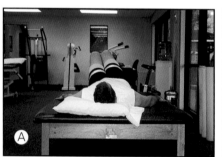

Figure 10.4
A. Supine torso rocking.
B. Supine torso rocking; notice the motion of the lower extremities and torso is small, with a relatively quick velocity.

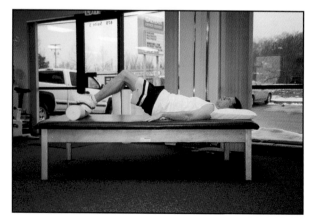

Figure 10.5
Bridging exercise. Use of a bolster roll under the feet may be omitted if the athlete reports pain during the exercise.

Figure 10.6
Pulley-resisted sidelying lumbar rotation. Range of exercise motion and resistance must occur without creating additional pain and muscle guarding of the injured spine segment.

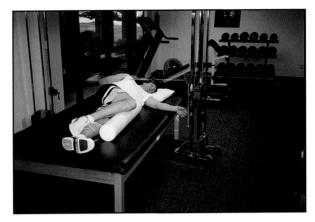

athlete can successfully complete 3–5 sets of 30 repetitions (Fig. 10.6). Based on the Holten diagram, and supporting research by Odvar Holten et al,[22,23] exercise with 30 repetitions (60% of 1 RM) causes multiple positive effects to tissue in the initial stages of healing. Of most importance is an increase in blood flow to muscle, prevention of atrophy without causing additional muscle trauma, flushing of metabolites from the injury region, and stimulation of Type I and II mechanoreceptors, which influence joint control and inhibit nociceptor input to the dorsal horn.[20]

Phase II

Goals

As acute symptoms lessen, due to manual techniques and exercise stress on recovering tissue, and pain-free lumbar active motion returns, therapeutic exercise goals change. New goals include:

- Progression from only unloaded supine and sidelying exercise positions, to both prone and standing during exercise.
- Progression from resistance and repetition levels designed to flush injury metabolites and stimulate tissue regeneration, to exercise resistance and repetition levels that challenge weakened muscular and connective tissues.

Therapeutic exercise

- Standing resisted torso rotation combined with a forward flexion component (Fig. 10.7) begins to recoordinate and strengthen synergistic trunk control. Forward flexion and rotation reinitiate the combined synergistic action of the abdominal rotatory groups primarily. Exercise is performed at 75–80% 1 RM (11–16 repetitions per set).
- Mid-range torso reverse rotation in a backward rotary direction primarily forces the lumbar rotary muscle groups to initiate and control torso motion, with the abdominal rotary muscles combining to keep the motion in the axial plane (Fig. 10.8). Exercise is again performed in the 11–16 repetitions per set range.
- Isolation of the lumbar rotary groups can be accomplished by performing a sidelying reverse rotation against resistance using a spine pulley and strap placed so that the resistance vector is through the hip, not the shoulder (Fig. 10.9A and B). Exercise is performed at 60% 1 RM for 3–5 sets of 30 repetitions.
- Combined prone extension and rotation place a direct mechanical exercise stress through the weakened connective and muscular tissue. Initially, this motion should begin in a flexed torso/lumbar position, and end in the mid-range of lumbar extension (Fig. 10.10A–D). As the athlete progresses

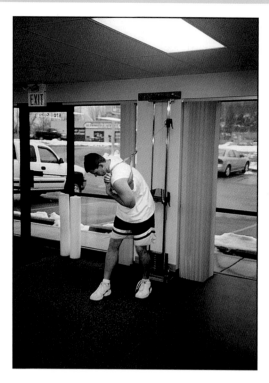

Figure 10.7
Standing resisted forward torso rotation using a spine pulley.

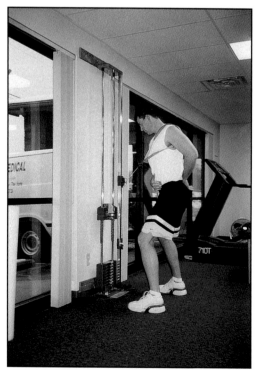

Figure 10.8
Mid-range torso reverse rotation using a spine pulley.

Figure 10.9

A. Recovery exercise of the lumbar rotary muscle groups at the injured area of the lumbar spine.

B. Exercise range of motion is small, isolating primarily the lumbar multifidi and quadratus lumborum muscle groups.

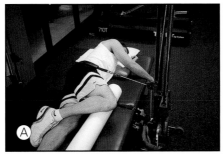
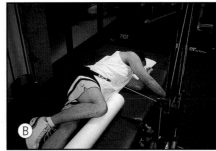

Figure 10.10

A. Initial lumbar extension exercise beginning in a flexed lumbar position and ending prior to moving past a neutral position.

B. Progression of the lumbar extension exercise into a full extension motion.

C. Initial phase of combined lumbar extension with torso rotation.

D. Progression of aggressive lumbar extension with torso rotation into a greater extension range of motion.

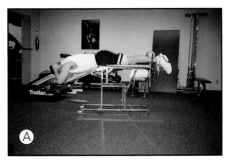
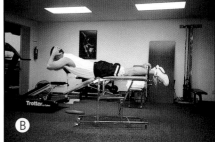
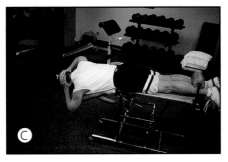
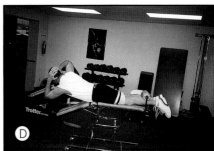

in tolerance to a resisted load into lumbar extension and rotation, the movement can begin to move through the full range of lumbar motion.

• Slideboard (Fig. 10.11) lateral drills in which the athlete is required to maintain a mid-range, lordotic lumbar spine while lateral, full-speed dynamic strength and coordination is developed is an excellent activity that assists the athlete in regaining proprioceptive awareness of a strong lumbar position during dynamic lower extremity movement. Usually the slideboard is performed for aggressive 1–2 minute intervals, often up to 5–6 sets.

• Progression back into basketball drills, but not into actual practice at full speed against other players.

Phase III

Goals

Phase III is a return to full practice and play. Prior to participation in an actual game situation, the athlete must demonstrate a full capability to perform in his designated position during full-court, full-speed

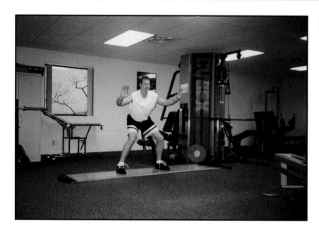

Figure 10.11
Slideboard position drills.

practice sessions against a practice team. Goals of the third phase of rehabilitation include:

- full-trunk AROM symptom free
- full return of proprioceptive control of the lumbar spine during dynamic movement
- full-speed individual basketball drills
- full-speed, full-court capability.
- return of pre-injury trunk and lower extremity strength levels.

Therapeutic and sport-specific exercise

- Continuation of slideboard exercise.
- Use of speed pulleys, which allow resistance to full-speed dynamic drills that simulate basketball activities (Fig. 10.12A–C).
- Inertial Trainer for coordinated high-speed lumbar synergistic gains (Fig. 10.13).
- Progression into full practice activities, no limitations.
- Progression back into competitive basketball.

CONCLUSION

Most spine-related basketball injuries involve hyperextension, loading of the spine due to player contact, and to a lesser extent, hyperflexion injuries. Isolated lumbar hyperextension dysfunction is fairly common, and relatively simple to diagnose and treat in basketball players. Many times, the mechanism of injury involves a combination of a compressive load during a combined rotation and extension motion that generates a much more complicated injury. Taking the time to complete a full physical examination of the lumbar spine and surrounding joints is imperative in order to fully address the potentially complicated multi-tissue type injury. It is very easy to rationalize how other related pathology, such as SI joint dysfunction, or isolated acute intervertebral disc herniation could occur, especially with a compressive overload due to player contact. Rehabilitation can be grouped into three separate phases with three separate goals of therapeutic exercise. Phase I involves unloading the tissue of compression during full-weight-bearing loads by exercising in the supine or sidelying position. Goals of treatment are the flushing of metabolic byproducts due to tissue breakdown, control of acute symptoms, and stimulation of tissue regeneration through appropriately dosed therapeutic exercise. Manual therapy techniques are used initially if the facet intra-articular fat pad and meniscoid structure is determined to be impinged or entrapped. Exercise is dosed around 30% of the contractile tissue's 1 RM, for 3–5 sets of 30 repetitions. All exercise is dosed and performed at a level that does not increase acute symptoms of pain or guarding. The time frame of Phase I is mostly dependent on the severity of acute tissue damage from the injury.

Figure 10.12
A. Straight line acceleration simulation using speed pulley.
B and **C.** Reproduction of the movement that created the initial injury, full speed against pulley resistance.

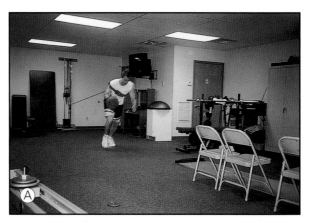

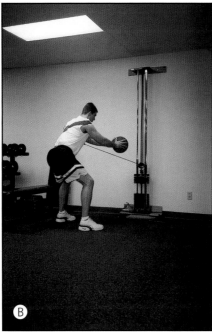

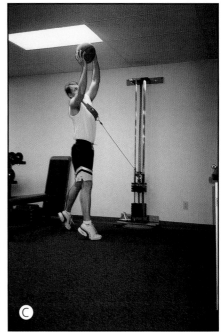

Mild connective tissue damage may only require 3–7 days of Phase I exercise and manual intervention, prior to progressing onto more loaded and resistive Phase II activities. More extensive tissue damage may require the athlete to spend a period of weeks performing tissue regeneration level activities before a level of tissue integrity is reached that will handle a more compressive or resistive load that leads to Phase II activities.

Phase II of the rehabilitation involves progression from levels of resistance and repetition necessary to stimulate tissue regeneration and remove injury metabolites, to providing a specifically dosed amount of tissue stress through exercise necessary to progress healing, weak tissue back to normal levels of contractile strength and connective stability. Exercise doses are changed from light-resistance, high-repetition, mid-range activities to appropriately heavy, lower-repetition, full-range activities that challenge tissue through multiple planes of torso movement. Ultimately, Phase II activities should return the athlete to a level of preparedness to begin individual sport-specific drills, initially at less than full speed, but quickly progressing to full-speed drills.

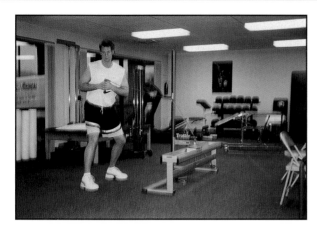

Figure 10.13
Inertial Trainer used as a high-speed lumbar/abdominal synergist control exercise.

Phase III of the rehabilitation concentrates less on isolated tissue healing or strengthening, and more on neuromuscular recruitment and proprioceptive control of thoracolumbar and lumbosacral joint motion. Strengthening at this point is more of a conditioning of the athlete. Aerobic activities, short-burst anaerobic activities, and full-speed return to basketball practice are all incorporated. The athlete moves back into practicing full court with the team in game situations against a practice squad. Rehabilitation activities involve low-resistance, high-speed activities that simulate sport-specific movements, or high-speed trunk synergistic movements that force greater lumbar segmental control during dynamic motion. The actual rehabilitation of the athlete is slowly eliminated, with the physical therapist or athletic trainer at this stage primarily monitoring the athlete to insure a successful recovery and return to sport.

REFERENCES

1. National Athletic Trainers Association Injury Surveillance Study: A three year multi-sport surveillance study released Sept. 21, 1999 via multiple media sites, including NATA's web page: www.nata.org/publications/press_releases/resultof3yearstudy.htm

2. Watkins RG: The spine in sports. St Louis: Mosby; 1996:431.

3. Mitchell FL, Moran PS, Pruzzo NA: An evaluation and treatment manual of osteopathic muscle energy procedures. Valley Park, MO: Pruzzo; 1979.

4. Grimsby O: The Ola Grimsby Institute, San Diego, CA, 1980.

5. Panjabi MM, Hausfield J, White A: Experimental determination of thoracic spine stability. Presented at the 24th Annual Meeting of Orthopaedic Research Society, Dallas, 1978.

6. Grimsby O: The Ola Grimsby Institute, San Diego, CA, 1980.

7. Miles M, Sullivan WE: Lateral bending at the lumbar and lumbosacral joints. Anat Rec 139:387, 1961.

8. Ola Grimsby Institute: MT-1, clinical and scientific rationale for modern manual therapy. Section 6. 1998:11, 12.

9. Ola Grimsby Institute: MT-1 clinical and scientific rationale for modern manual therapy. Section 5. 1998:15–19.

10. Dvorak J, Dvorak V: Manual medicine diagnostics, 2nd edn. New York: Thieme Medical; Table 2.1; 1990:47.

11. Gould J, Davies G: Orthopaed Sports Phys Ther. St Louis: CV Mosby; Table 2–1; 1985:53.

12. Ola Grimsby Institute: MT-1 clinical and scientific rationale for modern manual therapy. Section 5. 1998:26.

13. Bogduk N, Twomey L: Clinical anatomy of the lumbar spine, 2nd edn. Edinburgh: Churchill Livingstone; 1991:162–164.

14. Hall, Craigs: Anatomy as a basis for clinical medicine, 2nd edn. Baltimore: Urban & Schwarzenberg; 1990:47.

15. Bogduk N, Twomey L: Clinical anatomy of the lumbar spine, 2nd edn. Edinburgh: Churchill Livingstone; 1991:53, 54.

16. Bogduk N, Twomey L: Clinical anatomy of the lumbar spine, 2nd edn. Edinburgh: Churchill Livingstone; 1991:164, 165.

17. Bogduk N, Twomey L: Clinical anatomy of the lumbar spine, 2nd edn. Edinburgh: Churchill Livingstone; Figure 14.4; 1991:166.

18. Farfan HF, Cossette JW, Robertson GH, et al: The effects of torsion on the lumbar intervertebral joints: the role of torsion in the production of disc degeneration. J Bone Joint Surgery (Am) 52A:468–497, 1970.

19. Farfan HF: Mechanical disorders of the low back. Philadelphia: Lea & Febiger; 1973.

20. Dvorak J, Dvorak V: Manual medicine diagnostics, 2nd edn. New York: Thieme Medical; 1990:37, 38.

21. Wyke BD: The neurological basis of thoracic spinal pain. Rhem Phys Med 10:356, 1976.

22. Holten O: Medical exercise therapy. Holten Institutt (in coordination with the Sorlandets Fysikalske Institutt), 1986.

23. Ola Grimsby Institute: MT-1 clinical and scientific rationale for modern manual therapy: Section 5. 1998:26.

FURTHER READING

Bogduk N, Twomey L: Clinical anatomy of the lumbar spine, 2nd edn. Edinburgh: Churchill Livingstone; 1991:57, 70, 162–164.

Cyriax J: Textbook of orthopaedic medicine, Vol. 1: Diagnosis of soft tissue lesions, 8th edn. London: Ballière Tindall; 1978.

Gould J, Davies G: Orthop Sports Phys Ther II. St Louis: CV Mosby; 1985:114–116.

Gray, H: Gray's anatomy, 36th British edn. Philadelphia: WB Saunders; 1986.

Grieve GP: Common vertebral joint problems: Edinburgh: Churchill Livingstone; 1981: 253, 254, 256, 257.

Kandel ER, Schwartz JH, Jessell TM: Principles of neural science, 3rd edn. Norwalk, CJ: Appleton & Lange; Chap. 27; 1996:392–393.

Ola Grimsby Institute: MT-1 clinical and scientific rationale for modern manual therapy. Section 5. 1998:26.

Tillman R: Rehabilitation of the sacroiliac patient. Sci Phys Ther 3/4, 1992.

Wyke BD: Neurological mechanisms in the experience of pain. Acupuncture and electro-therapy Res 4:27, 1979.

11

Gymnastics and Spine Injuries

Heidi Prather
John Metzler

INTRODUCTION

Gymnastics is a popular sport that continues to grow in numbers of participants and fans. There are several forms of gymnastics, and gymnastic maneuvers are a central part of many sports outside of gymnastic competition. The Internationale Federation de Gymnastique oversees five different forms of gymnastics: men's artistic gymnastics, women's artistic gymnastics, rhythmic sports gymnastics, general gymnastics, and sports aerobics. The USA Gymnastics Organization reports there are 3 million recreational gymnasts and 85 000 competitive athletes in the United States supported by 4000 clubs.[1] This growing sport places high demands on the participants' musculoskeletal system. Special care in management of musculoskeletal problems as they arise is necessary to effectively return the athlete to participation. Understanding biomechanics and training techniques is essential for the healthcare provider managing gymnasts' musculoskeletal problems as well as devising a program to prevent injury.

Special considerations are necessary when managing an athlete with back pain. Gymnasts are at risk for spine injury and/or pain because of the high force load transmission that occurs across the trunk and the repetitive end ranges of motion that are required. Early diagnosis of the specific spine problem is important to avoid lengthy time away from sport. This chapter will discuss the biomechanics of the sport, common spine problems that occur in participants, sports-specific rehabilitation, and training techniques to help avoid future injury.

BIOMECHANICS

Gymnasts place demands on their musculoskeletal system to respond to large amounts of force transmission in short bursts, often repetitively with an accurate, controlled response (Fig. 11.1). These large forces and load transmissions are generated by muscles and tendons to control translation and rotation effects of large reaction forces.[2] If the muscle and tendons are unable to react effectively to these forces, ligaments, bones, and soft tissues will absorb the excess force. The ability of the muscles and tendons to produce an effective force may be compromised if the gymnast is unable to anticipate a load, if the muscle and tendon unit is weak because of inappropriate length, if poor muscle coordination is present, or if neuromuscular fatigue is a problem. Hence, any breakdown in this chain of required sequence of force generation and absorption will put the gymnast at risk for injury. A direct causal relationship between load and injury is difficult to determine because of the inability to measure the forces of the individual components of the musculoskeletal system.[3,4]

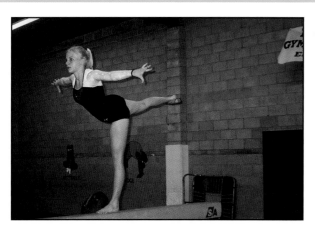

Figure 11.1
Gymnast on balance beam.

In competition, gymnasts perform before a panel of judges and are scored according to the Code of Points. This Code of Points is a document that continues to change with the sport. The evaluation process includes the gymnast's artistic presentation, routine composition and skill amplitude, originality, and difficulty. Gymnasts must continue to master more difficult skills in order to remain competitive. Therefore, as skill and difficulty increase, the total body center of mass velocity at contact and the level of reaction force experienced as a result of contact with the apparatus also increase.

Gymnasts develop skills to perform a variety of movements, including balance, agility, flexibility, strength, and coordination. Participants also learn to anticipate and control large reaction forces applied to the body in multiple directions during hand and foot interaction with mats or gymnastic apparatus. As a result, gymnasts learn to stabilize joints in order to resist external forces and/or limit body segmentation in order to improve movement aesthetics. In general, gymnasts tend to be small in stature. One study has shown that gymnasts also tend to be stronger relative to their body mass as compared to age-matched controls.[5] Claessens and colleagues also showed that gymnasts tend to weigh less and are shorter than age-matched controls. However, when segment lengths in relationship to stature were measured, gymnasts and controls were the same. Gymnasts' ability to generate muscle force consistently and control multiple joint movements simultaneously enables them to use effective compensatory mechanisms if one portion of the kinetic chain is inefficient or injured. As a result, gymnasts learn to stabilize joints in order to resist external forces and to limit body segmentation in order to improve aesthetics.

Male gymnasts compete on six apparatuses, whereas female gymnasts compete on four. These apparatuses will vary between events in height, shape, and mechanical properties, according to gender: for example the bar material suspension system, bar shape, and height are different in male and female bar events. Landing surface thicknesses also differ between male and female events. These differences are important when considering gender differences with regards to injury patterns. Male and female gymnasts may be required to execute the same skill but these differences in apparatuses apply different mechanical loads. In general, male gymnasts are often required to perform more upper extremity control reaction forces applied through the hands by the apparatuses such as on the rings, parallel bars, or pommel horse. Females participating in the uneven bar event are at a disadvantage as compared to their male counterparts because the low bar will reduce time and limits the distance the female gymnast can position her total body center of mass away from the bar during the downswing from a giant circle performed on the high bar. A male gymnast performs a giant swing on the high bar with an unrestricted downswing. In comparing these two differences the female gymnast may need to decrease the distance of her total body center of mass relative to the bar during the downswing. One means of doing so would be hyperextension at the lumbar spine. Recently, modifications were made to place the bars further apart to help reduce this mechanical disadvantage. This enables the gymnast to position her total body center of mass farther from the high bar for a longer period of time and reduces the need for compensatory responses. Even with these modifications, the female gymnast still has a relative mechanical disadvantage during the downswing of a giant swing as compared to males performing the same skill.[6]

The interaction between the gymnast's hand and foot with the apparatus occurs very quickly, often-times in less than 0.25 seconds. As a result, even a small difference in mechanical response to the apparatus between different venues may require the gymnast to modify his technique before or during a per-formance. Because total body momentum is generated throughout a performance through a series of skills, a missed interaction with one hand or foot contact in a series may have a detrimental effect on the final skill performed. As a result, the gymnast needs to be able to adapt to the variation in apparatuses that occurs in all events. Gymnasts need training in a manner such that it allows them to effectively control reaction forces in a multitude of conditions. If the gymnast is not able to adapt well, compensatory actions may be used to control changes in these reaction forces, which may then contribute to detrimental load distribution and possibly lead to injury.

Classification systems have been developed to break down the different movements involved in these skills for analysis purposes. One classification by Bruggeman[7] grouped skills into five categories:

1. takeoff and push off from solid or elastic surface
2. rotations in vertical plane about a fixed or flexible horizontal axis of rotation
3. rotations in a vertical plane about a vertical axis of rotation
4. airborne rotations
5. landings.

A significant number of studies[7–17] have analyzed different skills and requirements for the individual apparatuses. A few examples of concepts analyzed biomechanically include angular momentum, moment of inertia, torque, and kinetic energy. These concepts are analyzed for specific apparatuses. An example would be a study by Brown and colleagues[14] that specifically analyzed ground reactive forces on dismounts from a balance beam. They found the ground reactive forces of a simple dismount to be $10 \times$ body weight. A follow-up study of a more difficult somersault dismount was analyzed and was found to be $13 \times$ body weight. During landings and interactions with apparatuses, the trunk and pelvis absorb the forces that have not been attenuated through the extremities. The athlete may incur or aggravate trunk injuries when performing landings that include controlling large forces, rotation, or hyperextension.[18–20]

SPORT-SPECIFIC INJURIES

The spine is a commonly reported injury site in gymnastics. A 1980 review reported that 12.2% of injuries to female gymnasts were related to the spine.[21] Airborne dismounts, flips, and twists present the potential for acute neurologic injury. While traumatic injuries do occur, spine injuries related to gymnastics are more commonly due to chronic repetitive forces placed on the spine. Gymnastics imposes great demands on the strength and mobility of the spine. Most gymnasts reach the peak of their career, and are thus at the highest level of training during adolescence. Growth spurts experienced by adolescent gymnasts further increase the vulnerability to injury.[22] Sward et al, in their survey of elite Swedish athletes, found that 85% of the male gymnasts and 65% of the female gymnasts experienced back pain.[23]

Once a gymnast has suffered an injury, determining the specific structure or structures involved can be difficult. When possible, identifying the primary cause of injury and recognizing pain that occurs related to secondary adaptive changes is helpful. An example would be recognizing bony pain involved in an acute spondylolysis and secondary muscle pain related to muscle spasm and/or fatigue. If the muscle pain is not addressed, muscle shortening and inhibition may follow. When the spondylolysis achieves bony healing, if muscle imbalance continues the gymnast may be at risk for a second injury. Gymnastics demands the musculoskeletal system absorb and transmit forces in short high-velocity bursts as well as maintain positions that require significant muscle endurance and control. As a result, gymnasts are prone to specific injuries due to the unique demands of their sport.[24–26]

Gymnasts sustain injuries to the spine that are seen in other athletic and non-athletic populations. However, the relative frequency of these injuries can be much different in the gymnast. Micheli and Wood demonstrated a significant difference in the etiology of lower back pain in an adolescent athlete when compared with an adult.[27] The authors retrospectively reviewed files of 100 adolescents presenting with a complaint of low back pain. These findings were compared with files from an adult back clinic. The review demonstrated that discogenic pain was far more common in adults, with 48 of the 100 adult files reviewed listing discogenic pain as the etiology. In comparison, 11 of the 100 adolescents were diagnosed with discogenic pain. Spondylolysis and spondylolisthesis were the most common (47 of 100 cases) cause of adolescent back pain. In comparison, only 5 of the 100 adult cases were listed as spondylolysis or spondylolisthesis.[28] The incidences of spondylolysis and spondylolisthesis are further increased in the adolescent who participates in gymnastics.[29] Only limited data exist that document the incidence of pars interarticularis injuries in gymnasts.[26,29,30] Studies documenting the incidence of other spinal injuries (such as disc injuries) are even sparser and are generally limited to studies of small select populations.[22,26]

With regard to the adolescent complaining of back pain, abnormalities are commonly found on appropriate imaging studies.[28] Likewise, several studies[26,29,30] demonstrate that gymnasts, often have objective findings on imaging studies that may correlate with their complaints. In the gymnast with complaints of persistent back pain, one should be careful to avoid nonspecific diagnoses such as "lumbar strain" and "myofascial pain." Rather, a thorough history and examination with appropriate radiologic studies should be pursued.

Spondylolysis and spondylolisthesis

Spondylolisthesis and spondylolysis are common causes of lower back pain in adolescents and the incidence is further increased in adolescents who participate in gymnastics.[28,29] Patients will usually complain of vague low back pain that may radiate to the buttock or posterior thighs. The pain is typically worse with standing and further provoked by movements that incorporate extension or extension and rotation.[24]

The term "spondylolisthesis" was first used in 1854 and refers to the slippage of one vertebra forward on another.[25] The word comes from the Greek "*spondylo*," meaning vertebra and "*olisthesis*," meaning to slip or slide down a slippery slope. The Greek "*lysis*" refers to a loosening or coming apart.[25] Spondylolysis refers to dissolution at the pars interarticularis without slipping.[25] Spondylitic injuries are most common at the L5 level. Soler and Calderon found 84% of the lesions seen on X-ray to be located at L5, 12% were located at L4, with the rest being distributed over the remaining lumbar segments (Fig. 11.2).

Newman classified spondylolisthesis into five different subtypes: congenital (dysplastic), isthmic, degenerative, traumatic, and pathologic. An isthmic spondylolisthesis is most commonly seen in gymnasts and refers to a listhesis that has the underlying etiology as being a defect in the pars interarticularis. This defect may either be a lytic fracture or an elongated pars interarticularis.

Genetics and environmental stress both appear to be factors that have a role in the development of a pars defect. Genetic evidence comes largely from examination of the incidence of pars defects in a variety of different populations. The defect is rarely seen before the age of 5 years old.[31] A 5% incidence has been cited for those between the ages of 5 and 7 years old, with an increase to 6–7% seen in 18 year olds.[31] Gender and race both play a role in the likelihood of developing a pars lesion. In America white men have an incidence of 6.4%, black men 2.8%, white women 2.3%, and black women 1.1%.[32] Although the overall incidence is more common in males, a high-grade slip is four times more common in females.[31]

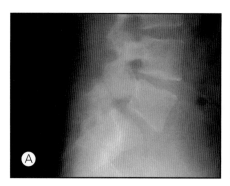
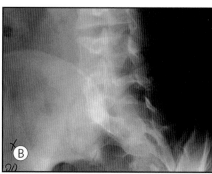

Figure 11.2
A and **B.** X-rays of spondylolysis with spondylolisthesis.

Although there is clear evidence for a significant genetic component, pars abnormalities cannot be completely attributed to genetics. Various athletic populations show an increased incidence of spondylolysis when compared to non-athletic populations, suggesting that repetitive loading of the pars interarticularis plays a role in the development of this defect. Jackson demonstrated an incidence of 11% in female gymnasts age 6–24 years.[29] Soler and Calderon examined the prevalence of spondylolysis in over 3000 elite Spanish athletes.[33] All athletes received a standard AP and lateral of the lumbar spine, regardless of a history or absence of lower back pain. Further radiographic studies were performed in additional cases when deemed necessary. The overall incidence of spondylolysis was 8%, which did not vary significantly from the quoted 3–7% in the general population. However, several sports showed a much higher incidence, including artistic gymnastics, with an incidence of 17%.[33] Jackson et al in a 1976 study obtained X-rays on a series of 100 gymnasts. These volunteers were selected without any knowledge of a history of back pain. Eleven of the 100 gymnasts demonstrated bilateral L5 pars interarticularis defects. Six of the 11 also demonstrated a Grade I spondylolisthesis of L5 on S1. This 11% incidence rate was four times higher than the previously documented rate of 2.3% reported in the general female Caucasian population.[34]

Not only is the incidence of spondylolysis increased in certain sports but also the likelihood of a spondylitic lesion being symptomatic is increased in athletes. In the general population, only 10% of those with spondylolysis are found to be symptomatic.[33] Soler and Calderon noted that 46% of the athletes with spondylolysis related some history of the existence of lower back pain.[33] This was in comparison to 24% of the athletes without evidence of spondylolysis who complained of lower back pain. Amongst the gymnasts, 53% of those found to have a spondylitic defect related a history of lower back pain. These findings correspond with data obtained by Jackson et al,[29] demonstrating that 55% of gymnasts with spondylolysis had a history of back pain, whereas 23% of those without evidence of a pars defect related a history of lower back pain.

Although epidemiologic evidence supports a role of repetitive stress in the development of a pars injury, there have been few radiographic reports to substantiate these findings. A recent case study reviewed two teenagers with complaints of lower back pain. X-rays taken at the time of those evaluations demonstrated defects in the pars interarticularis. These radiographs were compared with films taken several years earlier, which did not show any evidence of the lesion.[35] Wiltse reported seeing 17 patients presenting with lower back pain who initially demonstrated normal radiographic findings. Due to a persistence of symptoms, the X-rays were repeated and subsequently showed the development of pars interarticularis lesion.[36]

The overall likelihood of a spondylolisthesis progressing is low.[31] Various factors have been implicated, including age, sex, a rounded S1, and spina bifida.[37] Children and adolescents with a high-grade slip are at increased risk for further progression.[31] Women are more likely than men to show progression of a slip. Progression of a slip is rare after skeletal maturity. A 1996 study[37] of 77 athletes, between the ages of 9 and 18, examined radiographic risk factors for progression of a spondylitic lesion to spondylolisthesis. Not surprisingly, an advanced pars defects characterized as a wide defect with radioactive sclerosis and hypertrophy was more likely to progress than a hairline defect. Magnetic resonance imaging (MRI) analysis of cartilaginous and osseous endplates at the L5, S1 level demonstrated a much higher incidence of advance endplate lesions in the spondylolisthesis group when compared to the spondylolysis group. The authors felt that these changes in the endplates should be considered as a consequence rather than the cause of the listhetic process. They also noted that wedging of the L5 vertebral body and rounding of the upper endplate of S1 should be considered as sequelae of endplate lesions rather than the cause of spondylolisthesis.[37]

Discogenic pain

Although the posterior elements appear to be the most common cause of back pain in an adolescent gymnast, the disc is also at risk for injury. Gymnasts may suffer from both acute discogenic pain with or without radicular symptoms, as well as chronic discogenic pain related to degenerative changes.

No epidemiologic data exists that documents the frequency of disc herniations in gymnasts. In Micheli and Wood's review of 100 adolescent athletes, 9 of the 11 patients with discogenic pain were diagnosed with a disc herniation.[28] Micheli noted that the presentation of discogenic pain in a young gymnast might be different than that seen in an adult. A child may have minimal complaints of back pain. Rather, the complaints may focus on a loss of hamstring flexibility or possibly complaints related to a lumbar shift.[28]

Gymnastic maneuvers that involve repetitive flexion and torsion may create microtrauma that weakens the disc's inner annular fibers. Continued trauma leads to tears spreading radially and eventually leading to a disc herniation.[24] Callahan et al reported on an 11-year old with nerve root impingement at L5-S1. At surgery a "central protrusion of fibrocartilage and bone from the superior portion of the S1 vertebra" was found. The authors concluded that in a "subgroup" of patients with nerve root compression, the etiology may be an apophyseal fracture rather than a herniated disc.[38]

An intraosseous intervertebral disc herniation occurs when nuclear material extends through a fractured endplate and invades the cancellous bone of the vertebral body.[39] The type of disc injury sustained is thought to be a function of the position of the spine at the time of injury.[39] An intraosseous disc herniation occurs more commonly when the spine is in a neutral (or at least not fully flexed) position.[39] A posterior disc herniation appears to occur when the spine is in a fully flexed position.[39] Herniation of disc material through the endplate into the vertebral body manifests itself radiographically as a Schmorl's node. Schmorl's nodes may be found in both athletic and non-athletic populations.[26] The location of the Schmorl's node within the body, however, provides an important distinction between these two groups. Centrally located Schmorl's nodes are relatively common finding in non-athletes and can be associated with Scheuermann's disease. Hellstrom and colleagues reviewed radiologic images of top Swedish athletes, which included male and female gymnasts. Subjects were selected without knowledge of previous or present back injury or back symptoms. Radiologic findings were compared to non-athletes in a similar age group. Schmorl's nodes were commonly found within the central and posterior portion of the endplate in the non-athletic population. In comparison, the athletic population, including the subgroups of male and female gymnasts, demonstrated a much higher incidence of anterior Schmorl's nodes.[26]

Schmorl's nodes in a non-athletic population that are not related to trauma may be asymptomatic. Radiologic investigation of top athletics[22,39a] has shown a high degree of correlation between Schmorl's nodes and complaints of back pain. An acute injury to the vertebral endplate with the subsequent development of degenerative changes has been well demonstrated in two different case studies.[22,40] In a review by McCall,[40] eight patients ranging in age from 12 to 22 years old had sustained a variety of acute injuries, demonstrating radiologic features of an acute traumatic intraosseous disc herniation. The injuries typically occurred in the anterior portion of the disc space. Initially, a narrowing of the disc space with a slight kyphosis is seen at the effective level. Later, a defect in the anterior portion of the endplate is seen, with the subsequent development of sclerosis around the defect. Discography was performed in several of these individuals and demonstrated contrast flowing into the defect consistent with a disc herniation.[40] Sward et al reviewed progressive radiologic findings in two elite Swedish gymnasts.[22] Both gymnasts reported pain following an injury that involved hyperflexion and probable rotation of the spine. Initial radiographs in one subject were normal and in the other showed displacement of the anterior upper ring of T12. Serial radiologic evaluations over the next 10–12 months demonstrated, in both individuals, reduction in the T11, T12 disc height, and excavation of the upper anterior corner of T12. These findings demonstrated that injury of the vertebral ring might be traumatic and result in prolapse of disc material with subsequent disc degeneration.[22,39a]

Sacroiliac joint pain

The role of the sacroiliac joint as a pain generator remains controversial.[41] Several factors contribute to the controversy. The joint is narrow and has only a few degrees of motion, the biomechanics are complex, and there are no specific standards for evaluation of SIJ dysfunction. Physical examination techniques and imaging do not consistently distinguish a painful from non-painful joint. Reaching a diagnosis of sacroiliac joint pain is usually a diagnosis of exclusion and in an adolescent gymnast the clinician must perform a systematic and thorough evaluation to exclude other pain generators. A diagnostic fluoro-scopically guided sacroiliac joint injection can be helpful in confirming the diagnosis.

SIJ dysfunction may present in various patterns. Athletes commonly complain of pain in the low back or buttock near the posterior superior iliac spine. Pain may radiate down the posterior leg or anterior groin. Pain may be exacerbated with repetitive overload activity, transitional movements, and unsupported sitting. Gymnastics provides an opportunity for trauma as well as repetitive unidirectional pelvic shear and torsional forces. Both of theses are thought to be risk factors for the development of sacroiliac joint dysfunction.[42]

PHYSICAL EXAMINATION

The examination of the injured gymnast has several goals. A thorough neurologic examination appropriate to the nature of the injury should be performed. Provocative tests may be utilized to help localize the injured tissues (tissue injury complex). Further examination should then be geared toward determining the functional deficits which have lead to the injury, as well as identifying adaptations that have occurred in response to the injury.

The one-leg standing lumbar extension test is a provocative maneuver in which the patient stands on one leg and extends the spine. The test is repeated on the opposite side. Rotation toward the weight-bearing leg may be added to the extension. Reproduction of back pain is a positive response, suggesting the presence of a pars lesion on the off side of the weight-bearing lower extremity.[43]

Neural tension tests are an important component of any potential spine injury. A positive test suggests injury to neural tissue, which can be an important consideration in the diagnostic work-up and treatment of the injured gymnast. The straight leg raise is the most common neural tension test. By passively flexing the hip and extending the knee, the examiner places mechanical stress on the lower lumbar nerve roots and the sciatic nerve. Dorsiflexing the foot is a sensitizing maneuver that may produce symptoms in a previously negative test. Reproduction or an increase in symptoms with the addition of dorsiflexion can also be useful in differentiating hamstring tightness from neural injury. Plantarflexion combined with inversion will stress (or bias) the tibial portion of the sciatic nerve. The slump test is also utilized to assess the sciatic nerve and associated nerve roots. From a seated position, the patient is placed into a position of cervical, thoracic, and lumbar flexion (i.e., the patient is asked to "slump"). The knee is extended and similar sensitizing maneuvers added at the ankle. The femoral nerve stress test is performed placing the patient in the prone position and passively flexing the knee and, if necessary, extending the hip. Reproduction of anterior thigh pain is considered a positive test and suggests irritation of one or more of the L1–L4 nerve roots. Upper extremity neural tension test may also be performed and have similar sensitizing maneuvers. Motion at the shoulder, elbow, and wrist may be passively manipulated to produce neural tension that biases the median ulnar or radial nerve. For a detailed discussion of neural tension tests the reader is referred to the work of David Butler.[44]

A functional assessment of the gymnast is useful for determining areas of focus for rehabilitation as well as determining an individual's readiness for return to activity. Such an assessment may include traditional methods of isolating and evaluating muscle length and strength. However, evaluation of the functional movements necessary to participate in a given sport may provide more useful information. Assessment techniques should consider the quantity and quality of the entire kinetic chain and should make assessments of movement in the frontal, sagittal, and coronal planes.[45] The available range of motion for most gymnasts is likely to be well within "normal limits." Important findings in a functional examination are utilized to detect a relative restriction or weakness within the kinetic chain that may lead to mechanical overload or relative instability at a more proximal or distal segment. For example, a restriction of the right hip limiting internal rotation may lead to increased torsional stress in the lumbar spine with movements that employ extension and right-sided rotation.

SPECIFIC REHABILITATION

Acute management of spine problems in the gymnast starts with general principles used to treat many acute musculoskeletal disorders. Initially, acute inflammation, pain, and swelling can be controlled with topical ice and nonsteroidal anti-inflammatory drugs (NSAIDs). Relative rest is recommended. However, complete bedrest may be unnecessary, as it will facilitate deconditioning. Determining movement patterns or conditions in which movement patterns are relatively pain free is important. This may include abdominal bracing (concentric abdominal contractions) or pelvic tilt performed in a supine, sitting, or standing position. These abdominal exercises and range of motion of the hip and trunk might also be performed in water as to help alleviate pain related to compressive forces. Modifications in activities and relative rest should be individualized to the particular athlete and that athlete's specific injury. Range of motion should be performed within pain-free limits. The following sections suggest specific treatment options with respect to a particular injury.

Spondylolysis

A standard treatment for spondylolysis has not been determined. This is evident by literature currently available and is probably due to progress made in imaging technology and the uncertainty in how to apply this technology.[46] There is also an absence of large controlled trials in the management of spondylolysis. Goals for treatment should include obtaining bony healing of a fracture when possible, relieving pain, and optimizing physical function with return to sport safely. Treatment must be individualized to each gymnast.

Several studies do exist with regard to evidence of bony healing on imaging.[47–49] Blanda found that 37% of adolescent athletes (average age 15.5 years old) had radiographic union of their pars defect after treatment. Treatment consisted of bracing with a goal to maintain lordosis for 2–6 months, stopping sports participation, hamstring stretching, and abdominal strengthening as pain allowed. Fifteen percent of this patient population went on to have surgery. Daniel and colleagues used plain radiographs to follow military patients (average age 21 years old) treated with restricted duty and full-time bracing for 3 months. Only 2 out of 29 patients showed evidence of bony healing on radiographs. In another study by Yamane et al,[50] in patients whose pars defect did heal, it took 3–6 months for it to become evident on a computed tomography (CT) scan. The authors concluded that no fracture was completely healed within 2 months. Still, in another study by Steiner and Micheli,[49] 18% of patients (average of 16 years old) with spondylolysis and a low-grade spondylolisthesis showed evidence of healing on plain radiography after conservative treatment that was instituted for 6–12 months. Conservative management included the use of a modified Boston brace to prevent lordosis. The percentage of evidence of healing actually increased to 25% when the study population was restricted to patients with only spondylolysis. Multiple variables probably affected the outcome variations between these studies, including the participants age, position and timing of bracing, and lack of control for physical therapy. Also these studies did not show the use of a CT or single-photon emission computed tomography (SPECT) scan to diagnose or follow pars fractures. In general, unilateral pars defects have been shown to have higher rates of healing than bilateral defects, as noted in several studies.[47,51–53]

Other studies[53,54] have followed rate of healing in correlation with the stage of the pars fracture. These stages were classified as early, progressive, and terminal. Pars lesions were followed on plain radiographs and CT or CT alone. Morita and colleagues[53] studied 185 patients with the average of 13.9 years old. Treatment consisted of bracing with a nonspecific lumbar corset for 3–6 weeks, cessation of sports, with the use of an extension limiting corset for 3–6 months, simultaneous with rehabilitation once healing had occurred. They found that 37.9% of all pars defects showed apparent healing. Healing was found in 73% of early-stage as compared to 38.5% of those with progressive-stage pars fractures. No patients with the terminal defects healed. Katoh[54] studied 134 patients with spondylolysis who were aged 18 years old or younger. All patients underwent CT scan before and after treatment. Treatment consisted of relative rest, and no bracing. Sixty-two percent of the early-stage defects healed and none of the terminal defects healed. Three reports[55–57] involving six cases have shown bony healing with the use of external electrical stimulation in patients who failed conservative treatment.

Several studies[58–61,61a] have looked at correction of the pars defect by surgical fusion. O'Neill and Micheli[58] reported 90% healing rates of their pars defect treated with fusion. Those patients with non-healing defects were found to have a significantly longer course of preoperative symptoms (mean 48 months) as compared to those in whom bony healing was found on radiographs (mean 12 months). In a study by Pellise,[59] CT scanning was used to follow 7 patients 12–78 months after fusion. All reported improved clinical outcome on questionnaires despite 2/7 showing persistent pars defect on CT. Prasartritha[61] reported that in the 2/16 failing fusion for repair of pars defects, both had maldevelopment of the neural arch. Wu and colleagues[60] utilized diagnostic pars injections to determine if a patient was a good surgical candidate after failure of conservative management: 275 patients were reviewed. Ninety-three patients were symptomatic after conservative management with negative bone scans and relief of symptoms with Marcaine (bupivacaine) injection. These patients underwent autogenous bone grafting with internal fixation of the pars defect. Average follow-up was 30 months. A successful fusion rate of 87% was noted by plain radiographs.

Most patients experience good pain relief and functional recovery with conservative treatment. Blanda[62] reported 97% of patients treated for spondylolysis returned to strenuous activities with little or no back pain. However, some of these patients were treated surgically; 21 of the 52 patients reporting excellent results had bony healing on radiographs. Steiner and Micheli reported a 78% success rate with conservative treatment of spondylolysis and low-grade spondylolisthesis. Similarly, 12 of 42 patients with good or excellent results had bony healing. Blanda recommended using a brace to maintain lordosis, whereas Micheli recommended an anti-lordotic brace. Despite these differences, they had similar clinical results. In contrast to these studies, Jackson[63] treated 25 adolescent athletes with spondylolysis with only activity restriction. Only 50% of the patients completed follow-up. Of those, only 12 of 15 returned to unrestricted activity. O'Sullivan and colleagues[64] demonstrated improvement in pain scores and disability rating in adults with spondylolysis and spondylolisthesis treated with specific spinal stabilization exercises as compared to controls receiving non-specific exercise recommendations. The treatment group showed improvement in hip flexion and extension mobility.

Much of the uncertainty of conservative management of spondylolysis stems around bracing. There are a number of studies that support rigid bracing, whereas others advocate activity restriction.[46] The goals of bracing are to achieve bony healing and control pain. As just reviewed in the literature here, bony healing has been found to occur with rigid,[65,66] soft,[67] and no bracing.[54] Excellent and good clinical outcomes have been noted in the absence of bony healing.[62,65] These varied approaches with similar outcomes can make the decision to brace or not to brace complex. In general, the biomechanics of lumbar bracing are confusing. Lantz and Shultz[68] studied myoelectric activity during 19 functional tasks in five healthy adult men wearing three different types of lumbar braces. When the lumbosacral corset was worn, myoelectric signal levels ranged from 9% reduction to 44% increase in activity as compared to when the brace was not worn. In a second study, the authors determined that these same braces restricted some gross body motion as compared to values when no brace was worn. They concluded that lumbar bracing is often ineffective in reducing segmental motion and can be counterproductive.

In general, specific treatment for spondylolysis is difficult to state, based on the current literature as described above. Specific treatment should be individualized to the athlete, the length of time of the problem, and the future plans for sports participation. Follow-up studies may be needed for ongoing treatment. A CT may be needed to identify the stage of fracture according to pathology, and may result in a positive finding on a bone SPECT scan such as arthropathy, osteoarthritis, or osteoid osteoma. Restriction from provocative activities such as gymnastics during the acute stage is necessary to achieve optimal pain relief. However, restriction in activity needs to be performed in such a way as to continue to maximize aerobic conditioning when possible. Evidence from the literature shows that bracing is not necessary to achieve healing in all cases. In fact, bony healing is not the only goal for using a brace, as the literature shows that not all successfully conservatively treated injuries achieve bony healing. Instead, bracing may be used as a form of treatment to control pain and assist in activity restriction. Coordination of using bracing with therapeutic exercise is key. A physical medicine and rehabilitation program is essential in restoring function in order to return to competition and sports participation. Physical therapy should focus on range of motion (ROM) and quality of motion in the adjacent structures during the initial phase. This can be coordinated with bracing, for example. Assessing, maintaining, and or advancing hip ROM and control is essential in deterring further repetitive overload to the spine. Initiation of abdominal strengthening can start even in the acute stages of rehabilitation. The subacute stage of rehabilitation begins around 3–7 days after presentation to a healthcare provider. The acute pain has been addressed and activity restrictions have been implemented. Abdominal, gluteal, and hamstring length and strength must be balanced. There are a variety of therapeutic exercises with which to accomplish this. In the gymnast, special attention needs to be paid to loading the spine, and upper and lower extremities through multiple planes. For example, strengthening the gluteus medius in only a frontal plane can be achieved with sidelying hip abduction or resisted sitting abduction will not allow the athlete to achieve maximal function when landing a dismount from a rotated position. Lunges with rotation in multiple planes may be a way in which to bring the therapeutic exercise to better simulating the gymnast's plans to return (Fig. 11.3A and B) Careful examination of the athlete's training program, techniques, and equipment used should also be evaluated during this phase. Identifying timing and frequency and types of repetitive activities that facilitate back extension should be evaluated. Spacing activities or limiting the number of repetitive extension activities a gymnast performs at one interval may help prevent recurrence of or future injury. The maintenance phase of rehabilitation begins when the pain has resolved and muscle strength and functional activities have returned to 75–80% of baseline values. Advancing sport-specific activities and modifying the flexibility and strengthening program that the gymnast will use as part of their warm-up and cool-down activities is compiled at this time. Although we do have evidence that specific conservative therapeutic exercises are better than nonspecific intervention,[62,64,65] exactly what is best has not been disclosed in the literature. Therefore, individualizing treatment for gymnasts in relation to their symptoms, injury, chronicity or acuity, and specific activities they wish to return to seems key to effective treatment.

Lumbar discogenic pain

Axial low back pain with or without buttock or lower extremity pain attributed to lumbar disc pathology can be quite debilitating for the injured gymnast. The following includes rehabilitation recommendations for gymnasts whose pain is attributed to the lumbar disc. The imaging studies might reveal a variety of scenarios, including annular tear, disc protrusion, disc extrusion, or degenerative disc changes. Rehabilitation for these injured gymnasts should be guided by the patients symptoms and provocative activities and/or positions.

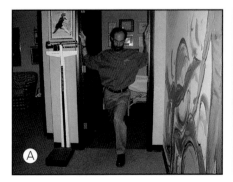 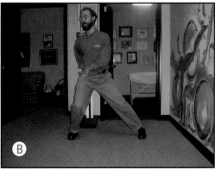

Figure 11.3
A. Sagittal plane lunge.
B. Frontal plane lunge.

Acute phase

During the first 1–3 days of onset of symptoms, the gymnast should avoid provocative activities, use ice and anti-inflammatory medications to facilitate pain improvement, and reduce inflammation. Pelvic tilts can facilitate maintaining segmental motion and pain control. Range of motion and muscle flexibility should be maintained through a stretching program within pain-free limits. Educating the gymnast regarding the expected recovery course and time frame is essential to make sure the gymnast is aware of his active roll in the treatment process. During the acute phase, the goal is to facilitate centralization of pain. The gymnast should be taught to recognize which postures or activities centralize pain and which make buttocks or lower extremity pain worse. Activities that provoke peripheral pain should initially be avoided.

Recovery phase

After appropriate rest and pain is in better control, recovery of the *functional biomechanical deficit* and *tissue overload complex*[69] becomes the focus of the treatment program. The use of anti-inflammatory medications should continue, based on the gymnast's symptoms and tapered accordingly. The goal of therapeutic exercise at this point is to facilitate improvement of symptoms by off-loading painful structures, and improving endurance and efficiency of loading and unloading of the lumbar spine. A place to start is to find the relative deficits in flexibility and strength in the muscle and surrounding fascia that stabilize the spine. This group includes the thorocolumbar fascia, abdominal, paraspinal, gluteal, hip, and pelvic muscles. Also, the nervous system structures in the lumbar spine and involved myofascial groups should be evaluated and, if they provoke pain, should be treated coincidingly. An example is the gymnast with back and lateral hip pain that can be provoked with adverse neural tension signs directed with a peroneal bias stretch. In addition to addressing the balance of abdominal and gluteal strength, adding neuromobilization may facilitate reduction of symptoms more quickly and allow the muscles innervated by the involved nerve root to respond more quickly to the strengthening program. Muscles remaining inhibited by pain are not able to respond efficiently to a strengthening program.[70,71] Muscle endurance must also be improved to better withstand repetitive activities as well as static postures. McGill's[72] work suggests that muscle endurance to maintain stability within the "margin of safety" rather than absolute muscle strength is most important. Muscles tested and found to be weak are often opposed by structures of relative stiffness or inflexibility. In the lumbar spine, muscles that typically can be involved in a discogenic pain syndrome can include the iliopsoas, hip external rotators, and hamstrings. Correcting inflexibility or stiffness patterns in these muscles will facilitate improving stabilization. Manual medicine has a long history of being beneficial in the treatment of low back pain but has been met with some controversy. Manual medicine may be of particular use in the gymnast as adjunct treatment.[73,74] This approach incorporates a wide variety of "hands on" techniques that facilitate lumbar segmental motion, improve nerve gliding within myofascial structures, and thereby reduce pain as an adjunct treatment to therapeutic exercise. We caution that recurrent mobilizations over a period of months may in fact not completely resolve the biomechanical deficit, but in fact be harmful as it may facilitate joint hypermobility. Applying a specific manual medicine technique for a specific effect is important.

Another therapeutic approach developed by McKenzie divides back pain into three categories: postural, dysfunctional, and derangement syndromes.[75] The derangement category involves the disc as being part of the breakdown. The derangement is described as an internal displacement, such as a herniated nucleus pulposus, leading to pain, loss of function, and possible deformity. The complex set of maneuvers described by this theory aims to identify postures and ranges of motion that "centralize" and/or reduce pain. Commonly, these positions include spinal extension but are not exclusionary to this. The exercise given is tailored to the patient.

Recently, incorporation of the above theories in devising therapeutic programs that incorporate the kinetic chain, the musculoskeletal system links from the lower extremity through the trunk to the upper extremity and vice versa, has become popular. This is often referred to as core stabilization. The purpose is to focus beyond the painful structure and devise a program that corrects the *functional biomechanical deficit* and *tissue overload complex*.[69] Several studies[76–78] have demonstrated how the joints of the lower extremity work together to transfer forces through the limb during motion. These studies have also shown that a compromised joint will lead to proximal or distal joint dysfunction. In the gymnast, correcting a scewed subtalar inversion to eversion ratio at the foot may reduce overload at the hip that is leading to low back pain. The "core muscles" include the lumbar paravertebral, abdominals, quadratus lumborum, diaphragm, pelvic floor, and lower extremity muscles.[79,80] The principles involve facilitating eccentric loading prior to concentric contraction, combining muscle stretching and strengthening. Balance is addressed by attempting to control the center of gravity as it moves through various planes of motion. The goals of the therapeutic program are to improve multifidi activity and endurance, restore the control of deep abdominal muscles, restore coordination and position sense, restore mobility, restore gluteal muscle activity, and lumbo-pelvic rhythm, and make the therapeutic exercise functional. In other words, the treatment needs to simulate the activity the athlete needs to return.

If lower extremity pain continues despite medications, modalities, and therapeutic exercise, lumbar epidural steroid injections may enhance pain management and expedite recovery. Injections focus to reduce inflammation associated with compressive and/or chemical radiculopathy. The use of fluoroscopic guidance to perform these procedures is recommended to prevent the potential 30–40% miss rate of injections completed without radiographic confirmation.[81,82] Epidural injections may be administered via a translaminar, caudal, or transforaminal approach. The transforaminal approach allows a high concentration of the solution injected to be delivered to the anterior epidural space at a desired target level. The translaminar approach delivers a high concentration of the injected solution to the posterior epidural space and may not consistently effect the nerve root at that level. There is a greater risk of wet tap and subsequent spinal headache with this approach. The caudal injection is less specific for a particular vertebral level but will affect the L4–L5, L5–S1 intervertebral levels.[83] The athlete's response to injection is usually evaluated at 2 weeks. A second injection may be recommended if partial relief has been noted. In general, more than three epidural injections within a short period of time are not recommended.[84] No studies have confirmed the therapeutic benefit of lumbar epidural injections in the actively participating gymnastic population. We recommend using these injections in the injured gymnast only when all other attempts to provide relief have been unsuccessful. Again, this treatment modality should be used in adjunct to correcting the biomechanical deficit through therapeutic exercise.

Return to sport

Once the biomechanical deficit has been corrected and pain has been eliminated, advancing sport-specific exercises for the gymnast is completed. At this point, the gymnast should have incorporated a core therapeutic program that incorporates strengthening, flexibility, proprioceptive, and plyometric training. For the gymnast, advancing the repetitive motions should be approached with gradual increase in frequency and speed. For example, initially limiting the number of repetitions of activities that require spinal extension should be slowly advanced with regard to number of spinal extensions performed during a session and the speed at which they are performed. Slowly advancing the frequency and speed of repetitions should help facilitate building endurance as well as correcting form errors as they might occur at a higher performance level. This author recommends that the gymnast should return to sport when full ROM is pain-free, sport-specific agility exercises can be performed in a neutral spine position, and muscle strength has been restored to perform both endurance tasks as well as manage rapid load absorption. By achieving these requirements, the intent would be to prevent reinjury or further injury to another link in the musculoskeletal system.

Sacroiliac joint treatment

Acute phase (1–3 days)

Acute injury is often associated with a direct trauma such as a fall or marked increase in intensity, frequency, or duration of a specific activity. In gymnastics, a direct fall landing on the pelvis or repetitive landings or take-off that involve loading through just one lower extremity may be an etiology for pain. Often, sacroiliac joint pain presents as a progressive problem with fluctuations in symptoms. During the acute phase anti-inflammatory medications and icing are helpful. Relative rest after an acute injury assists with pain control. This includes restricting running or excessive walking, as these activities often provoke sacroiliac joint pain. An activity restriction may include limiting repetitive landings. The relative rest prescription needs to be individualized with respect to the gymnast's training program. Identifying the activity that may aggravate symptoms is important, especially in those with progressive onset of symptoms. Correcting asymmetries in muscle length or stiffness should start as soon as possible and progress within pain-free limits. Muscle energy techniques are particularly helpful, as they require patient activation of muscle groups and therefore pain tolerance is easily monitored. Mobilization of the SIJ has become a more accepted form of treatment and can be quite helpful in restoring function. Care should be taken in which patients should receive this type of treatment. Treatment for athletes with significant muscle weakness and/or poor endurance may need to focus on stabilization through strengthening rather than recurrent mobilization.

Recovery phase (3 days to 8 weeks)

Once pain has been controlled and the injured area has been rested, correction of the *functional biomechanical deficit* and *tissue overload complex*[69] becomes the focus of rehabilitation. Balancing lower extremity muscle length and strength is important because of direct and indirect force transmission across the ilium and sacrum. Muscle length must first be restored. For example, if the iliopsoas is in a shortened position, it leads to an anteriorly rotated ilium. Hamstring strengthening cannot be accomplished until the iliopsoas is restored to activating at a biomechanically efficient length as an anterior pelvic tilt forces the hamstring to work in a lengthened position. The hamstring is a key muscle to provide stability to the sacroiliac joint because of its direct attachment and/or fascial connections to the sacrotuberous ligament, and therefore restoration of appropriate strength is a key to successful outcome. Other muscles commonly found to be working in a shortened position include the rectus femoris, tensor fascia lata, adductors, quadratus lumborum, latissimus dorsi,[45] and obturator internus. Achieving appropriate muscle flexibility may require several weeks of stretching two to three times per day. As muscle length and/or reduction of muscle stiffness are accomplished, strengthening of muscles that are inhibited by the biomechanical deficit can be completed. Neuromuscular re-education and facilitation techniques are helpful with this process. Closed kinetic chain strengthening should be attempted first and incorporated into the lumbopelvic stabilization program. As trunk strengthening improves, adding multiplanar strengthening exercises will facilitate return to functional activities. Muscles commonly found to be weak include the gluteus medius, gluteus maximus, lower abdominals, and hamstrings.

SIJ belts can be used to provide compression and thereby proprioceptive feedback to the gluteal muscles (Fig. 11.4). Vleeming et al[85] reported that SIJ belts applied to cadaver models reduced SIJ rotation by 30%. Clinically, it makes sense that sacroiliac joint belts can be especially helpful in patients with SIJ hypermobility or significant muscle weakness. Care must be taken to insure that the patient is able to

Figure 11.4
SIJ belt.

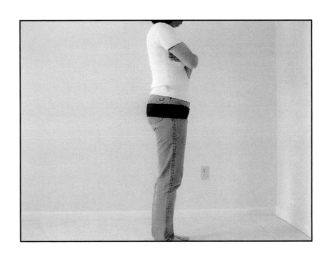

apply the belt appropriately. The SIJ belt should be secured posteriorly across the sacral base and anteriorly, inferior to the anterior superior iliac spines. Patients are often recommended to wear the belt during walking and standing activities. However, athletes with significant pain and weakness often find the belt helpful in reducing symptoms when worn during sedentary activities as well.

Other treatment considerations include orthotics and shoe modifications A shoe lift to correct a functional leg length discrepancy can be helpful in the acute setting to manage pain with weight-bearing or ambulation. Shoe lifts should be approached with caution, as functional leg length discrepancy should be corrected with muscle rebalancing and not orthotic intervention. An inappropriate shoe lift can promote adaptive muscle imbalances, which may initially be asymptomatic but cause problems because of a shift in force transmission which ultimately can change wear and tear pattern in the future. Of course, anatomical leg length discrepancies should be determined as early in treatment as possible so that the appropriate modifications can be completed.

SIJ injections can be used as an adjunct to a physical therapy program if the patient's progress plateaus or the program cannot be advanced because of pain provocation. The injections can also be used diagnostically if done under fluoroscopic guidance (Fig. 11.5). Maigne et al[86] reported 18.5% of 54 patients diagnosed with SIJ pain responded to double SIJ block under fluoroscopic guidance. This study did not control for other treatments given and therefore does not accurately report the success of injection alone. SIJ injections should only be used as an adjunct to the comprehensive pain management program.

During this phase of rehabilitation the focus turns to correcting the functional biomechanical deficits and adaptive patterns that have developed. Recognizing the adaptations that have occurred in response to the injury is essential to prevent further injury on return to normal activities, exercise, and sports. A common example includes the role of the gluteus maximus to stabilize the pelvis posteriorly via attachments at the ilium and sacrotuberous ligament. If the sacroiliac joint dysfunction involves an anteriorly rotated ilium, correction of the inflexibility of the iliopsoas alone will be insufficient. If the gluteus maximus contractions are too weak to stabilize posteriorly, then stretch will be placed on the iliolumbar ligament as well. The piriformis muscle length should be assessed with the hip flexed greater and less than 90 degrees. Stretching applied with the hip in either or both directions is necessary. Continued inflexibility of this muscle is often thought to be part of the source of recurrent pain. Although maintaining individual muscle flexibility and strength is important, retraining of multiple muscle groups to fire in coordination is key to a successful recovery. This can be facilitated with lumbopelvic stabilization, advanced proprioceptive re-education, plyometrics, and exercise or sport-specific activities. Education regarding proper ergonomics in activities of the daily living and work environment should be included. Careful attention to training techniques must also be incorporated into the program for those active in sports and exercise. Return to sporting activities is indicated when a pain-free state without medications is achieved. Proper muscle balance in flexibility and strength should remain a part of the maintenance program. Careful monitoring during initial return can prevent reinjury.

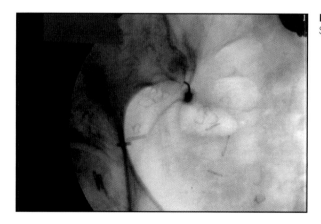

Figure 11.5
SIJ injection.

Advancement to the maintenance phase of treatment begins with an absence of pain, inflammation, functional joint and myofascial dysfunction, and return of approximately 75% of strength and flexibility as judged per the patient's pre-injury baseline. Normal activities of daily living, especially walking, should not provoke symptoms.

Maintenance phase

During this phase, therapy focuses on advancing the strengthening program while maintaining appropriate muscle length. The exercise program should be concise and specific to the individual's functional requirements. In other words, the maintenance exercise routine should simulate the individual's activities. Sidelying hip abduction as a form of gluteus medius strengthening may not be aggressive enough for a gymnast. The gymnast will need a gluteus medius strengthening exercise that incorporates multiple planes in a weight-bearing position. Aerobic conditioning is also advanced while monitoring return to usual sport/exercise activities. The exercise prescription should fit the individual.

Special consideration should be given for the individual with joint hypermobility. SIJ arthrodesis[87] and percutaneous fixation[88] have been utilized for instability. Long-term outcome studies thus far have not been completed and it is unknown what happens to surrounding articulations with the lumbar spine, contralateral SIJ, and hip years after SIJ fusion. Other therapy such as prolotherapy has been proposed as an invasive but less permanent option. Prolotherapy is described as the provocation of the laying down of an increased volume of normal collagen material in ligament, tendon, or fascia in order to restore function of the tissue at a specific site.[89] Provocation is achieved by provoking an inflammatory response at the location. A wide variety of agents have been used to provoke inflammation locally, from high-concentration glucose solutions to phenol alcohol. Often it is a combination of agents. Although the safety[90] and clinical outcomes have been reported,[91] no prospective, controlled studies exist to date on the specific use of prolotherapy and SIJ dysfunction.

For athletes with low back pain, posterior pelvic or gluteal pain, and groin pain, SIJ pain should be considered as part of the differential diagnosis. Because there are no good gold standards for diagnosis or treatment of this condition, it is often approached from the examiner's experience. The healthcare provider needs to have a good understanding of the integrated biomechanics of the spine, pelvis, and hips in order to guide both the evaluation and treatment. Research describing the biomechanics of the SIJ continues to add to our understanding of its function. Further research into the relationship between SIJ function and that of the hip, pelvis, and spine is needed.

SPORT-SPECIFIC TRAINING

It is well documented that gymnasts are at risk for sustaining low back injuries that can impair sports participation[92,93] and lead to low back problems that can last years beyond sports participation.[94,95] We could find no reference to sport-specific training for gymnasts directed solely at prevention. The following recommendations are based on literature and the authors' experience in the treatment of low back pain in the gymnastic population.

A key element in preventing musculoskeletal injuries in the gymnastic population is the balance of muscle length and muscle strength. Maintaining muscle flexibility insures that the muscle can perform to its best mechanical advantage. A shortened or lengthened muscle cannot perform at its maximal advantage. Gymnasts must be able to load joints while muscles perform both concentric and eccentric contractions. The training program should reflect these specific needs. Training must include both strength and endurance activities, with the joint loaded in multiple plane. This should enhance muscle strength, maintain muscle length, and facilitate proprioceptive feedback. Because many of the spine injuries that occur in gymnasts are related to repetitive motion, it seems logical that monitoring and even limiting the number of repetitive moves such as lumbar extension might reduce risk of injuries. The initial step would be to count the number of lumbar extensions performed per practice session. Once a base number is established, progressing this number in small increments such as 10% per week when aggressively training for a competition might decrease the risk of injury due to repetitive motion.

REFERENCES

1. The USA gymnastics organization. http://www.usa-gymnastics.org, 2002.

2. McNitt-Gray JL, Irvine DME, Eagle J: Relative work of net joint moments during landings of front and back saltos. In: Proceedings of the XIXth American Society of Biomechanics Meeting. Stanford, California: American Society of Biomechanics; 1995:132–133.

3. Nigg BM, Denoth J, Neukomm PA: Quantifying the load on the human body. Problems and some possible solutions. Biomechanics 8:88–98, 1982.

4. Nigg BM, Bobbert M: On the potential of various approaches in load analysis to reduce the frequency of sports injuries. J Biomech 23:3–12, 1990.

5. Claessens AL, Lefevre J, Beunen G, et al: Physique as a risk factor for ulnar variance in elite female gymnasts. Med Sci Sports Exerc 28(5):560–569, 1996.

6. McNitt-Gray JL: Gymnastics. In: Garrett WE, Lester GE, McGowan J, Kirkendall DT, eds. Women's health in sports and exercise. Rosemont, IL: American Academy of Orthopaedic Surgeons; 2001:209–228.

7. Bruggeman GP: Biomechanics of gymnastic techniques. In: Nelson R, Zatsiorsky V, eds. Sport science review. Champaign, IL: Human Kinetics 3:79–120, 1996.

8. Markolf KL, Shapiro MS, Mandelbaum BR, Teurlings L: Wrist loading patterns during pommel horse exercises. J Biomech 23:1001–1011, 1990.

9. McNitt-Gray JL, Nelson RC: Segment and joint kinematics of Olympic vault landings. Med Sci Sport Exerc 20:S48, 1988.

10. Hwang I, Seo G, Liu ZG: Take-off mechanics of the double backward somersault. Int J Sport Biomech 6:177–186, 1990.

11. Kerwin DG, Yeardon MR, Lee SC: Body configuration in multiple somersault high bar dismounts. Int J Sport Biomech 6:147–156, 1990.

12. Takei Y, Kim EJ: Techniques used in performing the handspring and salto forward tucked vault at the 1988 Olympic Games. Int J Sport Biomech 6:111–138, 1990.

13. Takei Y, Nohara H, Kamimura M: Techniques used by elite gymnasts in the 1992 Olympic compulsory dismount from the horizontal bar. Int J Sport Biomech 8:207–232, 1992.

14. Brown E, Witten W, Espinoza D, Witten C: Attenuation of ground reaction forces in dismounts from the balance beam. In: Bauer T, ed. Proceedings of the XIII International Symposium on Biomechanics in Sports. Lakehead University, Thunder Bay, Ontario, Canada; 1996:114–166.

15. King MA, Yeadon MR, Kerwin DG: A two-segment simulation model of long horse vaulting. J Sports Sci 17(4):313–324, 1999.

16. Arampatzis A, Bruggemann GP, Klapsing GM: Leg stiffness and mechanical energetic processes during jumping on a sprung surface. Med Sci Sports Exerc 33(6):923–931, 2001.

17. McNitt-Gray JL, Hester DME, Mathiyakom W, Munkasy BA: Mechanical demand and multijoint control during landing depends on orientation of the body segments relative to the reaction force. J Biomech 34(11):1471–1482, 2001.

18. Weber MD, Woodall WR: Spondylogenic disorders in gymnasts. J Orthop Sports Phys Ther 14:6–13, 1991.

19. Goldstein JD, Berger PE, Windler GE, Jackson DW: Spine injuries in gymnasts and swimmers. An epidemiological investigation. Am J Sports Med 19:463–468, 1991.

20. Micheli LJ, Wood R: Back pain in young athletes: significant differences from adults in causes and patterns. Arch Pediatr Adolesc Med 149:15–18, 1995.

21. Garrick JG, Requa R: Epidemiology of women's gymnastics injuries. Am J Sports Med 8:261–264, 1980.

22. Sward L: The lumbar spine in young elite athletes. Sports Med 13:357–364, 1992.

23. Sward L, Hellstrom M, Jacobsson B, et al: Acute injury of the vertebral ring apophysis and intervertebral disk in adolescent gymnasts. Spine 15:144–148, 1990.

24. Saal JA: Lumbar injuries in gymnastics. Spine: State of the Art Reviews 4:426–440, 1990.

25. Ciullo JV, Jackson DW: Pars interarticularis stress reaction, spondylolysis and spondylolisthesis in gymnasts. Clin Sport Med 14:95–110, 1985.

26. Hellstrom M, Jacobbson B, Sward L, Peterson L: Radiologic abnormalities of the thoraco-lumbar spine in athletics. Acta Radiologica 31:127–132, 1990.

27. Micheli LJ: Back injuries in gymnastics. Clin Sport Med 4:85–93, 1985.

28. Micheli LJ, Wood R: Back pain in young athletes. Arch Ped Adol Med 149:15–18, 1995.

29. Jackson DW, Wiltse LL, Cirincione RJ: Spondylolysis in the female gymnast. Clin Orthop Rel Res 117:68–73, 1976.

30. Sward L, Hellstrom M, Jacobsson B, Peterson L: Back pain and radiologic changes in the thoraco-lumbar spine of athletes. Spine 15:124–129, 1990.

31. Amundson G, Edwards CC, Garfin SR: Spondylolisthesis. In: Herkowitz HN et al, eds. The spine, 4th edn. Philadelphia: WB Saunders; 1999:835–885.

32. Rowe GG, Roche MB: The etiology of the separate neural arch. JBJS 35A:102, 1953.

33. Soler T, Calderon C: The prevalence of spondylolysis in the Spanish elite athlete. Am J Sport Med 28:57–62, 2000.

34. Douglas WJ, Leon LW, Cirincione RJ: Spondylolysis in the female gymnast. Clin Orthop Rel Res 117:68–73, 1976.

35. Reitman CA, Gertzbein SD, Francis Jr WR: Lumbar isthmic defects in teenagers resulting from stress fractures. Spine 2:303–306, 2002.

36. Wiltse LL, Jackson DW: Treatment of spondylolisthesis and spondylolysis in children. Clin Orthop Rel Res 117:92–100, 1975.

37. Ikata T, Miyake R, Katoh S, et al: Pathogenesis of sports related spondylolisthesis in adolescents. Am J Sport Med 24:94–97, 1996.

38. Callahan DJ, Pack LL, Bream RC, Hensinger RN: Intervertebral disc impingement syndrome in a child. Spine 11:402–404, 1986.

39. McGill SM: Low back exercises. Phys Ther 78:754–765, 1998.

39a. Sward L, Hellstom M, Jacobssen B, Nyman R, Perterson L: Disc degeneration and associated abnormalities of the spine in elite gymnasts. A magnetic resonance imaging study. Spine 16(4):437–443, 1991.

40. McCall IW, Park WM, O'Brien JP, Cao V: Acute traumatic intraosseous disc herniation. Spine 10:134–137, 1985.

41. Prather H: Pelvis and sacral dysfunction in sports and exercise. Phys Med Rehab Clin N Am 11:805–836, 2000.

42. Portersfield JA: Conditions of weight bearing: asymmetrical overload syndrome. In: Vleeming A, Mooney V, Tilscher H, et al, eds. The most effective role for exercise therapy, manual techniques, surgery and injection techniques. Third Interdisciplinary World Congress on Low Back Pain, Vienna, Austria; 1998:253.

43. Magee DJ: Orthopedic physical assessment, 3rd edn. Philadephia: WB Saunders; 1997:398.

44. Butler DS: Mobilisation of the nervous system. New York: Churchill Livingstone; 1991.

45. Geraci MC: Rehabilitation of the hip and pelvis. In: Kibler WB, Herring SA, Press JM (eds). Functional rehabilitation of sports and musculoskeletal medicine. Maryland: Aspen, 1998:216–243.

46. Standaert CJ, Herring SA, Halpern B, King O: Spondylolysis. In: Young JL, ed. Phys Med Rehab Clin N Am 11(4):785–803, 2000.

47. Blanda J, Bethem D, Moats W, et al: Defects of pars interarticularis in athletes: a protocol for nonoperative treatment. J Spinal Disord 6(5):406–411, 1993.

48. Daniel JN, Polly DW, Van Dam BE: A study of the efficacy of nonoperative treatment of presumed traumatic spondylolysis in a young patient population. Mil Med 160(11):553–555, 1995.

49. Steiner ME, Micheli LJ: Treatment of symptomatic spondylolysis and spondylolisthesis with the modified Boston brace. Spine 10(10):937–943, 1985.

50. Yamane T, Yoshida T, Mimatsu K: Early diagnosis of lumbar spondylolysis by MRI. J Bone Joint Surg 75B:764–768, 1993.

51. Lafferty JF, Winter WG, Gambro SA: Fatigue characteristics of posterior elements of vertebrae. J Bone Joint Surg 59A:154–158, 1997.

52. Letts M, MacDonald P: Sports injuries to the pediatric spine. Spine: State of the Art Reviews 4:49–83, 1990.

53. Morita T, Ikata T, Katoh S, et al: Lumbar spondylolysis in children and adolescents. J Bone Joint Surg 77B:620–625, 1995.

54. Katoh F, Ikata T, Fujii K: Factors influencing a union of spondylolysis in children and adolescents. In: Proceedings and Abstracts from North American Spine Society Meeting, New York; 1997:222.

55. Fellander-Tsai L, Micheli LJ: Treatment of spondylolysis with external electrical stimulation and bracing in adolescent athletes: a report of two cases. Clin J Sports Med 8(3):232–234, 1998.

56. Pettine KA, Salib RM, Walker SG: External electrical stimulation and bracing for treatment of spondylolysis. A case report. Spine 18(4):436–439, 1993.

57. Marharam LG, Sharkey I: Electrical stimulation of acute spondylolysis: 3 cases. Med Sci Sports Exercise 24(suppl):538, 1992.

58. O'Neill DB, Micheli LJ: Postoperative radiographic evidence for fatigue fracture as the etiology in spondylolysis. Spine 14:1342–1355, 1989.

59. Pelllise F, Toribio J, Rivas A, et al: Clinical and CT scan evaluation after direct repair in spondylolysis using segmental pedicular screw hook fixation. J Spinal Disord 12(5):363–367, 1999.

60. Wu SS, Lee CH, Chen PQ: Operative repair of symptomatic spondylolysis following a positive response to diagnostic pars injection. J Spinal Disord 12(1):10–16, 1999.

61. Prasartritha T: Surgical repair of pars defects in spondylolysis. J Med Assoc Thai 84(9):1235–1240, 2001.

61a. Dai LY, Jia LS, Yuan W, Ni B, Zhu HB: Direct repair of defect in lumbar spondylolysis and mild isthmic spondylolisthesis by bone grafting, with or without facet joint fusion. Eur Spine J February 10(1):78–83, 2001.

62. Blanda J, Bethem D, Moats W, et al: Defects of pars interarticularis in athletes: a protocol for nonoperative treatment. J Spinal Disord 6(5):406–411, 1993.

63. Jackson DW, Wiltse LL, Dingeman RD, et al: Stress reactions involving the pars interarticularis in young athletes. Am J Sports Med 9:304–312, 1981.

64. O'Sullivan PB, Phyty GD, Twomey LT, et al: Evaluation of specific stabilizing exercise in the treatment of chronic low back pain with radiologic diagnosis of spondylolysis or spondylolisthesis. Spine 22:2959–2967, 1997.

65. Steiner ME, Micheli LJ: Treatment of symptomatic spondylolysis and spondylolisthesis with the modified Boston brace. Spine 10:937–943, 1985.

66. Anderson K, Sarwark JF, Conway JJ, et al: Quantitative assessment with SPECT imaging of stress injuries of the pars interarticularis response to bracing. J Pediatr Orthop 20(1):28–33, 2000.

67. Morita T, Ikata T, Katoh, et al: Lumbar spondylolysis in children and adolescents. J Bone Join Surg 77B:620–625, 1995.

68. Lantz SA, Schultz AB: Lumbar orthosis wearing I: restriction of gross body motions. Spine 11:834–837, 1986.

69. Herring SA: Rehabilitation of muscle injuries. Med & Sci in Sports & Exerc 22:455, 1990.

70. Kaul M, Herring S: Rehabilitation of the lumbar spine injuries in sports. Phys Med Rehab Clin N Am 5:173–176, 1994.

71. Young J, Press J: The disc at risk in athletes: perspectives on operative and nonoperative care. Med Sci Sports Exerc 29:S222–S232, 1997.

72. McGill SM, Norman RW: Reassessment of the role of intra-abdominal pressure in spinal compression. Ergonomics 505:539–548, 1987.

73. Cherkin D, Deyo R: A comparison of physical therapy, chiropractic manipulation, and provision of an educational booklet for the treatment of patients with low back pain. N Engl J Med 339(15):1021–1029, 1998.

74. Andersson G, Lucente T: Comparison of osteopathic spinal manipulation with standard care for patients with low back pain. N Engl J Med 341(19):1426–1431, 1999.

75. Donnelson R, Silva G: Centralization phenomena: its usefulness in evaluating and treating referred pain. Spine 15(3):2111–2113, 1990.

76. Nadler SF, Shumko J, Galski T, Feinberg JH: Low back pain in college athletes: true incidence and proper screening. Proc N Am Spine Soc 10:62, 1995.

77. Osternig LR, Robertson RN: Effects of prophylactic knee bracing on lower extremity joint position and muscle activation during running. Am J Sports Med 21(5):733–737, 1993.

78. Knapik JJ, Baumana CL, Jones BH, et al: Preseason strength and flexibility imbalances associated with athletic injuries in female collegiate athletes. Am J Sports Med 16(1):76–81, 1991.

79. Gray GW: Total body functional profile. Adrian, MI: Wynn Marketing Inc.; 2001.

80. Press JM, O'Conner A: What is core rehabilitation. Proceedings American Academy of Physical Medicine and Rehabilitation Annual Meeting, Orlando, Florida; 2001.

81. White A, Derby R: Epidural injections for the diagnosis and treatment of lower back pain. Spine 5:78–86, 1980.

82. Metha M, Salmon N: Extradural block, confirmation of injection site by xray monitoring. Anesthesia 40:1009–1012, 1985.

83. Bryan BM, Lutz C, Lutz GE: Fluoroscopic assessment of epidural contrast spread after caudal injection. In: Syllabus of the 7th Annual Scientific Meeting of the International Spinal Injection Society, Las Vegas, Nevada; 1999:57.

84. Cooke P, Lutz G: Internal disc disruption and axial back pain in the athlete. Phys Med Rehab Clin N Am 11(4):837–865, 2000.

85. Vleeming A, Buyruk HM, Stoeckart R, et al: Towards an integrated therapy for peripartum pelvic instability: a study of the biomechanical effects of pelvic belts. Am J Obs Gynecol 166:1243–1247, 1992.

86. Maigne JY, Aivaliklis A, Pfefer F: Results of sacroiliac joint double block and value of sacroiliac pain provocation tests in 54 patients with low back pain. Spine 21:1889–1892, 1996.

87. Keating JG, Avillar MD, Price M: Sacroiliac joint arthrodesis in selected patients with low back pain. In: Vleeming A, Mooney V, Dorman T, et al, eds. Movement, stability and low back pain. New York: Churchill Livingstone; 1999:573–586.

88. Lippitt AB: Percutaneous fixation of the sacroiliac joint. In: Vleeming A, Mooney V, Dorman T, et al, eds. Movement, stability and low back pain. New York: Churchill Livingstone; 1999:587–594.

89. Dorman TA: Pelvic mechanics and prolotherapy. In: Vleeming A, Mooney V, Dorman T, et al, eds. Movement, stability and low back pain. New York: Churchill Livingstone; 1999:501–522.

90. Dorman TA. Prolotherapy: a survey. J Ortho Med 15:2, 1993.

91. Ongley MJ, Klein RG, Dorman TA, et al: A new approach to the treatment of chronic low back pain. Lancet 2:143–146, 1987.

92. Micheli LJ. Back injuries in gymnasts. Clin Sports Med 4(1):85–93, 1985.

93. D'Hemecourt PA, Gerbino PG, Micheli LJ: Back injuries in the young athlete. Clin Sports Med 19(4):663–679, 2000.

94. Soler T, Calderon C: The prevalence of spondylolysis in the Spanish elite athlete. Am J Sports Med 28(1):57–62, 2000.

95. Meeusen R, Borms J: Gymnastic injuries. Sports Med 13(5):337–356, 1992.

CHAPTER

12

Sports for Athletes with Physical Disabilities

James J Laskin

INTRODUCTION

Individuals with physical disabilities are not only becoming better integrated into mainstream society but they also have made significant achievements in the sporting world.[1–4] It is now routine for athletes with tetraplegia to complete the marathon in less than 2 hours.[3] Athletes with visual impairments and lower-limb loss compete on the same giant slalom course as their able-bodied peers.[3,5,6] In fact, in events such as bench press and solo yachting, there are competitions held that do not even discriminate between those who are able-bodied and those with a physical disability.[3] With these individuals pushing their physical limits, there comes associated injuries. Some injuries are merely an annoyance, whereas others without proper care and attention, can become career ending.[7,8] The intention of this chapter is to introduce you to the types of athletes and several sporting events that people with physical disabilities participate in. We will not only present the unique aspects of the care and prevention of sport-related injuries for people with physical disabilities but we also intend to demonstrate the able-bodied parallels. This chapter will provide you with the information needed to lessen the hesitation that many health professionals feel when treating a competitive athlete with a physical disability.

PARALYMPIC VERSUS SPECIAL OLYMPIC MOVEMENTS

The Special Olympics has become an institutional icon in the United States as well as internationally. Special Olympic programming has been developed for persons with developmental disabilities and utilizes strong local community support. The goal of Special Olympic programs is to provide sporting opportunities that facilitate the development of physical fitness and sports skills. Through sport the athletes have the opportunity to demonstrate courage, experience joy, and develop friendships. The primary aim is one of recreation versus truly elite competitive sport. Although diminished cognitive ability is the common denominator amongst these athletes, physical limitations and mobility impairments are present.[4] The Paralympic movement is based on a very different philosophy. The Paralympic Games are the ultimate competitive event for world class, elite athletes with physical disabilities. The "Para" in Paralympic is not a reference to paraplegia, but rather the parallel to the Olympic movement. Like any elite athlete "going for the gold," Paralympic athletes are committed to rigorous training regimes, are expected to meet strict qualification standards, and exist in an environment of excellence and personal best performances.[1,3,4]

HISTORY OF SPORT FOR ATHLETES WITH PHYSICAL DISABILITIES

Sports for people with physical disabilities had their start as a form of rehabilitation. Towards the end of World War II, Dr. Ludwig Guttmann, a neurosurgeon at the Stoke Mandeville Hospital in Aylesbury, England, suggested using sporting activities as part of his patients' rehabilitation. By 1948, the 1st Stoke Mandeville Games opened, with 16 WWII veterans who had a spinal cord injury or lower extremity amputation. Interestingly, the day that Dr. Guttmann picked for these inaugural games was July 28, 1948, the opening day of the XIV Olympic Games. Four years later, a team of Dutch wheelchair athletes came to Aylesbury for the 1st International Stoke Mandeville Games. These initial efforts to provide athletes with disabilities world-class competition resulted in the formation of the International Paralympic Committee and the 1st Summer Paralympic Games in 1960 in Rome. The 1988 Paralympic Games, held in Seoul, South Korea, were the first games to be endorsed by the International Olympic Committee and share the same venues several weeks after the able-bodied event.[3,4] The Seoul Games attracted 3000 athletes from 62 countries.[1] The most recent Summer Paralympic Games (2000) held in Sydney, Australia, drew 3800 athletes from 122 countries.[3] Currently, the Summer Paralympic Games allows competition in 18 sports, 14 of which are currently also Olympic sports (Table 12.1).[3] In conjunction with the development of the Summer Games, the Winter Paralympic Games have also grown dramatically. Although smaller than their Summer counterpart (416 athletes from 36 nations), the most recent Winter Paralympic Games were held in Salt Lake City, Utah, in 2002. The Winter Games feature athletes competing in ice sledge hockey, alpine and nordic skiing, and wheelchair curling.[3–6]

PARALYMPIC VERSUS NON-PARALYMPIC SPORTS

Not unlike the able-bodied games, the decision of which events shall be offered is mired in politics and history. The events given the Paralympic spotlight represent only a fraction of the recreational and competitive sporting opportunities afforded an individual with a physical disability.[3,4,8] Currently, in the United States there are competitive opportunities for handcycling, power soccer, water skiing, kayaking, golf, bowling, and square dancing to name a few. Recreational opportunities are only limited by one's imagination and ability to adapt the chosen activity to suit the individual's abilities. Activities such as hunting, fishing, rock climbing, softball, and skydiving are only a sample of what is available in the United States.[4,10]

TYPICAL CLINICALLY DEFINED CONDITIONS PARTICIPATING IN PARALYMPIC SPORT

Only athletes in the five disability-specific international organizations and their national and local affiliates are eligible to compete in Paralympic events.[2–4,10] These individuals tend to have a condition/disability that is relatively static in nature.[9] Athletes with a spinal cord injury, polio, or spina bifida are those represented by the International Stoke Mandeville Wheelchair Sports Federation.[11] Athletes with cerebral palsy, head injury, stroke, or other non-progressive brain injury are associated with the Cerebral Palsy – International Sport and Recreation Association.[12] Members of the International Sport Federation for the Disabled include those individuals with amputations, dwarfism, and other physically disabling conditions such as birth defects.[13] The International Blind Sports Federation represents athletes with visual impairments.[14] Finally, the International Sports Federation for Persons with Mental Handicaps promotes the inclusion of athletes with learning disabilities.[3] Although these organizations, especially at the local level, promote Paralympic sport, they also serve to facilitate the growth and development of other non-Paralympic endeavors. Historically, each of these organizations promoted and developed disability specific competitions. However, now with the majority of sports being multi-disability by design, the emphasis is

Table 12-1 Paralympic sports and the participating athletes[7,9]

Sport	Cerebral palsy, brain injury[5]	Spinal cord lesion	Amputee	Visually impaired	Les autres[6]
Archery		x	x		
Athletics	x	x	x	x[7]	x
Basketball	x	x	x		
Boccia	x				
Cycling	x		x	x[8]	x
Equestrian	x	x	x	x	x
Fencing	x	x	x		
Goal ball				x	
Judo				x	
Lawn bowls		x	x	x	x
Power lifting[1]	x	x	x		
Shooting	x	x	x		
Soccer	x				
Swimming	x	x	x	x	x
Table tennis	x	x	x	x	x
Tennis[2]		x	x		
Volleyball[3]	x	x	x		
Rugby[4]		x			

1. Bench press only. 2. Wheelchair users only. 3. Both standing and sitting versions. 4. For athletes with tetraplegia only. 5. Any non-progressive brain injury. 6. Any physical disability that does not fit into a specific category, e.g., dwarfism and extremity birth defects. 7. Some events allow a guide. 8. Uses a tandem bike and a sighted pilot.

placed on developing the sport versus focusing on opportunities for a given special interest/disability group.[4]

CLASSIFICATION

Many able-bodied sports use classification by gender, mass, or age to create an equitable competitive playing field. In sports for people with physical disabilities, classification is determined by lesion level, muscular strength, flexibility, balance, coordination, spasticity, sensation, or visual acuity.[3] The fundamental philosophy of classification is to allow athletes with similar functional abilities to compete such that the competition is deemed fair. As a classifier, one attempts to determine the innate functional ability of an athlete and not allow skill level (potential or developed) or athleticism bias their determinations.[4] Historically, when sports were disability specific, classification was primarily based on the type of lesion, lesion level, or amputation site. Presently, most sports have developed a sport-specific functional classification system that allows athletes, regardless of their medically defined condition, to compete against each other with similar functional abilities.[3,4]

INJURY PROFILE OF ATHLETES WITH PHYSICAL DISABILITIES

There has been a dramatic rise in the number of individuals with a physical disability participating in some form of recreational activity or competitive sport.[4,7,10,15] Legislative initiatives, technological advances, and changing social norms are three of the primary reasons for this increased participation.[4,7] Given the growth of participation in these recreational and sporting opportunities, it is surprising at the dearth of literature devoted to understanding the types and patterns of disability and/or sport specific injuries.[7,16] The challenge of documenting the patterns and types of injuries is enormous. As is evident in this text, there is a relatively large epidemiological literature base dealing with individual able-bodied sports. These studies only need to stratify the population by gender, age, and race or geographical region, as appropriate. Unfortunately, with the multiplicity of conditions, the wide range of activities, and the small number of participants, the challenges to the researcher interested in people with physical disabilities may be overwhelming.[7] However, there is a small body of literature, which focuses almost exclusively on wheelchair users and Paralympic sports.

In one of the earliest studies to document disability-specific injuries, 517 out of the 708 wheelchair users with spinal cord injuries responded to the authors' survey. Just over half (51.4%) reported pain in or around the shoulder.[17] The individuals that Nichols, Norman, and Ennis surveyed were not athletes; however, the authors documented a significant rate of injury from using a wheelchair for activities of daily living. Burnham et al,[18] followed by Ferrara et al,[19] found that the injury distribution for a given medical disability was consistent with the most active body parts. They observed that ambulatory athletes (visual impairments, upper and lower extremity amputations, and cerebral palsy/brain injury) reported primarily lower extremity injuries, whereas those who competed in a wheelchair (lower extremity amputation, spinal cord lesions, and cerebral palsy/brain injury) reported injuries to their upper extremities. A retrospective study by Ferrara et al[19] surveyed 426 athletes who attended the 1989 US National Championships: 137 responded. The authors documented a relatively equal distribution of injuries between the three main disability-specific categorizations (wheelchair users, visually impaired, and cerebral palsy/brain injury).[19] The injury rates observed were comparable to those reported in the literature for able-bodied athletes competing in similar sporting activities. Peck and McKeag reported 60% of the 1988 US Paralympic team seeking care for an injury/illness as compared to their Olympic peers at 75%.[20] Furthermore, these authors reported that the overall injury rate for athletes with disabilities was 32% versus a range of 24–40% for athletes participating in comparable able-bodied sports. Ferrara and Peterson reviewed the related epidemiological studies and concluded that the injury patterns for athletes with physical disabilities closely match those found in the able-bodied athletic population.[21] In examining data as far back as 1976 they confirmed that injury patterns are closely associated with disability type and the given sport. Ferrara and Peterson cited overall injury rates of 9.3/1000 for athletes with disabilities as compared to able-bodied American football (10.1/1000),[22,23] basketball (7.0/1000),[22] and soccer (9.8/1000).[22] In general, these and other studies consistently report that the most common injuries experienced by athletes with physical disabilities are either acute soft tissue abrasions, blisters, contusions, sprains, and strains to the extremities or chronic shoulder, elbow and/or wrist dysfunctions which are found primarily in the wheelchair users.[2,8,10,18,21,24–29] These findings were also supported by the first true longitudinal study in this area, authored by Ferrara et al.[15] This study was limited to US athletes attending international championships from 1990 to 1996. Besides this study's longitudinal design, it was unique in that it is the first to document a significant incidence (111 of the 728 non–illness-related reported injuries) in sprains and strains to the thorax and spine, particularly in the wheelchair users.[15] Although the severity of the spine injuries was low and the type of injury was typically a muscular strain versus actual joint dysfunction, discogenic, or fracture/dislocation, there is still reason to be concerned. This study only included elite athletes attending major international events. The athletes included in this study only represented a small percentage of those who participate in sport and did not include the sports that might have a higher incidence of trauma (e.g., wheelchair basketball, wheelchair rugby, nor any non-Paralympic activity).

Data in injury types and rates for winter sport athletes with physical disabilities is exceptionally limited. There is a paucity of literature available examining the injury rates, types, and patterns for any winter sport besides alpine skiing. The number of accidents per participant that required an emergency room inter-vention is comparable to other contact and/or high-velocity sports. Ferrara et al surveyed 68 athletes who represented primarily sit-skiers.[30] Of the chronic injuries reported, 73% were related to the upper extremity, whereas only 15% of the acute injuries were to the neck and head. Although small in number, the injuries of the lumbar spine were attributed to the sit-ski positioning, which causes excessive hip angulation and lumbar flexion. This position results in side-bending or rotation of the trunk to occur with the lumbar spine in its end range. Laskowski and Murtaugh reported retrospective injury rates for both physically disabled and able-bodied skiers of four ski areas located in California, Colorado, and Washington.[5] Across the four sites, approximately one-third of the physically disabled skiers were wheelchair users. The authors found that the injury rates for both physically disabled and able-bodied skiers were not significantly different. For example, one major Colorado resort reported that over a 4-year period there were over 64 000 disabled-skier visits, with an average injury rate of 3.7/1000 visits as compared to the able-bodied injury rate of 3.5/1000 skier visits. Petrofsky and Meyer's review of the literature specifically looked at the patterns of injury of individuals who use a monoski.[6] The monoskiers are wheelchair users who ski sit in a bucket-like apparatus attached to a single ski, with or without outrigger-style poles. The authors reported that two-thirds of the injuries that athletes with disabilities participating in winter sports athletes experience are chronic versus acute. Not surprisingly, of the injuries that do occur, they are primarily related to the upper extremities. This is largely because the monoskiing position requires the athlete to sit with the lumbar spine flexed to 80 degrees; the scapula is placed in a compromised inefficient position, putting the rotator cuff musculature and elbow at risk.

What is missing from this body of literature is the prospective style of epidemiological research. Of the studies that have been completed, there is no consistency regarding the definitions used for injury, which disabilities and/or sports being evaluated, level of competition, categorization of experience, training practices, and access to healthcare professionals.[7] In addition, the categorization used in many of the studies is so vague that at best one only knows that a certain percent of injuries were sprains of the thorax and spine, versus providing details as to the spinal level and/or the structures involved.[15] In fact, given that the majority of the research has been devoted to Paralympic sports and their associated athletes, the current state of the literature may not generalize well across the range of non-Paralympic sports nor to those individuals who do not fit into the strict definition of a Paralympic athlete. What is clear is that, in general, athletes with physical disabilities appear to be at no more risk for injury than their able-bodied peers.[31] The apparent lack of data related to spine injuries and dysfunction appear to be a limitation of the research and not an assertion that they do not occur in this population.[15] Another factor that could influence both the type and pattern of injuries reported in the physically disabled population is the fact that the literature reviewed almost exclusively dealt with elite or high-functioning athletes. It would be expected that those who achieve elite status are less predisposed to injuries and may in fact be less affected by disability-specific attributes such as spasticity, poor coordination, altered sensation, and ataxia.

SPINE INJURIES: DISABILITY-SPECIFIC CONCERNS

Given the literature reviewed and the author's experience, it appears that, while not of epidemic propor-tions, spine injuries do occur in this population. The types of spinal injuries reported seem to be soft tissue in nature following a pattern of chronicity. It has been noted that of the spinal injuries that do occur they tend to be chronic in nature.[7,21] Although there is an inherent risk in extrapolating the literature and clinical experiences reported from able-bodied sporting activities to their physically disabled analogue, it is a place to start. For any given activity, the primary difference between those athletes with a physical disability who ambulate and their able-bodied peers has more to do with disability-specific attributes versus the activity itself. One could anticipate that there would be little difference between the injuries observed and the prevention/rehabilitation measures taken when comparing able-bodied athletes and those with a visual impairment participating in judo or wrestling.[4] In addition to the disability-specific factors, for those who compete in a wheelchair or other seated device, the field of play and the rules may be similar to able-bodied sport, but the dynamics, movements, and sport-specific techniques may be substantially different. For example, the wheelchair marathon may take place on the same course as the able-bodied event, but the physiologic and biomechanical requirements are very different.[4] When working with an injured athlete with a physical disability, it is as important to understand the etiology, natural history, and pathophysiology of their condition as it is to have a clear understanding of the mechanism of injury and of the demands of their sport.[7,32,33] In addition to these components, it is also essential to have an appreciation for disability-specific issues such as altered sensation, altered reflexes, spasticity, hypotonicity, motor control issues, impaired balance or coordination, presence of contractures, and contributory/ concomitant disease.[11–13,32,33]

The types and patterns of spinal injuries that affect ambulatory athletes with visual impairments or amputations would be expected to be similar to those of the able-bodied athletic population.[4,7,13,14,34] Depending upon the degree and form of visual impairment, there may be compensatory alterations in gait, many of which are habitual and not functional. The same is true for both upper and lower extremity amputees. As the extent of limb loss increases, the greater the magnitude in the alterations of the individual's gait. These gait alterations are what put the spine at risk.[13,32–34] Regardless of the sport activity, injuries to the soft tissues, interverterbal discs, and facet joints can be expected. The challenge to the health professional or coach is to attempt to normalize the athlete's gait. For athletes with lower limb amputations the assistance of a prosthetist is essential.

Depending upon lower extremity function, those with cerebral palsy, brain injury, or stroke may compete as ambulatory or wheelchair athletes. Regardless of their mode of mobility, these athletes face the challenge of fluctuating tone.[12,32,35,36] These changes in tone may be diurnal in nature, but are also affected by stress, environmental conditions, fatigue, pain, and medication.[12,33,35,37,38] The typical scenario is one of some degree of increased tone in the extremities, with associated joint contractures, and decreased tone in the trunk. In addition, depending on the areas of the brain affected, these individuals may also present with ataxia, athetosis, impaired coordination, altered motor control, activation of primitive reflexes, hearing impairment, and cognitive delay. Some of the symptoms – such as altered tone, coordination, motor control, ataxia, and athetosis – may be temporarily exacerbated by strenuous exercise.[35] Given these movement challenges, specifically the decreased tone noted in the trunk, one would expect the lumbar spine and thoracolumbar junction to be primarily affected due to the poor stability of this region.[12] At risk would be the soft tissues and intervertebral discs.[7] In addition, it is important to note that the incidence of scoliosis and kyphoscoliosis is very high in this population.[35]

Although predominately wheelchair users, there are a few individuals with spinal cord lesions that compete as ambulatory athletes. Nevertheless, the risk to the spine varies with the level of lesion and the sporting activity.[7,21,25,27] Combinations of spasticity, flaccidity, altered sensation, and the variety of orthopedic surgical interventions further complicates the prediction of the type and pattern of spinal injuries.[11,27] Pain originating from the spine is commonly reported in the non-athletic wheelchair using population.[37–39] One cannot assume just because the individual may lack sensation that a spinal dysfunction at that or other referring levels may not be causing pain. The clinician must be watchful for the signs and symptoms of referred pain as well as associated changes in spasticity, hyperreflexia, and/or autonomic dysreflexia in those with tetraplegia.[11,27,32,39] The common denominator is the wheelchair design and setup, which is focused on maximizing performance and not prevention of upper extremity and spine injuries. An almost universal phenomenon of wheelchair users regardless of their medical condition is the kyphotic posture that they adopt. Not only does this posture put the thoracic and cervical spine at risk but also the head forward, protracted scapular position is a prime mechanism for rotator cuff impingement and other forms of shoulder dysfunction. The cause for this adopted kyphotic posture can be due to poor postural control, weak spinal musculature, or a premorbid condition. Due to the requirements of the sport-specific competitive wheelchair, not much can be done except to ensure that there is a balanced conditioning program that includes strengthening of the scapular retractors.[9,40] However, the setup of the athlete's everyday chair could significantly help mediate the problem.

Often in an effort to make wheelies easier (or forgetting to plan for a backpack hanging off the back of the chair), the center of gravity is set too far back. The center of gravity or balance point is determined by the positioning of the seat over the axles of the back wheels. The further back the center of gravity is set, the greater the "tipsiness" of the chair. If the tipsiness is excessive, the individual will compensate by leaning forward at the hips and adopting a head-forward position with excessive neck extension, and developing or accentuating a kyphotic posture. A second factor that may affect the wheelchair user's posture is the seat dump, which is the difference in seat height between the buttocks and the knees (Figs 12.1 and 12.2). Increasing the seat dump helps facilitate trunk stability, which helps with sitting balance and is a vital component of shoulder girdle stability. However, the cost of achieving trunk stability by increasing the amount of dump is the resulting kyphotic posture. The increased seat dump forces the trunk into flexion and results in the athlete adopting a head-forward, rounded-shoulder posture. A flatter seat may decrease trunk stability, but it will encourage a reduction in kyphosis.[9] By decreasing the forward lean and forward head posture, the flatter seat will "open up" the shoulders and help minimize the amount of impingement of the rotator cuff with overhead activities.[9,41] Modification of the chair's center of gravity and seat dump are just two of the simple alterations that can reduce the incidence of chronic spinal dysfunction.[9,32]

A final thought regarding the aging athlete, particularly one who is a wheelchair user. Osteoporosis not only of the lower extremities but also of the lumbar spine may have grave consequences as these athletes age.[11,39,42] The risk for osteoporotic changes taking place in these non-ambulatory individuals is

Figure 12.1
A flat seat dump.

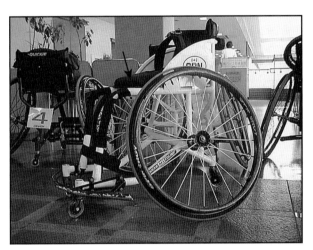

Figure 12.2
A steep seat dump.

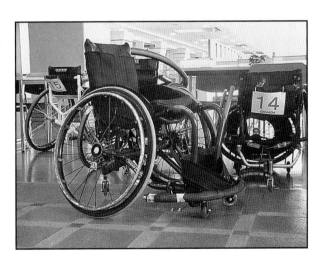

significantly greater due to the lack of weight bearing of the lower extremities.[11] Femoral fractures, spontaneous compression fractures of the vertebral bodies, and spinous process fractures are just a few of the possible sequelae.[42] Although more likely to occur in the older/retired athlete, the author is aware of two elite wheelchair basketball athletes where a spontaneous femoral fracture has occurred as a result of individuals with paraplegia performing their daily self-stretching routine.

SUMMARY

Given the lack of available literature and the enormity of the task, it was not the intention of this chapter to provide the sport-specific biomechanics, potential mechanisms of injury, and suggested preventive techniques for each disability. What we suggest is that readers familiarize themselves with the able-bodied activity and apply the information provided in this chapter to assist them with the sport medical care of their athletes. There is also a growing body of applied literature dealing with disability and sport-specific biomechanics and skill development. In addition, there is an increasing number of resources available that relate to disability-specific attributes, medical concerns/contraindications, and exercise adaptations. In a typical sports medicine setting it would not be surprising that many healthcare providers would initially feel hesitant when confronted with an individual who has a physical disability, but always remember that they are a competitive athlete first.

REFERENCES

1. Atlanta Paralympic Organizing Committee: Brief history of the Paralympic Games: Press packet. Atlanta, GA: APOC; 1996.

2. Bergeron JW: Athletes with disabilities. Phys Med Rehab Clin N Am 10(1):213–228, 1999.

3. International Paralympic Committee: Paralympic overview. Available from: URL: http://www.paralympic.org

4. Paciorek MJ: Adapted sport. In: Winnick JP, ed. Adapted physical education and sport, 3rd edn. Champaign, IL: Human Kinetics; 2000:33–46.

5. Laskowski ER, Murtaugh PA: Snow skiing injuries in physically disabled skiers. Am J Sports Med 20(5):553–555, 1992.

6. Petrofsky J, Meyer J: Causes and suggested preventives for injuries to monoskiers. Palaestra 19(1):28–37, 2003.

7. Harmer PA: Disability sports. In: Caine DJ, Caine CG, Lindner KJ, eds. Epidemiology of sports injuries. Champaign, IL: Human Kinetics; 1996:161–175.

8. Stopka C: An overview of common injuries to individuals with disabilities (part 1). Palaestra 12(1):44–51, 1996.

9. Laskin JJ: Aim high: conquering the primary and secondary disabilities of wheelchair athletes. Phys Ther Prod 14(5):10–14, 2003.

10. Schaefer RS, Proffer DS: Sports medicine for wheelchair athletes. Am Fam Physician 39(5):239–245, 1989.

11. Kelly L: Spinal cord disabilities. In: Winnick JP, ed. Adapted physical education and sport, 3rd edn. Champaign, IL: Human Kinetics; 2000:215–234.

12. Parretta DL: Cerebral palsy, stroke, and traumatic brain injury. In: Winnick JP, ed. Adapted physical education and sport, 3rd edn. Champaign, IL: Human Kinetics; 2000:181–198.

13. Parretta DL: Amputations, dwarfism, and les autres. In: Winnick JP, ed. Adapted physical education and sport, 3rd edn. Champaign, IL: Human Kinetics; 2000:199–214.

14. Craft DH, Lieberman L: Visual impairments and deafness. In: Winnick JP, ed. Adapted physical education and sport, 3rd edn. Champaign, IL: Human Kinetics; 2000:159–180.

15. Ferrara MS, Palutsis GR, Snouse S, et al: A longitudinal study of injuries to athletes with disabilities. Int J Sports Med 21:221–224, 2000.

16. Stopka C: Athletic therapy for athletes with disabilities. Part 2. Special conditions. Athl Ther Today 8(3):23–25, 2003.

17. Nichols PJ, Norman PA, Ennis JR: Wheelchair users shoulder? Shoulder pain in patients with spinal cord lesions. Scand J Rehab Med 11(1):29–32, 1979.

18. Burnham R, Newell E, Steadward RD: Sports medicine for the physically disabled: the Canadian team experience at the 1988 Seoul Paralympic Games. Clin J Sport Med 1:193–196, 1991.

19. Ferrara MS, Buckley WE, McCann C, et al: The injury experience of the competitive athlete with a disability: prevention implications. Med Sci Sports Exerc 24:184–188, 1992.

20. Peck M, McKeak DB: Athletes with disabilities: removing barriers. Phys Sportsmed 2(4):59–62, 1994.

21. Ferrara MS, Peterson CL: Injuries to athletes with disabilities: identifying injury patterns. Sports Med 30(2):137–143, 2000.

22. Buckley WE: Five year overview of sport injuries: the NAIRS model. J Phys Educ Rec Dance 17:36–40, 1982.

23. Buckley WE, Powell JP: NAIRS: an epidemiological overview of the severity of injury in college football. Athlet Training 18:279–282, 1982.

24. Bloomquist LE: Injuries to athletes with physical disabilities: prevention implications. Phys Sportsmed 14(9):96–100;102;105, 1986.

25. Curtis KA, Dillon DA: Survey of wheelchair athletic injuries: common patterns and prevention. Paraplegia 23(3):170–175, 1985.

26. Ferrara MS, Davis RW: Injuries to elite wheelchair athletes. Paraplegia 28(5):335–341, 1990.

27. Figoni SF, Kiratli BJ, Sasaki R: Spinal cord dysfunction. In: Myers JN, Herbert WG, Humphrey R, eds. ACSM'S resources for clinical exercise physiology. Philadelphia: Lippincott, Williams & Wilkins; 2002:48–67.

28. Subbarao JV, Klopfstein J, Turpin R: Prevalence and impact of wrist and shoulder pain in patients with SCI. J Spinal Cord Med 18(1):9–13, 1995.

29. Taylor D, Williams T: Sports injuries in athletes with disabilities: wheelchair racing. Paraplegia 33(5):296–299, 1995.

30. Ferrara MS, Buckley WE, Messner DG, et al: The injury experience and training history of the competitive skier with a disability. Am J Sports Med 20(1):55–60, 1992.

31. Dec KL, Sparrow KJ, McKeag DB: The physically-challenged athlete: Medical issues and assessment. Sports Med 29(4):245–258, 2000.

32. Curtis KA: Health Smarts Part 2. Strategies and solutions for wheelchair athletes: common injuries of wheelchair athletes – prevention and treatment. Sports 'n Spokes 22(2):13–19, 1996.

33. Curtis KA: Health Smarts Part 3. Strategies and solutions for wheelchair athletes: common medical problems – prevention and treatment. Sports 'n Spokes 22(3):21–28, 1996.

34. Pitetti KH, Manske RC: Amputation. In: Myers JN, Herbert WG, Humphrey R, eds. ACSM's resources for clinical exercise physiology. Philadelphia: Lippincott, Williams & Wilkins; 2002:170–178.

35. Laskin JJ, Anderson, MA: Cerebral palsy. In: Myers JN, Herbert WG, Humphrey R, eds. ACSM's resources for clinical exercise physiology. Philadelphia: Lippincott, Williams & Wilkins; 2002:16–28.

36. Rimmer J, Nicola TL: Stroke. In: Myers JN, Herbert WG, Humphrey R, eds. ACSM's resources for clinical exercise physiology. Philadelphia: Lippincott, Williams & Wilkins; 2002:3–15.

37. Bernardi M, Castellano V, Ferrara MS, et al: Muscle pain in athletes with locomotor disability. Med Sci Sports Exerc 35(2):199–206, 2003.

38. Boninger ML, Cooper RA, Fitzgerald SG, et al: Investigating neck pain in wheelchair users. Am J Phys Med Rehab 82:197–202, 2003.

39. Ehde DM, Jensen M, Engel JM, et al: Chronic pain secondary to disability: a review. Clin J Pain 19(1):3–17, 2003.

40. Stopka C: Prevention comes first! (Managing common injuries in individuals with disabilities, part 2). Palaestra 12(2):28–31, 1996.

41. Stopka C: Managing common injuries in individuals with disabilities: evaluation, treatment, & rehabilitation (part 3). Palaestra 12(3):32–33;35–38, 1996.

42. Curtis KA: Health Smarts Part 6. Strategies and solutions for wheelchair athletes: slowing down the hands of time. Sports 'n Spokes 22(6):53–60, 1996.

CHAPTER

13

The Martial Arts: Biomechanical Principles, Injury Prevention, and Rehabilitation

Robert E Windsor

Michael Furman

Ross Sugar

Ricardo Nieves

Stephen Roman

Unlike other contact and many non-contact sports, the martial arts enable individuals to participate in an athletic activity from childhood through retirement. Physical and mental flexibility, agility, and speed make up for relative weaknesses or small stature. Martial artists benefit from increased fitness, strength, concentration, self-confidence, and body awareness.[1] Serious participants go beyond the techniques, and martial arts philosophy becomes a way of life.

The mystique of the martial arts results from its history and recent popularization. Practice of the martial arts was shrouded in secrecy until the beginning of the 20th century, and knowledge of its specific origins is vague. About 1400 years ago, Bodhidharma, the founder of Zen Buddhism, used strength, endurance, and self-defense techniques as methods to promote his disciples' health and spiritual development. These techniques were taught in the monastery of the Shaolin Temple in China, where they were refined and developed into Shaolin boxing.

In the 16th century, Shaolin boxing found its way to Okinawa, Japan, where it was integrated into the region's native fighting techniques. During several periods in the coming years, Okinawans were prohibited from owning weapons and participating in self-defense training. This resulted in great advancements in unarmed combat techniques. Secret training flourished, and the styles became more efficient and deadly.

It was not until 1906 that the first public exhibition of martial arts (karate) was held. Master Gichin Funakoshi, widely held to be the father of modern karate, introduced martial arts to the rest of Japan in 1922 at the first National Athletic Exhibition in Tokyo. Students of Master Funakoshi traveled to various countries, including the United States, and brought organized martial arts with them. These events signaled the transition of karate from a martial art into a sport.

There are hundreds of martial arts styles incorporating thousands of throwing, striking, kicking, blocking, and other techniques. Some involve weapons, and others use empty hand and foot techniques. Styles range from the slow, deliberate, non-contact motions of tai chi, to the grappling, wrestling-like judo, and so-called "hard" full-contact arts of karate and taikwondo. Other works are fully described in detail elsewhere.[2-10] This chapter focuses on the hard styles, their biomechanical principles, and their implications in injury prevention and rehabilitation. Since prevention obviates treatment, it must be emphasized that many injuries are avoidable when participants train and compete with the proper technique, equipment, focus, and attitude. Despite these measures, injuries are inevitable. The most common injuries are identified, and suggestions are made for their treatment and rehabilitation.

MARTIAL ARTS TRAINING

Training occurs in a well-lit, ventilated gym (dojo) with a flexible wooden or matted floor. Mats are typically used if the style relies heavily on floor techniques and throws, as judo does. Most classes are performed in group settings led by an instructor (sensei). The training is commonly broken into three interrelated parts: basic techniques (kihon), forms (kata), and sparring (kumite). The emphasis on each area differs between the many martial arts styles and even between schools of the same style. Tai chi, for example, has no sparring, and judo does not use forms.

Basic techniques (Kihon)

All levels of participants practice drills that emphasize distance, timing, speed, precise technique, and other fundamental skills as part of kihon. Basic techniques are first learned without partners, often using a mirror for self-observation and correction. Techniques must be practised repeatedly an equal number of times on each side so they become second nature. The participant's goal is to block or attack from any angle.

Forms (Kata)

Forms are prescribed sequences of movements against imaginary attackers and always begin with a defensive maneuver. Through the centuries these movements have earned different interpretations in the martial arts schools. Despite the diversity in styles, forms used by the various schools share similar series of movements, illustrating their common origin.

Sparring (Kumite)

At basic levels, sparring consists of offensive and defensive techniques and stances (Fig. 13.1A and B). As individuals progress through the ranks, sparring becomes less structured, which allows participants more freedom to incorporate different stances in kumite and work on distance: i.e., the appropriate space between an individual and his opponent, so that both offensive and defensive maneuvers can be performed effectively. At advanced levels there are no restrictions on sparring techniques as long as they are executed in a controlled manner, observing acknowledged protocols to prevent injuries (Fig. 13.2A and B).

Many masters in martial art styles encourage participants to get the feel of free sparring early in their training. More traditional stylists argue that trainees should first master basic techniques and stances and

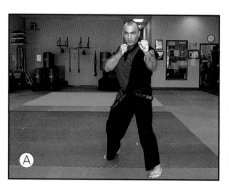
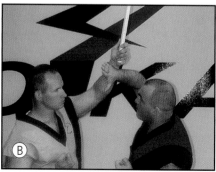

Figure 13.1
A. Demonstration of a three-quarter forward fighting stance.
B. Demonstration of an upward block of an assault with a weapon.

Figure 13.2
A. Demonstration of a round kick to the head and an upward block.
B. Demonstration of an axe kick with an upward block. With an axe kick, the aggressor's hip is maximally flexed with the knee extended and the heel is brought down on the defender's head, neck, shoulder, or upper extremities.

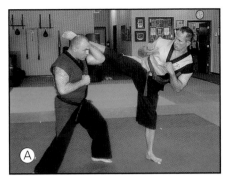
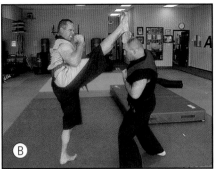

get an appreciation for distance before being permitted to free spar. It is hoped that this approach will reduce the likelihood of developing improper or uncontrolled techniques.

Today, market forces can influence teaching protocols. With many different styles and classes available, certain consumers will choose the less-traditional schools so that they can fight sooner. The authors recommend choosing a school that balances fundamental techniques and well-controlled sparring and where safety is the primary concern.

Ancient and modern ancillary training techniques

There are several ancillary activities that trainees practice independently, usually before or after class, to improve their techniques. A punching bag may be used to practice hand and foot striking techniques and to develop a sense of timing and distance. (Fig. 13.3A–C)) Punching the padded makiware board builds

Figure 13.3
A. Forward round kick to the heavy bag.
B. Side kick to the heavy bag.
C. Jab to the heavy bag.

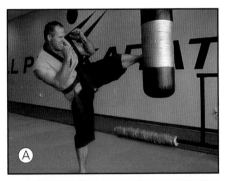
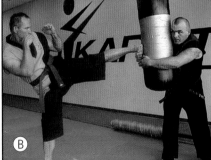
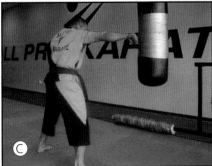

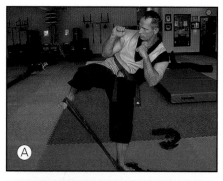
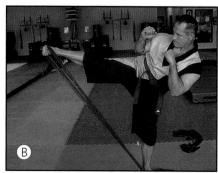
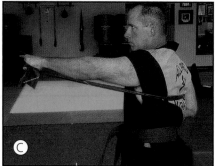

Figure 13.4
A. Beginning position of forward leg side snap kicking against Theraband resistance.
B. End position of forward leg side snap kicking against Theraband resistance.
C. Jab against Theraband resistance.

calluses over the metacarpophalangeal joints and increases tolerance to punching. In addition, it develops power generation through strengthening shoulder, elbow, and wrist stabilizing musculature. After years of makiware use, some participants advance their practice to striking packed sand or gravel. Despite the remarkable visible changes sometimes seen in the overlying soft tissue, significant bony changes at the site of impact have not been demonstrated by radiographs in limited, non-controlled studies.[11,12] However, hypertrophic infiltrative tendinitis, with resultant entrapment of the long extensor tendon, has been reported from attempting to accelerate the hand-toughening process too rapidly.[13]

Board breaking, while dramatic, is not a component of most martial artists' training. It is performed to demonstrate control in striking techniques. Improper technique in board breaking may result in injury. Depending upon the technique used, when improperly performed fifth metacarpal fracture, radial fracture, and/or traumatic neurapraxia of the ulnar nerve may result.[14,15] Despite some expectation to the contrary,[16] limited non-controlled studies have failed to demonstrate that board breaking, makiware use, or knuckle push-ups lead to accelerated degenerative arthritis or traumatic bursitis.[11,12] Some martial artists incorporate resistance work into punching and kicking training by connecting the extremity to a stable object with an elastic material (Fig. 13.4A–C). This changes what are usually open kinetic chain activities to closed kinetic chain activities. Closed kinetic chain exercises work agonist and antagonist muscles simultaneously during training, and are believed to be a safer training modality due to enhanced stabilization of the involved joints.[17]

EXERCISE PRINCIPLES

The nature of martial arts practice requires aerobic and anaerobic fitness combined with superior flexibility, agility, and balance. The warm-up period helps the participant to prepare physically and mentally for the demands of the sport. Diligence in performing a sport-specific warm-up and cool-down program, taking into consideration the trainee's medical conditions, is central to prevention of injury. Stretching has been demonstrated to result in an increased number of muscle fiber sarcomeres.[18] Stretching is particularly important for older athletes, because tissues tend to lose compliance with age. The importance of a good flexibility program for participants in the martial arts cannot be over-emphasized.

Warm-up

The warm-up period begins with cardiovascular exercise, often taking the form of jumping jacks, jogging around the dojo, jump rope, or an activity more specific to the sport, such as repetitive punches or kicks (Fig. 13.5A–C). Although commonly done as part of the warm-up, serial high kicks should be reserved until after the participant has stretched to prevent muscle strains. Once the participant has warmed up, it is common to perform attack and defend sequences prior to sparring (Fig 13.5D–F).

When stretching, one should target muscles about joints requiring extremes in range of motion, such as at the hips and two-joint muscles. These muscles – including rectus femoris, the hamstrings, and gastrocnemius – are most prone to strains. Connective tissue adapts to imposed demand of prolonged stretching by gradual elongation, which is known as creep. The desired elongation of fibers of the myotendinous unit is most effective after the target tissue has warmed.[17] Thus, warm-up stretching is optimally timed to follow mild cardiovascular conditioning. The authors do not intend that the athlete should begin a training session with extreme cardiovascular activity, but rather perform mild conditioning to the point of breathing hard and sweating prior to flexibility exercises. This assures that the muscular blood flow and core temperature have increased. For stretching to be effective, it must become a regular and integrated part of the exercise program.

Post-training cool-down

Cool-down stretching should concentrate on the individual's hard-to-stretch regions and the regions specifically exercised during the preceding session. Cool-down stretching is arguably as important as the pre-exercise stretch. With the muscles still warm from the work-out, stretching is optimally effective. Delayed muscle soreness may be reduced with adequate cool-down activities and when cryotherapy precedes stretching.[19] The cool-down period may help to prevent post-exercise syncope, a hypotensive phenomenon resulting from blood pooling in the exercised extremities after an abrupt halt to strenuous exertion.[20]

Stretching techniques

Ballistic stretching should be avoided because tissue damage may occur from the abrupt force applied by bouncing. Further, it may cause activation of the stretch reflex, resulting in contraction rather than elongation of the targeted muscles. A controlled, slow stretch is safer and results in greater tissue elongation.[21] Stretching is applied parallel to the orientation of the muscle fibers, with stretch maintained for at least 30 seconds per stretch for 2–4 repetitions or until maximum elongation has occurred.

Contract–relax techniques are sometimes used to facilitate stretching. A training partner often provides assistance. The target muscle is passively stretched and, while still in the stretched position, isometrically contracted. After a momentary pause during which time the muscle may be allowed to shorten slightly, the muscle is passively stretched further, and the cycle is repeated. Several variations on this scheme are used. Some participants make use of isometric contraction of the antagonist muscles when the target muscle is in the stretched position, whereas others use antagonist concentric contraction. It is reasoned that reciprocal inhibition relaxes the target muscle, further facilitating its subsequent stretch.

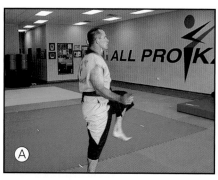

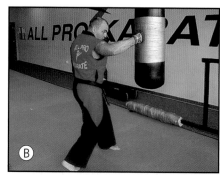

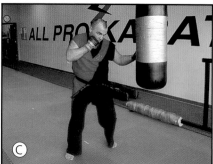

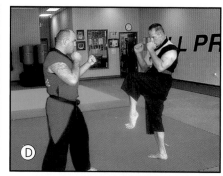

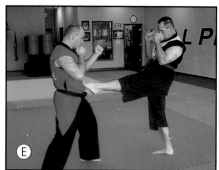

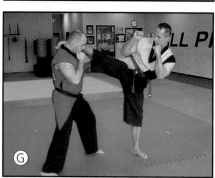

Figure 13.5
A. Speed rope jumping as a warm-up exercise.
B. Right upper hook to the heavy bag.
C. Left middle hook to the heavy bag.
D. Knee pointing to target during mid left rear forward snap kick.
E. Left foot making contact during rear left forward snap kick.
F. Left foot is placed down perpendicular to right foot during transition to round kick to the head.
G. Round kick to the head is executed.

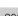

Specific stretches

Attention to form is essential to isolate the intended muscles and to avoid injury from the exercise itself. For example, during early hamstring stretching activities, the stretch should be performed in the seated position. This unloads the spine and reduces stress on weight-bearing joints and postural muscles, making the overall stretch less stressful (Fig. 13.6A and B). During this stretch, the knees should be fully extended and the back kept reasonably straight while flexing the torso over the hips; in other words, bending should come from the hips and not the back. A partner may assist, taking care to avoid bending or twisting the spine and using steady pressure at the low back to facilitate the stretch.[22]

The hurdler's stretch effectively stretches the hamstring muscles of the forward limb but may place undue stress on the flexed knee and should be avoided by individuals with known knee pathology or tight hip external rotators (Fig. 13.6C). As an advanced succession to the traditional hurdler's stride, the

Figure 13.6
A. Straight-backed bilateral hamstring stretch. This is the appropriate stretching technique, since it does not apply stress to the lumbar spine.
B. Bilateral hamstring stretch with flexed lumbar spine. This is an inappropriate method of stretching.
C. Hurdler's stride.
D. Lay back on a hurdler's stride.
E. Figure of 4 stretch.

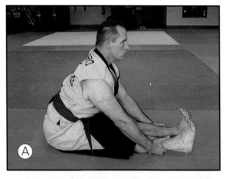

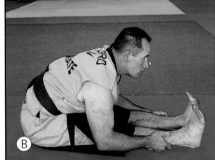

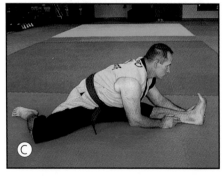

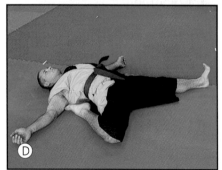

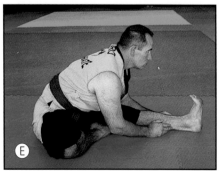

participant may "lay back" on the stretch, which accentuates the internal rotational stress on the hip capsule and supporting musculature (Fig. 13.6D). This is an advanced stretch and if the participant's hip is modestly tight, or if there is known lumbar spine pathology, then this stretch should be avoided or performed with assistance. An alternate stretch is the "Figure of 4" stretch in which the contralateral knee is flexed and the contralateral hip is externally rotated (Fig. 13.6E).

Safe performance of side kicks requires hip adductor and external rotator flexibility. Strains occasionally occur but can be largely prevented through stretching before working out. Martial artists routinely stretch the hip adductors, flexors, and extensors by doing front ("American") and side ("Chinese") splits (Fig. 13.7A and B). The front splits place passive extension (lengthening) forces on the anterior hip capsule and hip flexors of the posterior hip, extension forces on the lumbar spine, and flexion (lengthening) forces on the posterior hip musculature and hamstring of the anterior lower extremity. The hip capsule, hip external rotators, and quadriceps muscles crossing the hip may be further stretched by flexing the posterior knee while in the front splits (Fig. 13.7C). An alternate to the front splits may be easily accomplished by the participant taking a posterior knee, anterior-foot posture and gently rocking forward supporting himself on the anterior knee (Fig. 13.7D). This easily stretches the anterior capsule and iliopsoas of the posterior hip and the groin muscles of the anterior hip. The side splits are accomplished by pressing the pelvis forward while keeping the hips maximally abducted and externally rotated. The lumbar spine is maintained in neutral position. This also places extreme stretch on the anterior and medial hip capsule as well as a posterior and medial gliding force on the ilium over the sacrum. Alternatively, the anterior groin muscles and internal rotators may be addressed with the Butterfly stretch (Fig. 13.7E), the Sumo stretch (Fig. 13.7F), or the Lotus position (Fig. 13.7G).

The upper extremities and neck musculature should be stretched, since fluidity of movement requires agility and flexibility throughout the kinetic chain. Shoulder girdle musculature should be stretched with the shoulder in flexion, internal and external rotation, and horizontal adduction and abduction. A wooden dowel or broomstick held behind the back may be used to assist shoulder stretching. When using ancillary equipment, it is particularly important to observe the above principles to prevent injury.

Strengthening

Most strengthening occurs through performing the classroom drills described above. Spot strengthening should be saved until after the work-out to avoid over-fatigue of the specific muscles. It is important to include muscles supporting the back and trunk to increase their effectiveness in spine positioning and their ability to accept loading without injury at intervertebral segments. One should avoid exercises that demand extremes of spine flexion or extension, particularly if loading is involved, because they increase intervertebral disc pressure. Abdominal muscles support the back in everyday activity as well as give trunkal support and protect internal organs by contracting in anticipation of an attack. If the participant has a back injury or is not accustomed to strengthening the abdominal muscles, full sit-ups should be avoided. Crunches and cross-over crunches minimize stress to the spine while effectively isolating abdominal muscles. These muscles are secondarily worked while performing exercises that require active hip flexion, such as running, kicking, or jumping rope. Limb girdle and extremity muscles are best strengthened through closed kinetic chain exercises. Scapular stabilizers and upper extremity muscles, for instance, are worked with push-ups.

Some authors have described evidence that range can be lost during strengthening and endurance exercise programs if it is not specifically maintained.[23] For this reason, many martial artists discourage weight training, believing it inevitably results in loss of flexibility. In 1997, Violan et al reported a statistical increase in strength, flexibility, and balance in 14 boys ages 8–13 after 6 months of karate training.[24] The authors advocate cross-training with resistance exercises in addition to martial arts training because it balances muscle development with aerobic conditioning. If the strength training incorporates proper stretching into the program, along with balanced attention to antagonist muscle groups, flexibility is not lost.

Figure 13.7
A. Front ("American") splits.
B. Side ("Chinese") splits.
C. Front splits with flexed posterior knee.
D. Alternate to front splits.
E. Butterfly stretch.
F. Sumo squat.
G. Lotus position.

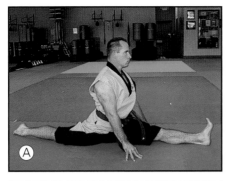

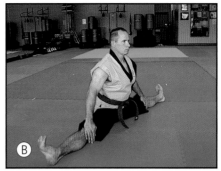

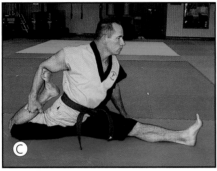

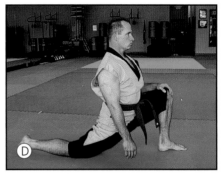

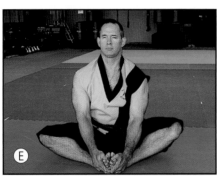

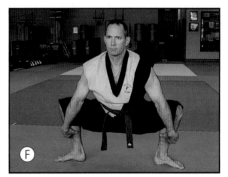

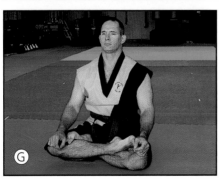

STANCE

Physiologic and biomechanical principles

By understanding the mechanics of power generation using the hips, one can design sport-specific training, conditioning, and rehabilitation programs while optimizing performance and injury prevention. Trained martial artists learn that power comes from the hips.[5] Limited high-speed electromyographic and videographic analyses of basic karate techniques objectively confirm this. Cavanagh and Landa investigated muscle activity in the upper extremity and trunk during the pre-impact phase of breaking boards.[25] Using cinematography, accelerometry, and electromyography, they identified a sequence of muscle activation starting in the trunk and progressing proximal to distal from the shoulder girdle through the upper extremity.

Analogous studies have been done for swinging a baseball bat[26] and golf club[27] and for pitching a baseball.[28–30] These activities show similarities in the muscle activation sequence from the pelvic stabilizers into the extremities. Shaffer et al analyzed the relationship between different muscle groups used in swinging a bat.[26] They separated the sequence into wind-up ("trigger"), pre-swing, swing, and follow-through. Swing phase is further divided into early, middle, and late stages. A coordinated power transfer is described, starting at the hips, followed by the trunk, and terminating in the upper extremities. Although not formally defined, "coiling" is understood to be the mechanism of storing energy in the hips during wind-up, analogous to a watch spring. Similarly, the terms "cocking" and "un-cocking" refer, respectively, to energy storage and transfer by the striking or blocking extremity.

In wind-up, most of the muscle activity is noted in the trailing lower extremity as the knee is flexed and the muscles tensed in preparation for the swing. In pre-swing, hip stabilizers (including bilateral pelvic, abdominal, and paraspinal muscles) show high levels of activity as the pelvis is moved slightly towards the back leg and rotated from an "open" position (slightly facing the pitcher) to a "closed" position (slightly towards the catcher). Stated another way, the batter first twists, or coils, the hips in the direction opposite to that in which the pelvis will rotate during the swing of the bat. In early swing, the vastus medialis oblique (VMO) muscles prevent collapse of the trailing knee as the leg pushes against ground reaction forces. Later in swing, weight transfers onto the lead leg. Hip stabilizers maintain a high level of activity throughout pre-swing and swing as force is generated. As the body uncoils, power is transferred from the hips, through the trunk, and into the upper extremities. Upper extremity muscles actually show a decrease in activity during swing, suggesting they are helping more with positioning than with power generation. In follow-through, the VMO and trunk stabilizer activity remain high. DiGiovine et al describe similar muscle activity in pitching, with momentum transferred from the pelvis, through the trunk, and finally into the upper extremity.[28] The pitching extremity is moved into a cocked position to store energy. During un-cocking, the shoulder internally rotates and the elbow actively extends to accelerate the hand forward. Other upper extremity muscle function is largely for joint stabilization.

Analogous momentum transfer mechanisms appear to exist in martial arts striking and blocking techniques (Fig. 13.8A–C). Energy is stored in the lower body by coiling the hips and, in upper extremity techniques, by also cocking the limb into the pre-release movement. As the uncoiling occurs, the lower extremity pushes against ground reaction forces and the momentum is transferred through the pelvis and trunk into the striking or blocking extremity. Unlike the act of throwing or swinging, karate techniques have a moment when contact with the opponent is made. Therefore, all body musculature must be contracted at the moment of impact to maintain a strong base of support, with maximal power transfer to the attacking or defending limb. Subsequent to the block or attack, the participant needs to instantaneously relax to facilitate returning to a safe defending or attacking position.

Power versus protection

In traditional styles, a powerful attack is produced by maintaining a broad stance (with feet slightly wider than shoulder width, depending upon the technique to be used), with a low center of gravity (CG), and

Figure 13.8
A. Opponents are squared off in fighting stance.
B. One participant generates force through the hips while throwing a straight cross and the other participant blocks the strike.
C. One participant moves from a defensive block position to executing a straight cross middle punch.

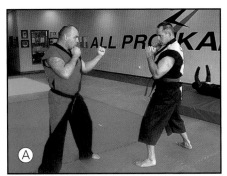
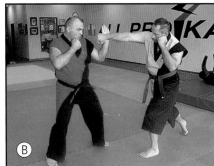
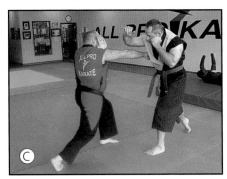

with the pelvis and trunk oriented almost en face to the opponent (Fig. 13.9A). This, however, results in less mobility and a larger potential target area (Fig. 13.9B). Less stability is required during blocks and in close fighting and therefore a narrower base of support may be used. Power is still transferred via the coiling and uncoiling of the pelvis, through the trunk, and into the defending extremity as it deflects the attack from vital structures. In true self-defense or combat situations where the intent may be to actually break the opponent's striking extremity, a more powerful stable stance would be used.

The kiai

The kiai is a guttural noise produced while strongly contracting the abdominal muscles during rapid exhalation. This technique increases trunk stability and is said to concentrate mental energy, thereby facilitating more force transfer when executing moves. It is used to intentionally startle or intimidate the

Figure 13.9
A. Traditional straddle leg stance.
B. Traditional back stance.

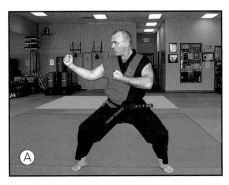
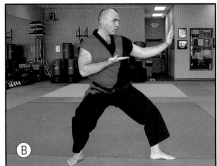

opponent and to dramatically reduce the perception of pain when being struck. It is interesting that this technique has become popular in other sports, such as tennis.

Advanced aspects of technique

The biomechanical essence of a well-executed technique is to use a strong base of support, swift coiling–uncoiling hip mechanism, and synchronized cocking–un-cocking of the striking or blocking extremity. Joint stabilizing musculature must contract through the kinetic chain at the time of striking or blocking. A rigid connection is formed from the stable stance, through the pelvis, torso, and extremity, to the point of contact.

Many traditional stances are used in the martial arts (Fig. 13.10A–C), and each has different uses and advantages. When advanced participants spar, they often use a higher fighting stance (Fig. 13.11), which

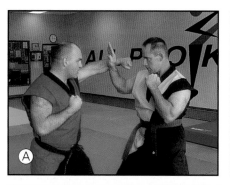

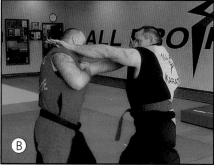

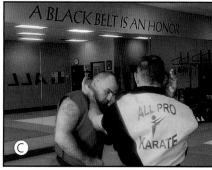

Figure 13.10
A. Knife hand block.
B. Ridge hand to the neck.
C. Knife strike to the neck.

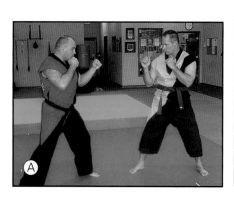

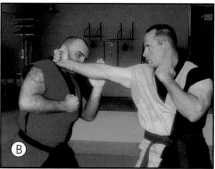

Figure 13.11
A. Fighting stance.
B. Back fist.

can be easily adjusted to accommodate change from attacking to defending postures. One gradually learns to make subtle changes in stance to accommodate the opponent's height, build, style, and technical expertise. Trained martial artists develop the ability to accomplish all the above principles quickly and efficiently by adjusting their own style to meet the situation. In free sparring, i.e. sparring without regard to style, these techniques are all smoothly executed as one takes stances appropriate for attacking or defensive techniques. Another strategy is to transfer the momentum generated by the opponent's attack into one's defensive technique. This is commonly seen in soft styles such as aikido.

DISTANCE

An imaginary circle surrounds all people. Theoretically, when opponents are outside this circle, they pose no threat. When within the circle, they may potentially execute a successful attack. Participants in the martial arts use this concept with the understanding that no offensive or defensive maneuvers can be executed unless the opponent is in that space. Practitioners grow to understand which distance is close enough for attack yet far enough for defense. The distance is a function of the individual participant's build and changes with level of experience. For example, a person with long legs strives to keep shorter opponents far enough away both to enable leg technique execution and to maintain a safe distance from attack. Conversely, shorter individuals prefer to stay closer to their opponents to some extent mitigating effective use of the opponent's longer extremities. Style also dictates the distance maintained by participants, with grappling techniques requiring shorter distances than striking and kicking techniques. While improper stance or distance is not likely to lead directly to injury, it may make one less able to thwart an attack or mount a defense, thus compromising safety.

HAND POSITIONS

A tightly closed fist minimizes hand injuries. It is formed by fully flexing the second through fifth fingers and opposing the thumb across the middle phalanges. In karate, the striking surface is limited to the heads of the index and middle metacarpals.[31] In contrast to Western boxing where force is dissipated through a relatively large surface area, karate techniques allow transmission of large forces through small areas of contact.[32]

The knife hand strike is made by tensing the hand with the fingers extended and the thumb adducted tightly against the radial aspect of the second metacarpal (see Fig. 13.10C). The striking surface is usually the medial edge of the fifth metacarpal.[5,6] Injury is prevented by keeping the hand tensed upon impact. When using the hand to break boards, the hand is maintained in a slightly radially deviated position and the only bony surface making contact is the ulnar border of the pisiform.[6,33]

ARM MOVEMENT

Straight punch

In a straight punch, power is generated in synchrony, starting from the ground–foot interface and moving up through the hips and ultimately through the striking upper extremity as discussed above. Although little power is generated by the upper extremity, its musculature stabilizes the joints and keeps the punching arm moving in a direct line. Ideally, the extremity is recoiled immediately after striking to limit the opponent's ability to injure the extremity or striking the portion of the body the extremity was protecting prior to the strike. This permits immediate resumption of a more easily defensible posture by the aggressor. During the punch, the upper extremity is kept in a straight line by maintaining the forearm in supination until just before striking, at which time the forearm pronates (see Fig. 13.8A–C). Although some practitioners feel that this sequence adds rotational force to the punch, Walker demonstrated that it is statistically negligible.[9] Rather, this sequence ensures that the fist and forearm follow an almost linear path by keeping the elbow from deviating laterally while it extends, as it would if the forearm were prematurely pronated. This method of punching also allows the participant to apply more force through the extremity without concern for injuring the elbow.

Back fist strike

Unlike the direct forces that go into a straight punch, the back fist strike uses a whip-like mechanism. The participant takes a stance that is oriented perpendicular to the opponent, with the striking arm initially kept close to the body. As the hip uncoils, the upper extremity is rapidly abducted while the upper body thrusts toward the opponent (Fig. 13.11A and B). The elbow flexors contract only to decelerate the fist, creating a snap as the elbow is pulled back from the opponent. As described for other martial arts techniques, the force transmitted by a back fist strike originates in the hips and is transmitted through the torso to the arm. In competition, when the goal is to complete a quick controlled technique to the face, some practitioners may lead with the arm rather than initiate the movement from the hip.

BLOCKING TECHNIQUES

When blocking, the goal is to deflect the opponent's attack and at the same time minimize one's available target area (Fig. 13.12A–C and Fig. 13.1B). Most blocking techniques use the upper extremities. The arm is cocked by bringing it to the contralateral ear, shoulder, or waist, for upper, middle, or lower blocks, respectively. The force for the blocking technique is generated through coiling and uncoiling at the hip

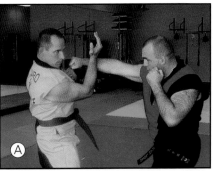

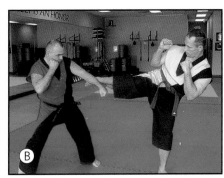

Figure 13.12
A. Left peri-block of a straight cross.
B. Downward block of a forward round kick.
C. Shin block is used for a kick or implement used against the legs.

and torso, similar to the upper extremity striking techniques described earlier. The arm is swiftly brought from the cocked position to the final position using the power that has been generated. Just prior to contacting the opponent's attacking extremity, the blocking forearm is swiftly pronated or supinated for additional torque and stability. Typically, the opponent's extremity is blocked during a "hard block" with the mid-shaft of the ulna ("blade of the ulna") (Fig. 13.12B). This focuses the force of the block through a small area of hard striking surface, promoting injury to the opponent's striking extremity. Alternatively, a "soft block" technique may utilize the palmar surface of the hand or other structure in combination with moving away from the force of the opponent's strike (Fig. 13.12A). Lower extremities may also block by deflecting the opponent's attacking technique using principles similar to those discussed below for kicking (Fig. 13.12C).

The blocking techniques often terminate with the athlete's stance oriented perpendicular to the opponent, decreasing the available target area. During free sparring, a frequently used strategy is to deflect the blow while moving away from the attacking technique and simultaneously launching an attack. Since some techniques may not be able to be blocked, the body should always be adequately conditioned to receive a blow. Additional preparation to absorb impact by making a kiai and contracting abdominal muscles is beneficial, as outlined before.

A successful block will deflect the attacking technique away from the defender's body or at least from vital structures. If the block is intended to be a hard block, then an additional metric of success may be breaking or injuring the opponent's striking extremity. Injury to the participant occurs when the defending block fails or is performed incorrectly by directly striking the opponent's arm or leg rather than deflecting the striking structure (i.e., hand or foot).

KICKING TECHNIQUES

Biomechanical principles used to generate force in kicking are similar to those of upper extremity techniques. However, here only one limb supports the body during execution of the technique unless the kick involves a jump in which the effort is unsupported.

Front snap kick

Ground forces are transmitted through the stance-leg and hip stabilizers into the kicking leg. The attacking limb is cocked by flexing both the hip and knee while aiming the flexed knee at the target (Fig. 13.13A). As the pelvis is uncoiled and thrust forward, the hip is kept in flexion and the knee is smoothly extended with the momentum that has been generated (Fig. 13.13B). As in upper extremity techniques, the muscles of the attacking limb are kept fairly relaxed and are used more for guidance of the extremity than for generation of force. Just before contact is made, the hamstring and gluteal muscles are simultaneously contracted to decelerate the leg and thigh and snap them back. Greater force is generated by delaying deceleration of the leg until the last moment, which allows maximum velocity of the extremity to be reached at the time of impact. Also, quickly snapping the leg back allows for reduced risk of it being injured by the opponent. The striking surface is the plantar aspect of the distal metatarsals of the first two rays, which are exposed by fully extending the digits.

Injuries associated with front snap kicking usually occur when the toes are incompletely extended or the opponent strikes the toes with his elbow while blocking. Either one of these mechanisms may force the toes into flexion, hyperextension, or a varus or valgus attitude, resulting in fracture or soft tissue injury. Unlike the metatarsals, the toes cannot tolerate the reaction forces generated by striking an unmoving object with a direct strong kick. The anterior tibia can be injured if the opponent blocks by striking the tibia directly rather than deflecting the kick. For this reason, many martial artists repeatedly condition the anterior tibia by striking it against wood or other hard surfaces to induce bony hypertrophy, cutaneous calluses, and desensitize the area.

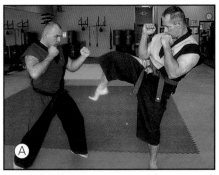

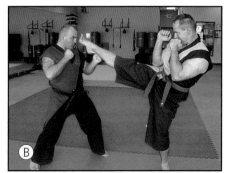

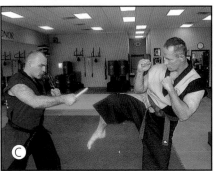

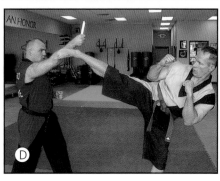

Figure 13.13
A. Forward knee and hip is flexed, pointing the forward knee at the target on the opponent's body.
B. Forward knee is extended during a forward snap kick. The distal metatarsals of the kicking foot strike the opponent in his face.
C. Forward knee and hip are flexed, pointing the knee at the weapon in the opponent's outstretched hand.
D. Knee is extended making contact with the opponent's forearm and moving the weapon to a less-threatening position.

Side snap and side thrust kicks

The side thrust and side snap kicks are related kicks with different mechanisms and striking surfaces. The striking surface of the foot with the side snap kick is the dorsolateral foot. The intent of this kick is usually to dislodge a gun, club, or knife from an opponent's hand (Fig. 13.13C and D). The mechanics of the side snap kick are similar to the whipping action of the front snap kick except that the force is generated laterally rather than forward. The cocked position is with the hip partially abducted, and the flexed knee aimed at a laterally located target. The pelvis is coiled and uncoiled by quickly shifting it toward the opponent. The momentum transfer of un-cocking the lower extremity results in simultaneous further hip abduction, hip internal rotation, and knee extension. During knee extension, the path of the foot moves in an arcing motion towards the opponent's hand holding the implement. The side snap kick protects the toes by curling them under the foot and supinating the ankle, also making the foot a hard striking structure. The side snap has the same feel as a back fist strike.

The side thrust kick starts in a similar side-cocked position as the side snap kick but it is executed so that the foot is thrust out in a straight line similar to the straight punch (Fig. 13.14A–C). While there are slightly varying themes on the execution of this kick, typically the foot is picked up from the ground to hip level by flexing the hip 120 degrees while simultaneously abducting and internally rotating the hip 30–45 degrees and flexing the knee 100–120 degrees to achieve the fully cocked position. To execute the kick, the hips are moved towards the opponent while simultaneously extending, abducting, and internally rotating the hip and extending the knee. The plantar aspect of the foot and heel is the striking surface and the kick has the feeling of a jab or straight cross. Injuries during side thrust and snap kicks usually occur when the target is missed or the technique is performed poorly.

Figure 13.14
A. Fighting stance.
B. Stance leg pushed off the floor, while kicking hip and knee are forcefully flexed, pulling the participant towards his opponent.
C. The kicking knee is extended while the stance hip is forcefully internally rotated, thus rotating the pelvis towards the ground and striking the opponent with the heel and posterior plantar aspect of the foot.

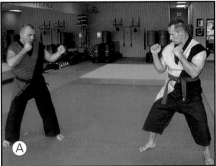
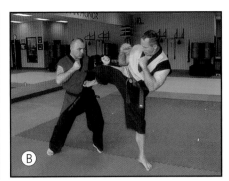

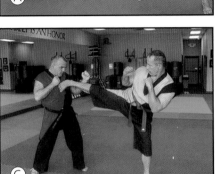

Front leg round kick

The front leg round kick is performed from the traditional three-quarter fighting stance (see Fig. 13.1A). To execute this technique, the participant must first decide if he wants to perform a sliding front round kick or a step-up front round kick. A sliding front round kick is performed by pushing toward the opponent with the stance leg and externally rotating the stance hip so that the stance heel is facing the opponent. Simultaneous with the push off from the stance leg, the kicking hip and knee are forcefully flexed, which literally helps pull the aggressor toward his opponent. The kicking hip is externally rotated 45–60 degrees and is flexed 90–120 degrees while the kicking knee is flexed 110–120 degrees and pointed at the intended target on the opponent's body. When the stance foot has securely landed on the ground, the kicking knee is explosively extended so that the foot or shin makes contact with the intended target (see Fig. 13.5G) If the aggressor intends to perform a step-up front round kick, then a similar procedure is used except that the weight is momentarily taken off the stance foot to move the stance foot into position immediately behind the kicking foot such that the heel is pointed toward the opponent. The time from onset of action until the termination of the kick is approximately one-half to three-quarters of a second.

If the experienced martial artist intends to make powerful contact with the opponent, then the knee is pointed 10–15 degrees past his target, which means that upon full knee extension the foot will move "through" the target by several inches. In addition, immediately prior to contact, the experienced martial artist may shift his center of gravity "past" the target by effectively internally rotating his stance hip. This will add an additional level of torque through the pelvis, resulting in increased force delivered through the foot or shin. Finally, an additional level of torque may be added through the kick by internally rotating the kicking hip immediately prior to contact, which in effect means that the striking foot, rather than striking the target horizontally, will strike it in a slightly downward trajectory, giving added power to the kick.

Striking surfaces on the kicking leg include the mid-shin, the dorsum of the foot, the extended great toe, and the distal first and second metatarsals. If the dorsum of the foot is to be used as the striking surface, then the ankle is forcefully plantarflexed and the toes are securely flexed under the foot. If the metatarsals are the intended striking surface, the ankle is in neutral and toes are extended. As in all techniques, if the opponent's defensive technique strikes the extremity rather than deflecting it, injury may occur.

The many other lower extremity techniques, too numerous to describe here, use biomechanical principles and injury mechanisms are similar to those discussed above.

WEAPONS TECHNIQUES

Weapons techniques use the same biomechanical principles as those of the upper extremities. For example, the stab of a knife or short sword may be likened to the thrust of a straight punch. The slashing motion of a knife or sword is similar to the motion used in a back hand strike. Injuries sustained during weapons use are notably rare but may include contusions, lacerations, broken bones, and, potentially, visceral injuries if caution is not taken.

MARTIAL ARTS COMPETITION

Only a fraction of time in martial arts is spent in competition; training makes up most of the experience for most participants. Many martial artists do not compete at all.

Competition varies, even within each specific style. Because of this variability, it is not possible to describe scoring in detail. Martial artists compete to optimize their score and will therefore adjust their style in competition accordingly. Typically, individuals and teams compete in forms, sparring, and weapons. Forms are judged numerically based on the judges' perception of proper technique and timing. Injuries during forms competition are no different from those that occur in training and include sprains and injuries that result from overuse or improper warm-up and fractures that result from improperly executed techniques.

Scoring in sparring is less consistent and varies according to style and the judges' and participants' experience. Injuries during competition depend on the spirit of the competition. If rules are strictly enforced and participants are warned and disqualified appropriately, competition need not include many injuries. In some karate competitions, for example, beginners (and children) limit sparring to single techniques in a stationary front stance announced prior to execution. As participants gain rank, there are gradually fewer restrictions, until the two individuals competing in free sparring (kumite) are moving within the ring and executing any allowed technique and wearing only hand protection. Scoring is based on clean techniques striking specific allowed areas.

Depending upon the style and forum, individuals who execute uncontrolled techniques to the head or repeatedly to illegal areas are not awarded points for the technique and are often warned and disqualified if they persist. The lead author has witnessed a competition in which a 5th degree black belt's head received an uncontrolled blow from an elbow strike, resulting in tetraparesis for several days. The lead author has also witnessed competition in which a participant received an uncontrolled blow and was knocked out. The individual knocked out was then declared the winner because the attacker was disqualified for using an unsafe technique. On the other hand, in one competition in which judges did not warn an individual after various infractions and illegal maneuvers were allowed, the attacker eventually grabbed, lifted, and dropped his opponent to the ground head-first. The dropped individual became a tetraplegic (C. Robinson, pers comm). Since the best rehabilitation is prevention, it is clear that during competition, safety should be the first consideration.

Trends in competition injuries

Multiple studies have found that the lower-ranking and less-experienced athletes tend to be injured both earlier and more frequently in competition;[34–36] however, Tuominen's[37] and Zetaruk's[38] studies draw the opposite conclusions. Some studies identify adult men as being most prone to injury,[34,36] which is attributed to their greater strength, mass, and aggression over women or younger men. In 1995, Pieter et al found that the round house kick was the most common maneuver injuring both men and women as a group; that men were most commonly injured by the round house kick; and that women were injured by the round house kick and the spinning back kick with equal frequency in the 1993 European Taekwondo Cup.[39] In 1997, Pieter and Zemper found that the lower extremities were the primary body parts injured in both boys and girls and that the number one reason for injury was unblocked techniques.[40]

Spine biomechanics and injury

There is a paucity of data related to spinal biomechanics in the medical literature. While the spine is stressed during all forms of martial arts, it has not been a primary site of injury in the kicking and striking styles; however, there have been a significant number of spine injuries related to the grappling forms of martial arts such as judo and jujitsu[41] (Figs 13.15A–D and 13.16A–E). In the styles which rely on kicking and upper extremity strikes, the primary forces placed on the spine while executing techniques are usually

Figure 13.15
A–D Thigh throw sequence. Note that if participant does not land correctly a spine injury may result.

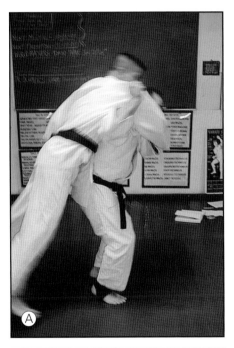
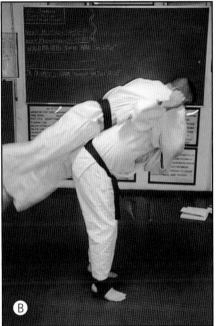
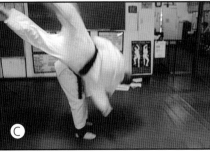
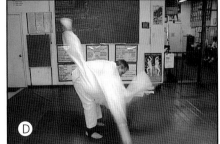

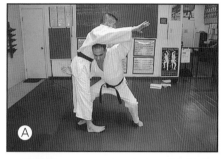
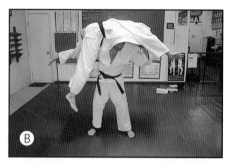

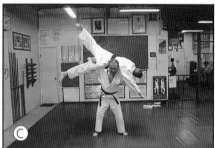
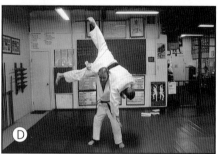

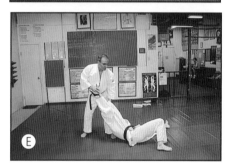

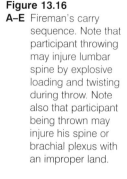

Figure 13.16

A–E Fireman's carry sequence. Note that participant throwing may injure lumbar spine by explosive loading and twisting during throw. Note also that participant being thrown may injure his spine or brachial plexus with an improper land.

rotational and to a lesser extent extension-based. In the majority of techniques in these types of styles, the primary object is to maintain a neutral spine posture and in no technique is the spine towards end-range.[22] The posture of the spine in a front leg round kick is in ipsilateral side bend. The spine may experience a slight extension force upon contact with the opponent but this force is largely dissipated by the ipsilateral hip. Front leg round kicks to the head may apply a posterior gliding force to the ilium on the sacrum but sacroiliac joint injuries are rare in martial arts.

While spine injuries in the kicking and striking forms of martial arts are rare, they can be severe. They usually occur from an upper extremity strike to the neck or kick to the neck. Neck injuries also occur when a participant has been rendered unconscious or dazed by a blow and falls to the floor striking his head on the floor and injuring his neck simultaneously. Neck injuries also occur when a participant is thrown and lands poorly. In grappling styles, neck injuries may occur from choke holds, bridging, or shooting techniques.[41]

Reducing injuries in competition

Protective gear, advocated by many as being essential to injury prevention,[37] may include a head guard; mouthpiece; padding for the wrist, forearm, foot and shin; and chest protection for women and a cup for men. In other styles, the attacker uses only cushioned gloves to protect the opponent or uses no protection at all. In 1999, Critchley et al reported that the injury rate in Shotokan karate national competitions in 1996, 1997, and 1998 in which protective equipment was prohibited compared favorably with injury rates reportedly in prior reports.[42] Medical coverage should be available at tournaments to triage and treat the inevitable injuries. Specific recommendations are offered by Liebert and Buckley.[43]

The use of protective padding is controversial. Some practitioners advocate wearing full gear during all sparring so that the participants can become accustomed to the feel of full contact.[44] Other practitioners argue that the use of full padding leads to development of uncontrolled techniques, less control in sparring, and a heightened and potentially dangerous sense of self-confidence that may adversely affect judgment in a dangerous situation.[36] McLatchie's recommendations regarding protective gear and adherence to strict rules on permissible contact resulted in a significant reduction in injuries, especially to the head, neck, and limbs.[45–47] Padding the fist, forearms, shins, and feet and using mouth and groin guards were felt to be most important in the reduction of the incidence of injury. Of note, in Schwartz et al's study of the biomechanics of full-contact karate,[48] acceleration of a dummy head during punching was decreased using a 10 ounce boxing glove but not decreased using karate-style hand padding.

In another study, whereas hand padding significantly reduced the incidence of severe injuries in Danish competition, there was an increase in the number of minor injuries.[49] The authors feel that excessive padding may lead to poor defensive skills. Severe injuries can be reduced if limited padding is used, rules are implemented that more fully reward techniques to the body rather than to the head, and potentially injurious moves are penalized.

REHABILITATION OF COMMON MARTIAL ARTS INJURIES

Sports medicine strives towards the prevention of injuries. Although some injuries are unavoidable in any sport, many can be prevented. By analyzing the biomechanics of the movements and understanding the causes of the most common injuries, steps can be taken to minimize their incidence. For the injuries that do occur, the consequences can also be improved. The rehabilitation period requires early identification and correction of training errors to obviate recurrence.

Injuries are sometimes described in terms of intrinsic or extrinsic elements, in which the cause is attributed, respectively, to factors associated with the athlete's body or to other athletes and the environment in which the activity takes place. Mismatch between an athlete's physical attributes and demand of the activity is an example of an intrinsic contributor to injury. Usually, an injury can be tied to an isolated mechanical event in which a single stress is applied to an otherwise normal system, as with fractures, or to repeated submaximal stresses such as tendinitis.

The inflammatory response – which relies on chemical, humoral, and cellular events – may be modified with the components of the acronym RICE: rest, ice, compression, elevation, and injury-specific treatments.

In a monumental retrospective study spanning 8 years, Birrer categorized more than 41 000 injuries sustained by 15 000 martial artists.[34] Most injuries were mild and involved contusions (43%), sprains and strains (27%), and lacerations and abrasions (13%). The lower extremities were the most common site of injury (40% of injuries), particularly the digits. Less common injuries involved fractures (6%) or dislocations (5%). The face and head sustained the most severe trauma and were more likely to be hurt in free sparring than in more controlled situations. These findings generally concur with those of earlier investigators.[36,46,47,50,51] Six fatalities, following blows to the head (4) or neck (1), or the chest (1) were recorded during this study.

Overall, three of every four injuries occurred during sparring. Although the incidence of injury was lower in competitions, competition-related injuries were more likely to be severe than the injuries occurring in non-competition settings. Concussion was the most common severe injury, followed by fractures of the long bones and skull. Injury rates and severity were highest in the absence of protective equipment. New trainees experienced both a higher rate and severity of injuries. In concurrence with Birrer's earlier findings, only a minority (32%) of participants reported their injuries at competitions.[52]

Among unreported incidents were concussions, shoulder and finger dislocations, unrecognized metatarsal and phalangeal fractures, and moderate and severe abdominal injuries. A similar proportion of observed incidents went unreported in training sessions. Ignorance of injury severity is common among athletes. Reinjury rates diminished with supervision, use of protective gear, availability of medical care, rehabilitation, and certified training staff.

Injury patterns differ among the martial arts schools. For instance, taekwondo is associated with a relatively high incidence of head injuries from high kicks.[53,54] Dental fractures are more common in karate than in other sports[31] but are rare in judo.[51] The most commonly reported injuries of judo matches are sprains, but there is also a relatively high rate of severe injuries (20%).[34,41,55]

Muscle strains

Muscle strains are common to martial artists and are graded according to the extent of the tear. While grade 1 tears generally resolve spontaneously in several days without formal medical intervention, some muscle tears can be quite debilitating and persistent. A grade 2 tear is characterized by partial disruption of muscle tissue, generally at the myotendinous junction. Ecchymosis and an appreciation of the muscle defect may be present, but the musculotendinous unit is intact. In distinction, a grade 3 tear represents a complete disruption of the muscle. A defect is frequently appreciated on physical examination immediately after injury, but it may later be obscured by edema or hematoma.

Muscle strains are treated with immediate icing for 15–20 minutes every hour while awake during the first 2–4 days. In addition, the injured muscle should be put to relative rest. Some practitioners use a pillow under the knee to provide comfort by maintaining a strained hamstring muscle in a shortened position. However, permitting rest with the muscle in a shortened position can result in tendon and joint capsule contracture and scar formation within the muscle. This limits lengthening when healed and increases the tendency for reinjury because of reduced distensibility at the scar. As a result, the authors recommend rest with the muscle in its physiologically lengthened state.

Aggressive stretching should be avoided for the first 7–10 days. Gentle stretching may be acceptable, depending on which muscle is torn and the extent of the tear. The affected area should be wrapped in a compressive bandage or neoprene sleeve for patient comfort and to provide functional assistance by adjacent muscles. When there is significant bleeding, elevation of the limb helps to limit edema. Crutches may be appropriate to assist mobility and to avoid developing an antalgic gait pattern. Strengthening exercises and deep massage are initially avoided as a precaution against further, inadvertent injury to the muscle or against rebleeding by disrupting the hematoma.

The optimal time at which to initiate rehabilitation is controversial. Some practitioners start almost immediately after injury, and others wait up to 6 weeks to begin any activity whatsoever. The authors advocate beginning gentle stretching after the acute period has resolved, usually 3–7 days after injury, with the goal of re-establishing full and pain-free range of motion. Isometric exercises help to maintain strength during the subacute recovery period. They can often be safely performed at home, while the patient is still immobilized, until it is appropriate to advance to concentric and eccentric strengthening. Aerobic cross-training maintains fitness during the recovery period, and may include single-limbed cycle ergometry of the uninvolved extremity. Aquatic exercise in a warm pool has the advantage of permitting the extremities to work in a buoyant environment.

Tears often linger due to the relatively poor vascular supply at the myotendinous intersection, thus increasing the risk of reinjury. The authors advise waiting until full painless range of motion and full strength is obtained before returning to full unrestricted activity.

Hand and digit injuries

Most of the injuries sustained in extremity striking techniques involve the hands or feet and often occur because unintended surfaces make contact (see the section on hand positions).

Uncomplicated toe and finger sprains are generally treated using similar principles and RICE. Buddy taping is often adequate to immobilize the affected joint, although splinting may be used. Whether the athlete may immediately return to training and competition is based on clinical judgment.

In cases of fracture or any joint instability resulting from sprain, undue stress on the injured area should be avoided until full active range of motion is achieved. In cases of prolonged instability after an adequate healing period, continued bracing during sports participation or even corrective surgery may be indicated. A reasonable anatomic position must be assured in finger fractures, particularly if the articular surface is involved, to avoid healing with fingers in a rotated posture, causing the fingers to overlap when making a fist.

Knee injuries

Knee injuries can occur through different mechanisms, resulting in a variety of problems. Direct impact to the lateral side of the knee by a misdirected kick can result in a medial collateral ligament sprain or disruption. If the knee is in full extension when it is struck, a posterior capsule tear combined with a posterior cruciate tear and tibial plateau injury may result.[56] The menisci are similarly prone to tears. Rotational forces through the joint can result in internal derangement. Internal rotation of the femur with the foot planted may tear the medial meniscus, whereas external rotation of the femur over a planted foot tends to preferentially involve the lateral meniscus. Bony contusions often accompanies these injuries.

Rehabilitation of specific knee injuries is beyond the scope of this chapter. However, several principles are generally observed. In a stable joint, there is rarely need for emergent intervention. Edema is controlled using RICE. Patients derive comfort early from the use of knee immobilizers. Their use after the first few days should be avoided and, if necessary, crutches substituted to keep patients from learning an antalgic gait.

If there is no specific contraindication, weight bearing is permitted as tolerated with the aid of an appropriate assistive device.

Rehabilitation focuses on maintenance of normal range of motion and strength. Lower extremity and hip girdle muscles are strengthened, with attention to closed kinetic chain exercises for the quadriceps and hamstrings strengthening. A low-impact aerobic exercise program is commenced early to maintain cardiovascular fitness. Consideration to draining effusions about the knee must be given, both for patient comfort and to prevent quadriceps (and especially VMO) atrophy. Anti-inflammatory medication should be considered as an important means of controlling inflammation.

Cranial trauma

Facial trauma – such as lacerations, contusions, and nasal pathology, including epistaxis and fractures – is among the most common injury in martial arts competition.[57] Loss of consciousness, change in vision, or any concern regarding neurologic status must be medically evaluated in a formal setting. McLatchie reports permanent partial field blindness from an orbital blow-out fracture and also a spinning back kick that resulted in cervical dislocation.[16] In other instances, deaths resulting from cerebral hemorrhage, cervical fractures, or dislocations followed throws.[55,58]

OTHER CONSIDERATIONS IN INJURY EVALUATION

In cases of severe joint or extremity pain, particularly after a direct blow, fracture or dislocation should be ruled out. Persistent pain should be re-evaluated, because early fractures are frequently missed in initial radiographs. One should also consider the possible evolution of myositis ossificans following hematoma formation in soft tissue, especially in the quadriceps muscle.

Special consideration must be given to possible injury to growth centers in young persons. Typically, there is relative instability at sites of maximal growth, and therefore this is where injuries frequently occur. Cianca notes that "children are particularly susceptible to injury during or just after a growth spurt, because of a lag in development of soft tissue tensile strength."[2]

Intense abdominal pain following a direct blow may be indicative of internal injury, including a ruptured spleen or contused other organ and should be medically evaluated. Liver laceration, ruptures of the liver, kidney, spleen, or lung, traumatic pancreatitis, rib fractures, testicular contusions, and myoglobinuria have been reported.[16,59–61] A study of injury potential from taekwondo kicks to the chest demonstrated the thoracic compression of 3–5 cm, and values of 200 J and 15 m/sec for basic swing (snap) kicks.[57] Several cases of cardiac contusion, rupture, and sudden death from cardiac arrest appear in the literature.[58,61,62] Despite the clear potential for soft tissue and skeletal injury, the efficacy of chest protection has not been demonstrated.

CONCLUSION

This chapter reviews the training and biomechanical principles behind many martial arts techniques. Understanding these principles, as well as the mechanism and incidence of injuries, will help to produce positive preventive and treatment outcomes by clinicians who treat these athletes. Martial arts have proven to be an excellent form of conditioning and a relatively safe sport when appropriate controls are maintained. Teachers of the martial arts and physicians should become familiar with high-risk activities and techniques so that catastrophic injuries may be prevented during competition and training.

REFERENCES

1. Massey P: Medicine and the martial arts. A brief historical perspective. Altern Complement Ther 4:438–445, 1998.

2. Cianca J: Sports injury. In: Garrison S, ed. Handbook of physical medicine and rehabilitation basics. Philadelphia: JB Lippincott; 1995: 369–390.

3. Jaffe L, Minkoff J: Martial arts: a perspective on their evolution, injuries, and training formats. Orthop Rev 17:208–221, 1988.

4. Kodansha: Illustrated Kodokan Judo. Tokyo: Kodansha; 1962.

5. Nakayama M: Dynamic karate. New York: Kodansha International/USA; 1980.

6. Okazaki T, Stricevic M: The textbook of modern karate. New York: Kodansha International/USA; 1984.

7. Reid H, Croucher M: The way of the warrior: the paradox of the martial arts. Woodstock: The Overlook Press; 1991.

8. Vos J, Binkhorst R: Velocity and force of some karate arm-movements. Nature 211:89–90, 1966.

9. Walker J: Karate strikes. Am J Physiol 43:845–849, 1975.

10. Westbrook A, Ratti O: Aikido and the dynamic sphere. Rutland: Charles E. Tuttle; 1970.

11. Crosby A: The hands of karate experts. Clinical and radiological findings. Br J Sports Med 19:41–42, 1985.

12. Larose J, Kim D: Karate hand-conditioning. Med Sci Sports 1:95–98, 1969.

13. Gardner R: Hypertrophic infiltrative tendinitis (HIT syndrome) of the long extensor: the abused karate hand. JAMA 211:1009–1010, 1970.

14. Chiu D: "Karate Kid" finger. Plast Reconstr Surg 91:362–364, 1993.

15. Neiman E, Swann P: Karate injuries. BMJ 1:233, 1971.

16. McLatchie G: Karate and karate injuries. Br J Sports Med 15:84–86, 1981.

17. Young J, Press JM: The physiologic basis of sports rehabilitation. Phys Med Rehab Clin North Am 5:9–36, 1994.

18. Herring S, Grimm A, Grimm R: Regulation of sarcomere number in skeletal muscle: a comparison of hypotheses. Muscle Nerve 7:161–173, 1984.

19. Meeusen R, Lievens P: The use of cryotherapy in sports injuries. Sports Med 3:39–44, 1986.

20. Bjurstedt H, Rosenhamer G, Balldin U, et al: Orthostatic reactions during recovery from exhaustive exercise of short duration. Acta Physiol Scand 119:25–31, 1983.

21. Smith R: A complete guide to judo. Rutland: Charles E. Tuttle; 1958.

22. Schauer G: Spine defense and the martial arts. In: White AH, Schofferman JA, eds. Spine care: diagnosis and conservative treatment. Mosby: St. Louis; 1995.

23. Joynt R: Therapeutic exercise. In: DeLisa JA, Gans BM, eds. Rehabilitation medicine: principles and practice. Philadelphia: JB Lippincott; 1993:346–371.

24. Violan M, Small E, Zetaruk M, et al: The effect of karate training on flexibility, muscle strength, and balance in 8 to 13 year old boys. Pediatr Exerc Sci 9:55–64, 1997.

25. Cavanagh P, Landa J: A biomechanical analysis of the karate chop. Res Q 47:610–618, 1976.

26. Shaffer B, Jobe F, Pink M, et al: Baseball batting: an electromyographic study. Clin Orthop 292:285–293, 1993.

27. Pink M, Jobe F, Perry J: EMG analysis of the shoulder during the golf swing. Am J Sports Med 18:137–140, 1980.

28. DiGiovine N, Jobe F, Pink M, et al: An electromyographic analysis of the upper extremity in pitching. J Shoulder Elbow Surg 1:15–25, 1992.

29. Jobe F, Moynes D, Tibone J, Perry J: An EMG analysis of the shoulder in pitching: a second report. Am J Sports Med 2:218–220, 1984.

30. Jobe F, Tibone J, Moynes D, et al: An EMG analysis of the shoulder in throwing and pitching: a preliminary report. Am J Sports Med 11:3–5, 1983.

31. Kelly D, Pitt M, Mayer D: Index metacarpal fractures in karate. Phys Sportsmed 8:103–106, 1980.

32. Feld M, McNair R, Wilk S: The physics of karate. Sci Am 240:150–158, 1979.

33. Fahrer M: Anatomy of the karate chop. Bull Hosp Jt Dis Orthop Inst 44:189–198, 1984.

34. Birrer R: Trauma epidemiology in the martial arts: the results of an eighteen year international survey. Am J Sports Med 24:72–79, 1996.

35. McLatchie R: Analysis of karate injuries sustained in 295 contests. Injury 8:132–134, 1976.

36. Stricevic M, Patel M, Okazaki T, et al: Karate: historical perspective and injuries sustained in national and international competitions. Am J Sports Med 11:320–324, 1983.

37. Tuominen R: Injuries in national karate competitions in Finland. Scand J Med Sci Sports 5:44–48, 1995.

38. Zetaruk M, Violan M, Zurakowski D, et al: Safety recommendations in Shotokan karate. Clin J Sports Med 32:421–425, 2000.

39. Pieter W, Ryssegem G, Lufting R, et al: Injury situation and injury mechanism at the 1993 European taekwondo cup. J Human Movement Stud 28:1–24, 1995.

40. Pieter W, Zemper E: Injury rate in children participating in taekwondo competition. J Trauma 43:89–95, 1997.

41. Nakamura N: Judo and karate-do. In: Schneider RC, Kennedy JC, Plant ML, et al, eds. Sports injuries: mechanisms, prevention, and treatment. Baltimore: Williams & Wilkins; 1985:417–430.

42. Critchley G, Mannion S, Meredith C: Injury rate in Shotokan karate. Br J Sports Med 33:174–177, 1999.

43. Liebert P, Buckley T: Providing medical coverage at karate tournaments. J Musculoskel Med 9:23–30, 1992.

44. Johannsen H, Norregaard F: Prevention of injury in karate. Br J Sports Med 22:113–115, 1988.

45. McLatchie G: Recommendations for medical officers attending karate competitions. Br J Sports Med 13:36–37, 1979.

46. McLatchie G, Davies J, Caulley J: Injuries in karate: a case for medical control. J Trauma 20:956–958, 1980.

47. McLatchie G, Morris E: Prevention of karate injuries. A progress report. Br J Sports Med 11:78–82, 1977.

48. Schwartz M, Hudson A, Fernie G, et al: Biomechanical study of full-contact karate contrasted with boxing. J Neurosurg 64:248–252, 1986.

49. Norregaard F, Johannsen H: Byskyttelseshandskers skadeforebyggende effekt ved de individuelle Danmarksmesterskaber i karate. [The prophylactic effect of protective fist pads in the individual Danish karate championships.] (summary in English). Ugeskr Laeger 150:354–356, 1980.

50. Birrer R, Halbrook S: Martial arts injuries: the results of a five year national survey. Am J Sports Med 16:408–410, 1988.

51. Norton M, Cutler P: Injuries related to the study and practice of judo. J Sportsmed Phys Fitness 5:149–151, 1965.

52. Birrer R, Birrer C: Unreported injuries in the martial arts. Br J Sports Med 17:131–134, 1983.

53. Siana JE, Borum P, Kryger H: Injuries in taekwondo. Br J Sports Med 20:165–166, 1986.

54. Zemper E, Pieter W: Injury rates during the 1988 US Olympic trials for taekwondo. Br J Sports Med 23:161–164, 1989.

55. Fetto J: Judo and karate-do. In: Fu FH, Stone DA, eds. Sports-specific injuries: mechanisms, prevention, treatment. Baltimore: Williams & Wilkins; 1994:455–468.

56. Tria A, Hosea T, Alicea J: Clinical diagnosis and classification of ligament injuries. In: Scott WN ed., The knee. Mosby: St. Louis; 1994:651–672.

57. Serina E, Lieu D: Thoracic injury potential of basic competition taekwondo kicks. J Biomech 24:951–960, 1991.

58. Koiwai E: Fatalities associated with judo. Phys Sportsmed 9:61–66, 1981.

59. Cantwell J, King J: Karate chops and liver laceration. JAMA 224:1424, 1973.

60. Russell S, Lewis A: Karate myoglobinuria. N Engl J Med 293:941, 1974.

61. Schmidt R: Fatal anterior chest trauma in karate trainers. Med Sci Sports 7:59–61, 1975.

62. Maron J, Poliac L, Kaplan J, et al: Blunt impact to the chest leading to sudden death from cardiac arrest during sports activities. N Engl J Med 333:337–342, 1995.

FURTHER READING

Buschbacher R: Martial arts. PMR Clini N Am 1:35–47, 1999.

Corcoran J, Farkas E: Martial arts. Traditions, history, people. New York: WH Smith; 1983.

Koh J: Injuries at the 14th World Taekwondo Championships in 1999. IJASS 1:33–48, 2001.

Kujala U, Taimela S, Antti-Poika L, et al: Acute injuries in soccer, ice hockey, volleyball, basketball, judo, and karate: analysis of national registry data. BMJ 311:1465–1468, 1995.

VanBrocklin J, Ellis D: A study of the mechanical behavior of toe extensor tendons under applied stress. Arch Phys Med Rehab 46:369–373, 1965.

Windsor R, Dreyer S, Lester J, et al: Weight lifting. In: White AH, Schofferman JA, eds: Spine care: diagnosis and conservative treatment. Mosby: St. Louis; 1995:746–761.

Index